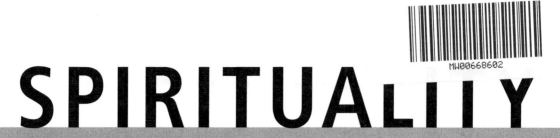

SPIRITUALITY

AND OCCUPATIONAL THERAPY

A MODEL FOR PRACTICE AND RESEARCH

Edited by

TAMERA KEITER HUMBERT, MA, DED, OTR/L

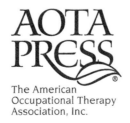

AOTA PRESS

The American
Occupational Therapy
Association, Inc.

AOTA Centennial Vision
We envision that occupational therapy is a powerful, widely recognized, science-driven, and evidence-based profession with a globally connected and diverse workforce meeting society's occupational needs.

Mission Statement
The American Occupational Therapy Association advances the quality, availability, use, and support of occupational therapy through standard-setting, advocacy, education, and research on behalf of its members and the public.

AOTA Staff
Frederick P. Somers, *Executive Director*
Christopher M. Bluhm, *Chief Operating Officer*

Chris Davis, *Director, AOTA Press*
Caroline Polk, *Digital Manager and* AJOT *Managing Editor*
Ashley Hofmann, *Development/Acquisitions Editor*
Barbara Dickson, *Production Editor*

Rebecca Rutberg, *Director, Marketing*
Amanda Goldman, *Marketing Manager*
Jennifer Folden, *Marketing Specialist*

American Occupational Therapy Association, Inc.
4720 Montgomery Lane
Bethesda, MD 20814
Phone: 301-652-AOTA (2682)
TDD: 800-377-8555
Fax: 301-652-7711
www.aota.org
To order: 1-877-404-AOTA or store.aota.org

Disclaimers
This publication is designed to provide accurate and authoritative information in regard to the subject matter covered. It is sold or distributed with the understanding that the publisher is not engaged in rendering legal, accounting, or other professional service. If legal advice or other expert assistance is required, the services of a competent professional person should be sought.
—From the Declaration of Principles jointly adopted by the American Bar Association and a Committee of Publishers and Associations

It is the objective of the American Occupational Therapy Association to be a forum for free expression and interchange of ideas. The opinions expressed by the contributors to this work are their own and not necessarily those of the American Occupational Therapy Association.

ISBN: 978-1-56900-380-0

Library of Congress Control Number: 2016933301

Cover artwork "The Return" by Robert Avon Lees. Used with permission.
Cover design by Debra Naylor, Naylor Design, Inc., Washington, DC
Composition by MidAtlantic Publishing Services, Baltimore, MD
Printed by Automated Graphic Systems, Inc., White Plains, MD

DEDICATION

To my mother, Nancy L. Keiter, and all of the others who showed me glimpses of their own spirituality through life and death. —T. K. H.

CONTENTS

ACKNOWLEDGMENTS

My desire for this book was to provide some foundational context in understanding spirituality within occupational therapy. It helps, I believe, to answer the questions how is spirituality understood within the profession and how might it be attended to within practice. It is not a book about how to become more spiritual or a guidebook as to how to actually do therapy. However, it is my hope that the text will further conversations about spirituality and prompt us to consider expanding our knowledge about spirituality, our working relationships with those attending to spirituality, and our appreciation for the depth and complexity of the topic.

This book could not have been completed without the work and dedication of so many others. It was a labor of love, and it is fitting to acknowledge the many people who have given voice to this text and contributed in some way to its completion.

First and foremost, to Dr. Mary Ann McColl, who took a stance more than a decade ago to write about spirituality and occupational therapy with candor and thoughtfulness. Her previous work and publications opened the door for practitioners and students to not only consider the topic but to expand concepts and ideas about how spirituality could be imagined within the therapeutic context. In this text, Dr. McColl challenges us to further consider what client-centered care should mean in consideration and delivery of occupational therapy services.

To the many occupational therapy authors who were part of the conversations about spirituality and provided insights and perspectives on the topic over the past 30 years, thank you. I have tried my best to acknowledge and reference your perspectives throughout this book. My sincerest apologies for any oversights.

To Dr. Mary Egan and Dr. Suzette Brémault-Phillips, my deepest gratitude for your work and passionate scholarship related to spirituality. You have been in the forefront of moving the profession along by asking us what is next or what we should further consider about this topic. In this text, Drs. Egan and Brémault-Phillips offer images of humility to consider how we can grow as practitioners and develop deep listening. Joëlle Richard provides a real-world example of living that humility.

To the many occupational therapy scholars and writers who have encouraged us to consider the value in embracing diversity and being open to consider how culture impacts lives and understanding, my sincerest thanks. I have tried to incorporate the ideas of cultural sensitivity along with spirituality within the text, hoping to convey ideas of openness and humility.

Within this book, the Rev. Dr. Priscilla Denham provides insights into the role of the chaplain and does so with tender stories of those who demonstrated and shared their own spiritual awareness. She elucidates the challenges and turmoil many clients experience so that we, as occupational therapy practitioners, may become more aware and recognize and attend to spiritual aspects of life. Thank you, my friend.

To the many graduate students over the past decade who have challenged me to consider new insights and ideas about spirituality and who have worked diligently in their scholarship related to this topic, thank you for your inspiration: Lauren Rossi, Amanda Sedlack, Jaclynn Bess, Abby Mowery, Katharine Huylebroeck Engelman, Courtney Lang Miller, Kathryn Karoly, Laurel Taylor, Corrine Zannetti McGrail, Christine Maley, Nicole Pagana,

Christa Velenger, Rachel Turkovich, Elizabeth Van-Buskirk, Kelly Van Clief, Rebecca Anderson, Kendra Beittel, Emilia Costa, Abigail Mitchell, Emily Peters, Sarah Williams, and all of the other students, past and present, who have made me a better teacher, mentor and scholar.

To my colleagues at Elizabethtown College who supported this work by honoring my sabbatical and providing additional awareness and resources when needed, it is a privilege working with you.

I wish to thank the many people who have reviewed portions of this text, in its various conceptions and offered insights and feedback, formally and informally. Rev. Dr. Tracy Sadd, Dr. Lisa Ruth-Sahd, Dr. June Hanks, Rabbi Leah Wald, and Rev. Dr. Trace Haythorn.

To my family and friends, especially Phil, who supported this work in so many ways, too numerous to count.

And certainly, my greatest appreciation and thanks goes to Ashley Hofmann, Acquisitions/ Development Editor at AOTA Press, who provided great care, compassion, and dedication in making the simple words come to fruition.

—**Tamera Keiter Humbert**

ABOUT THE EDITOR

Tamera Keiter Humbert, MA, DEd, OTR/L, is an Associate Professor of Occupational Therapy at Elizabethtown College, Elizabethtown, PA. She earned her master's and doctorate degrees in education at Penn State.

Dr. Humbert is a teacher, mentor, and scholar, addressing topics related to health and wellness, spirituality, international occupational therapy practice, clinical reasoning, and women overcoming violence. She has provided occupational therapy services within adult rehabilitation, mental health and wellness arenas, and early intervention. Additionally, she has been a clinical supervisor, fieldwork educator, administrator, and private practitioner.

Spirituality has been centered in Dr. Humbert's personal and professional life. In 2010, Dr. Humbert completed a master's degree in religion at Lancaster Theological Seminary in Lancaster, PA, focusing on spiritualty and pastoral care.

CONTRIBUTORS

Suzette Brémault-Phillips, PhD, OT(C)
Assistant Professor
Rehabilitation Medicine
University of Alberta
Edmonton, AB, Canada

Priscilla Denham, MDiv, DMin
Senior Pastor
Hummelstown United Church of Christ
Hummelstown, PA

Mary Egan, PhD, OT(C)
Professor
School of Rehabilitation Sciences
University of Ottowa
Ottowa, ON, Canada

Tamera Keiter Humbert, MA, DEd, OTR/L
Associate Professor
Department of Occupational Therapy
Elizabethtown College
Elizabethtown, PA

Mary Ann McColl, PhD, MTS
Professor
School of Rehabilitation Therapy
Queen's University
Kingston, ON, Canada

Joëlle Richard, MScS, OT(C)
Occupational Therapist
Extramural Program
Vitalite Health Network
Sainte-Anne-de-Kent, NB, Canada

FIGURES, TABLES, EXHIBITS, CASE EXAMPLES, AND APPENDIXES

FIGURES

TABLES

EXHIBITS

CASE EXAMPLES

APPENDIXES

INTRODUCTION

Tamera Keiter Humbert, MA, DEd, OTR/L

I recently became aware of the importance of occupational therapy practitioners melding our personal and private selves with the public ones. I believe that it is in this integration of doing and becoming, being, and belonging that brings wholeness to our lives. Some would say this is the essence of spirituality—the ability to express our truest and most complete presence. It also reflects principles of occupational therapy.

This text intends to further the conversation about spirituality as it has been articulated throughout the contemporary occupational therapy literature. It continues already expressed ideas and reflects the hope that spirituality can be part of the human existence. Spirituality is valued by many who are dealing with life challenges and transitions. It is more than an avenue for coping but often a tremendous source of hope and a means for transformation. Spirituality also can be—and is—part of the therapeutic process.

Why Study Spirituality?

The question may be asked, Why are we spending so much time and effort with the topic of spirituality? Are there not more important aspects in the occupational therapy profession that need our attention? I believe that spirituality is at the heart of life, and attending to it moves us closer to that center. Paying attention to spirituality demonstrates interest in the topic as well as deeming it worthy of value. Part I, "General Considerations for Spirituality in Occupational Therapy and Health Care," provides practical arguments that support occupational therapy practitioners taking an interest in and being involved with spiritualty, including the necessity of

attending to the values and desires of clients during the therapeutic process.

Conversations About Spirituality in Occupational Therapy

This is also a text that is not finished. It was created to facilitate conversation and further open dialogue. It should be explicitly noted that the ideas presented throughout the text come out of our own epistemology or knowing. Those who have been fortunate, or have been in the right places at the right times to have their perspectives published have glimpsed how the term *spirituality* is understood.

More voices need to share in that conversation, but the politics of doing so is tricky. It suggests humility and openness to other possibilities while still presenting what is known or has been expressed. Pollard and Sakellariou (2012), in their new text, *Politics of Occupation-Centred Practice: Reflections on Occupational Engagement across Cultures,* warns of the danger in innocence when we suppose that our understanding, based on our particular lives, supersedes others' experiences.

Multiple Points of View: How This Text Is Organized

This work comes from a constructivist lens that recognizes that multiple voices strengthen, not diminish, points of truth. I have tried to offer a collective perspective about the topic of spirituality without taking any particular stance, even though I have one.

Part I, "General Considerations for Spirituality in Occupational Therapy and Health Care," focuses on the historical and preliminary groundwork for understanding this complex and diverse topic. There is no set definition of *spirituality* but an assortment of definitions and descriptions. Within the chapters, the term is used to highlight a process either currently engaged or evolved over time. It is also presented as something that individuals can and do hold metaphorically and can access. The term encompasses the active connection between all living things. It is also used in association with our fundamental beliefs and ideals. I have tried to represent all of these aspects as they are represented in the literature.

Part II, "Understanding Spirituality Through Occupational Therapy Literature," gives readers a conceptual model for practice. This section provides both a general theoretical perspective and grounding of the concepts of spirituality and then elaborates on phenomenology, one particular construct of spirituality as it relates to occupational therapy practice. Ideas of occupation and spirituality, as well as client and practitioner perspectives, provide depth to the model.

When I think about the model, an image of a kaleidoscope comes to mind in which some images are brought to the forefront, while other images are in the background. With the turn of the kaleidoscope the focus shifts. The images that were in the background are now brought to focus, and the previously viewed images have faded into the background. All of the images are important for the depth and richness of the viewing experience. As it applies to spirituality and occupational therapy, within these multiple aspects, one image is always in the foreground but gradually recedes to the background as our "lens" shifts perspectives.

Part III, "Further Considerations and Challenges," provides even further conversation about the diversity and richness of spiritualty in occupational therapy. This section conveys the openness needed to expand and dig deeper into what should come next and how others have made sense of this important and timely subject. It adds breadth and depth to some of the principles set forth in the first two sections and promotes consideration of new possibilities in attending to practice and research.

Conclusion

I thank Dr. Mary Ann McColl for her dedication and work related to this topic. She provided the profession with foundational perspectives with her formative books, *Spirituality and Occupational Therapy* (2003, 2011). In a way, she gave occupational therapy practitioners permission to talk about spirituality openly and evoke personal thoughts that were translated into public discourse. Mary Ann truly brought the conversation on spirituality to life, and I am eternally grateful for her energy, drive, and passion. This text reflects her thoughtful approach in presenting multiple voices and gently nudging us back to consider others' perspectives.

I also wish to thank all of past authors who have contributed to this vital discussion. May the conversation continue to expand and flourish.

References

McColl, M. A. (2003). *Spirituality and occupational therapy.* Ottawa, ON: CAOT Publications.

McColl, M. A. (2011). *Spirituality and occupational therapy* (2nd ed.). Ottawa, ON: CAOT Publications.

Pollard, N., & Sakellariou, D. (2012). *Politics of occupation-centred practice: Reflections on occupational engagement across cultures.* Hoboken, NJ: Wiley–Blackwell.

Part I.

GENERAL CONSIDERATIONS OF SPIRITUALITY IN OCCUPATIONAL THERAPY AND HEALTH CARE

CHAPTER 1.

ADDRESSING SPIRITUALITY IN OCCUPATIONAL THERAPY

Tamera Keiter Humbert, MA, DEd, OTR/L

Chapter Highlights

✧ Defining *spirituality*
✧ Student and practitioner perspectives on spirituality
✧ Challenges in integrating spirituality in practice
✧ Positive client perspectives of spirituality
✧ Caution: spirituality in practice and research
✧ Client-centered care.

Key Terms and Concepts

✧ Awareness
✧ Client-centered care
✧ Coping
✧ Culture
✧ Intrinsicality

✧ Negative religious coping
✧ Religion
✧ Resiliency
✧ Spiritual awakening
✧ Spirituality

Why consider the topic of spirituality in occupational therapy practice? Should occupational therapy students and practitioners take on this complex subject? Furthermore, should they use spirituality within practice?

When I talk about spirituality to occupational therapy students or practitioners, some people are keenly interested in the subject and openly share their perspectives about it, some appear interested and curious but reserved, and others are skeptical. Such responses have also been consistently reflected in the literature during the past 20 years as authors

have supported or challenged the use of spirituality in occupational therapy practice.

This chapter introduces the topic of spirituality by offering three rationales, in succeeding conviction, for a dialogue about spirituality and occupational therapy. First, although occupational therapy practitioners may be unsure of how to incorporate spirituality into practice, it is valued by many practitioners and deemed important to consider when providing therapeutic intervention. Second, clients and families often seek to incorporate spirituality into their lives when dealing with health-related concerns. Third, because practitioners support client-centered intervention, they need to be aware of this topic and have an appreciation for how spirituality may be lived out by the people they engage in practice.

Defining *Spirituality*

Spirituality pertains to the fundamental aspect, enlivened presence, or essence of a person (Egan & DeLaat, 1994; McColl, 2011). It encompasses foundational beliefs and perspectives, providing meaning and purpose to life (Boswell, Hamer, Knight, Glacoff, & McChesney, 2007; Williams, 2008). Spirituality may be observed while doing occupations but may also be instrumental in the process of becoming, belonging, and being (Kang, 2003; Wilcock, 1998) and may entail seeking the sacred or transcendent (Koenig, 2013).

According to the *Occupational Therapy Practice Framework* (3rd ed.; *Framework;* American Occupational Therapy Association [AOTA], 2014), *spirituality* is defined as "the aspect of humanity that refers to the way individuals seek and express meaning and purpose and the way they experience their connectedness to the moment, to self, to others, to nature, and to the significant or sacred" (p. S7). Moreover, *religion* is "an organized system of beliefs, practices, rituals, and symbols designed to facilitate closeness to the sacred or transcendent" (Moreira-Almeida & Koenig, 2006, p. 844). Religion is often a formal collective but is also an individualized framework in which spirituality is lived out or that is informed by one's spirituality (Koenig, 2013).

Student and Practitioner Perspectives on Spirituality

The concept of *spirituality* within the occupational therapy profession is not new but has been magnified over the past 20 years. Students and practitioners have identified the importance of attending to spirituality within the scope of practice and increasingly believe that spirituality does have a place within the profession or are willing to consider that possibility.

In one of the first studies to assess therapists' comfort with the topic, 500 randomly selected occupational therapists from the United States shared their perspectives about spirituality and practice (Engquist, Short-DeGraff, Gliner, & Oltjenbruns, 1997). Although 89% of the respondents indicated that spirituality was an important aspect in practice, 63% were undecided about whether occupational therapists should address this topic or did not agree that they should.

Farrar (2001) later conducted a survey with randomly chosen occupational therapists from both Canada ($n = 78$) and the United States ($n = 80$), again seeking their perspectives on spirituality. Of the 158 participants, 88.1% indicated that spirituality was an appropriate concern for occupational therapists to address and 58% reported having incorporated spirituality into practice.

In a more current study, Morris et al. (2014) surveyed a conveniently sampled group of U.S. occupational therapists ($n = 97$) and reported a 90% rate of agreement that spirituality is "an integral part of the human experience" (p. 4), with 60% of the respondents agreeing or strongly agreeing that occupational therapists should address spirituality.

In Farrar's (2001) study, 23% of participants indicated that the client's religion should not be addressed in therapy, making a distinction between spirituality and religion. In addition, survey respondents expressed concern regarding the imposition of therapists' own religious beliefs onto clients. They also acknowledged not fully comprehending the term *spirituality* and confusion about the difference between religion and spirituality.

Challenges in Integrating Spirituality in Practice

Despite the expressed, and slightly increasing, value of practitioners and students in supporting the incorporation of spirituality into practice, legitimate concerns and challenges also need to be recognized. Some question whether practitioners are adequately prepared to address spirituality (Bursell, 2010) or use modalities associated with spirituality (Christiansen, 2008; Peloquin, 2008), and from a larger perspective, whether the profession has a legitimate role in assessing and incorporating spirituality into regular routines (Wilson, 2010).

Johnston and Mayers (2005) discussed the challenges of occupational therapists to thoroughly understand the concept of spirituality and deal with conflicting definitions of *spirituality* and *religion*. In addition, they referenced the dearth of information on how to address spirituality with clients. More specifically to practice, a study by Morris et al. (2014) found that 85% of respondents indicated that they did not use any assessments related to spirituality and that only 6% knew of any specific instruments to use. Moreover, incorporating spirituality in occupational therapy practice presents other, practical, problems, including

- How to bill for such services (Collins, Paul, & West-Frasier, 2001),
- Lack of student education and preparation for addressing spirituality in practice (Collins et al., 2001; Morris, 2013; Rose, 1999),
- Lack of institutional time and support in addressing spirituality (Wilding, 2002), and
- Interpersonal barriers to incorporating spiritual occupations into practice (Mollineux, 2006).

Student Preparation

Sufficient attention has not been given to occupational therapy students' understanding of spirituality or preparation for addressing the topic in practice. For example, Kirsh, Dawson, Antolikova, and Reynolds (2001) reported on the curriculum of Canadian occupational therapy programs and identified an expressed value by faculty to address spirituality but a low level of satisfaction in preparing students to address it in practice. In addition, Meredith (2010) identified a lack of preparation of students to take on roles within palliative care, including addressing the spiritual aspect of such care.

Csontó (2009) echoed the lack of preparation for students as well as a lack of clear definitions and constructs related to spirituality as barriers to engagement of spirituality in student clinical practice. In addition, students reported practical clinical issues such as a lack of assessment options and perceptions of other staff as negatively influencing their use of spirituality in fieldwork education; however, they did discuss spirituality with some clients (Csontó, 2009). Although some evidence has suggested that facilitating a reflective practice assisted students in understanding and

feeling more confident in exploring spirituality, it did not necessarily prepare them for using the constructs of spiritual assessment and intervention within practice (Barry & Gibbens, 2011). Conversely, Morris (2013) acknowledged that practitioners who had educational experiences preparing them to define *spirituality* and consider the topic thoughtfully had more favorable attitudes in using spirituality in client care.

Debates Among Scholars

Occupational therapy scholars have presented arguments about whether or not to incorporate the term or the ideals about spirituality into practice (Hammel, 2001; Unruh, Versnel, & Kerr, 2002; Wilson, 2010). The larger philosophical debate about occupational therapy's role within the realm of spirituality seems to be more compelling than whether practitioners value spirituality. Beagan and Kumas-Tan (2005) presented an argument for occupational therapy practitioners to recognize that spirituality is an inherent part of practice and acknowledge that they already use spirituality in practice, making it a legitimate element of practice:

> It seems clear that although occupational therapists do not name their work as spiritual, they are in practice addressing aspects of the spiritual: holism, respect for client's personhood, attention to meaning, relationships and connection, and inclusivity. In fact, it is difficult to imagine authentic occupational therapy practice that does *not* attend to such basic and all-encompassing elements.... It appears that occupational therapists may need to be urged to name what they are already doing in everyday practice as attending to the spiritual, in order to recognize and legitimate those aspects of practice. (pp. 22–23)

Wilson (2010) highlighted the inherent challenges when engaging spirituality in the occupational therapy process, arguing that the diversity in the ways spirituality is articulated, expressed in daily life, and experienced through life challenges and transitions needs to be recognized and respected by occupational therapy students and practitioners. Potential conflict within and among such diverse expressions may underlie the therapeutic relationship and affect intervention. Practitioners are encouraged to recognize differences; be tolerant of conflicting values, practices, and ideals of spirituality; and assess their own skills and abilities in knowing when and how to use spirituality in practice. This task is challenging and should be taken seriously if pursued.

Hammel (2001) contended that the focus of spirituality as described in the Canadian Model of Occupational Performance (Fearing, Law, & Clark, 1997) is related to people's motivation or the reasons why they engage in occupations. She proposed using the term **intrinsicality,** instead of *spirituality,* to convey this concept and eliminate potential confusion with matters of religion and spirituality. Unruh et al. (2002) also expressed concern that the use of the term *spirituality* linked to occupational therapy may lead to practitioners engaging in tasks and roles associated with chaplaincy. They argued for the concept of occupational identity (vs. spirituality) as the central component in the Canadian Model of Occupational Performance:

> Understanding the client's spirituality may provide the occupational therapist with insight about the meaningfulness of occupations in the client's daily life and the way the client has constructed an occupational identity. Listening to the client will enable the therapist to understand what resources the client uses to manage daily occupational needs during health crises and challenges. Listening with sensitivity and respect to the client will support rather than hinder a person's spiritual struggle in such circumstances. Asking about spirituality, listening and understanding reflect a caring occupational therapy process rather than outcome goals of occupational therapy. Targeting spirituality as an intervention goal may be beyond the occupational goals of evidence-based occupational therapy. (p. 14)

Although some students, practitioners, and scholars believe that spirituality should be addressed within occupational therapy—and the term *spirituality* is found in AOTA (2014) and Canadian Association of Occupational Therapists (2007) publications—others are concerned about the many challenges that can occur when discussing and using the concepts of spirituality (Bray, Egan, & Beagan, 2012; Hess & Ramugondo, 2014). Using the argument that many students and practitioners value the use of spirituality in practice as the sole justification for promoting its use in practice is a precarious position for practitioners. Therefore, practitioners must consider and investigate alternative reasons why spirituality should be part of occupational therapy.

Positive Client Perspectives on Spirituality

Just as some occupational therapy practitioners have acknowledged the importance of spirituality within daily life and occupations, clients, caregivers, and others have done the same (Schulz, 2004). Moreover, small but increasing evidence within the occupational therapy literature (and applicable allied health literature) also shows that clients value religious practices and engagement in spirituality during life challenges and transitions (Table 1.1).

The evidence-based articles listed in Table 1.1 provide a rich understanding of how the authors, and various clients and family members, described concepts of spirituality. In some articles, spirituality was identified as a source beyond the person (Hattie & Beagan, 2013; Humbert, Bess, & Mowery, 2013), an impetus for or an appreciation of comfort (Schwarz & Fleming Cottrell, 2007; White, 1998), a way or source for connection with God or a spiritual power (Glover-Graf, Marini, Baker, & Buck, 2007; Griffith, Caron, Desrosiers, & Thibeault, 2007; Schulz, 2005; Wong-McDonald, 2007), or a way to connect with others (Glover-Graf et al., 2007; Martins Silva, Sampaio, Mancini, Luz, & Alcantára, 2011; Selman et al., 2011; White, 1998; Wilding, 2007). Spirituality provided compassion (Lorenzo, 2003), the strength to offer forgiveness (Wong-McDonald, 2007), and the possibility of peace to the world (Simó-Algado, Mehta, Kronenberg, Cockburn, & Kirsh, 2002).

Spirituality was associated with an internal sense of being. For example, it was described as a sense of inner well-being (Egan et al., 2011), satisfaction with or interest in life (McPhee & Johnson, 2000), and a feeling of being at peace (Fieldhouse, 2003; Selman et al., 2011; Tryssenaar, Jones, & Lee, 1999). It also offered a sense of hope and optimism (Faull et al., 2004; Revheim, Greenberg, & Citrome, 2010; Schwarz & Fleming Cottrell, 2007; Simó-Algado et al., 2002; Sinclair, Pereira, & Raffin, 2006; Tryssenaar et al., 1999; White, 1998; Wong-McDonald, 2007).

Table 1.1. Evidence of the Value of Spirituality During Life Challenges and Transitions

Article Title	Author/Link	Focus/ Population	Country/Link
Health and wellness outcomes for members in a psychosocial rehabilitation clubhouse participating in a healthy lifestyle design program	Okon et al. (2015)	Severe mental illness/rehab clubhouse members	United States http://bit.ly/ 1ZVVzCr
Exploring occupation roles of hospice family caregivers from Maori, Chinese and Tongan ethnic backgrounds living in New Zealand	Angelo & Wilson (2014)	Hospice caregiving/ caregivers	New Zealand http://bit.ly/ 23vXmCZ
Beyond the clinical model of recovery: Recovery of a Chinese immigrant woman with bipolar disorder	Kwok (2014)	Bipolar disorder/a Chinese woman	Canada/Hong Kong
Occupational competence strategies in old age: A mixed-methods comparison between Hispanic women with different levels of daily participation	Orellano, Mountain, Varas, & Labaut (2014)	Aging/elderly	Puerto Rico
Anxiety and depression in care homes in Malta and Australia: Part 2	Baldacchino & Bonello (2013)	Transitions/elderly	Malta/ Australia http://bit.ly/ 1VuqtRh
Reconfiguring spirituality and sexual/ gender identity: "It's a feeling of connection to something bigger, it's part of a wholeness"	Hattie & Beagan (2013)	Gender identity/ women	Canada http://bit.ly/ 1P02B3Q
Exploring women's perspectives of overcoming intimate partner violence: A phenomenological study	Humbert, Bess, & Mowery (2013)	Overcoming violence/women	United States http://bit.ly/ 1PleN2M
Spirituality and substance abuse recovery	Morris, Johnson, Losier, Pierce, & Sridhar (2013)	Substance abuse/treatment program patients and staff	United States http://bit.ly/ 1QGHMiF
"With God in our lives he gives us the strength to carry on": African Nova Scotian women, spirituality, and racism-related stress	Beagan, Etowa, & Bernard (2012)	Occupational justice and racism/African Nova Scotian women	Canada http://bit.ly/ 23vZ1bw
Assessment of religious and spiritual capital in African American communities	Holt et al. (2012)	Health benefits and depression/ African Americans	United States http://bit.ly/ 1RPaG1e
"It's not what you were expecting, but it's still a beautiful journey": The experience of mothers of children with Down syndrome	Pillay, Girdler, Collins, & Leonard (2012)	Down syndrome/ mothers and caretakers	Australia http://bit.ly/ 1Kd9CSn
Religious and/or spiritual practices: Extending spiritual freedom to people with schizophrenia	Smith & Suto (2012)	Schizophrenia/ people with schizophrenia	Canada http://bit.ly/ 1JIBoWW
What is spirituality? Evidence from a New Zealand hospice study	Egan et al. (2011)	Terminal cancer/ clients and family members	New Zealand http://bit.ly/ 1nqy2gD

(Continued)

Table 1.1. Evidence of the Value of Spirituality During Life Challenges and Transitions (*Cont.*)

Article Title	Author/Link	Focus/ Population	Country/Link
Role of religious involvement and spirituality in functioning among African Americans with cancer: Testing a mediational model	Holt et al. (2011)	Cancer/African Americans	United States http://bit.ly/ 1PDeyvM
A qualitative study of workers with chronic pain in Brazil and its social consequences	Martins Silva, Sampaio, Mancini, Luz, & Alcántara (2011)	Chronic back pain/ Brazilian workers	Brazil http://bit.ly/ 23vZCdi
Patient perceptions of an art-making experience in an outpatient blood and marrow transplant clinic	Mische Lawson et al. (2012)	Bone and marrow transplants/adult patients	United States http://bit.ly/ 1Kdac2l
Quality of life among patients receiving palliative care in South Africa and Uganda: A multi-centred study	Selman et al. (2011)	HIV and cancer/ palliative care patients	South Africa/ Uganda http://bit.ly/ 1Ut9QoC
Exploring the meaning of making traditional arts and crafts among older women in Crete, using interpretative phenomenological analysis	Tzanidaki & Reynolds (2011)	Well-being/retired women	Crete http://bit.ly/ 1PVsGRB
Religious and spiritual beliefs in stroke rehabilitation	Giaquinto, Sarno, Dall'Armi, & Spiridigliozzi (2010)	Cerebrovascular accident/stroke patients	Italy http://bit.ly/ 1QGKEfn
Spirituality, schizophrenia and state hospitals: Program description and characteristics of self-selected attendees of a spirituality therapeutic group	Revheim, Greenberg, & Citrome (2010)	Schizophrenia/ therapeutic group attendees	United States http://bit.ly/ 1RPcabP
Exploring the relation of health-promoting behaviors to role participation and health-related quality of life in women with multiple sclerosis: A pilot study	Tyszka & Farber (2010)	Multiple sclerosis/ women with multiple sclerosis	United States http://bit.ly/ 1NDi6Nq
Self-identity in an adolescent a decade after spinal cord injury	Webb & Emery (2009)	Spinal cord injury/ an adolescent	United States http://bit.ly/ 1KdaIxq
Children's spiritual development in forced displacement: A human rights perspective	Ojalehto & Wang (2008)	Occupational justice/children	Global http://bit.ly/ 1PVtS7w
Religious and spiritual beliefs and practices of persons with chronic pain	Glover-Graf, Marini, Baker, & Buck (2007)	Chronic pain/ patients	United States http://bit.ly/ 1lXdQC6
Defining spirituality and giving meaning to occupation: The perspective of community-dwelling older adults and autonomy loss	Griffith, Caron, Desrosiers, & Thibeault (2007)	Autonomy loss/ older adults	Canada http://bit.ly/ 1Kdb6vQ
Art and recovery in mental health: A qualitative investigation	Lloyd, Wong, & Petchkovsky (2007)	Mental health recovery/ art program participants	Australia http://bit.ly/ 23w0QFt

(*Continued*)

Table 1.1. Evidence of the Value of Spirituality During Life Challenges and Transitions (*Cont.*)

Article Title	Author/Link	Focus/ Population	Country/Link
What older people do: Time use and exploring the link between role participation and life satisfaction in people aged 65 years and over	McKenna, Broome, & Liddle (2007)	Life satisfaction/ community-dwelling elderly	Australia http://bit.ly/ 1KI2PuQ
The value of spirituality as perceived by elders in long-term care	Schwarz & Fleming Cottrell (2007)	Long-term care/ elderly	United States http://bit.ly/ 20vpTWA
Prayer warriors: A grounded theory study of American Indians receiving hemodialysis	Walton (2007)	Renal failure/ Native Americans	United States
Spirituality as sustenance for mental health and meaningful doing: A case illustration	Wilding (2007)	Mental health diagnosis/one man	Australia
Spirituality and psychosocial rehabilitation: Empowering persons with serious psychiatric disabilities at an inner-city community program	Wong-McDonald (2007)	Psychiatric disabilities/ Psychosocial rehab program participants	United States http://bit.ly/ 1JJ469X
Religion, spirituality, and career development in African American college students: A qualitative inquiry	Constantine, Miville, Warren, Gainor, & Lewis-Coles (2006)	Racism and occupational justice in academic and career development/ African American college students	United States
An occupational journey: Narratives of two women who divorced a spouse with alcoholism	Lee & Kirsh (2006)	Occupational justice/women overcoming violence	Canada http://bit.ly/ 1nBbuup
Critical elements as identified by adolescent mental health clients	MacGillivray, Sumsion, & Wicks-Nicholls (2006)	Mental health/ adolescents	Canada http://bit.ly/ 1WQ2Y6s
A thematic review of spirituality literature within palliative care	Sinclair, Pereira, & Raffin (2006)	Palliative care/ professionals and patients	Canada http://bit.ly/ 1nRLsCP
Understanding the experience of HIV/ AIDS for women: Implications for occupational therapists	Beauregard & Solomon (2005)	HIV and AIDS/ women	Canada http://bit.ly/ 1RPrGUU
Positive consequences of surviving a stroke	Gillen (2005)	Cerebrovascular accident/stroke survivors	United States http://bit.ly/ 1QHuTVp
The meaning of spirituality for individuals with disabilities	Schulz (2005)	Disabilities (childhood and adult onset)/adults	United States
Spirituality: A coping mechanism in the lives of adults with congenital disabilities	Specht, King, Willoughby, Brown, & Smith (2005)	Congenital disabilities/adults	Canada http://bit.ly/ 1ZWVvSS

(*Continued*)

Table 1.1. Evidence of the Value of Spirituality During Life Challenges and Transitions (*Cont.*)

Article Title	Author/Link	Focus/ Population	Country/Link
Achieving a restorative mental break for family caregivers of persons with Alzheimer's disease	Watts & Teitelman (2005)	Alzheimer's disease/caregivers	United States http://bit.ly/ 1WQd4nR
Wellness in Tillery: A community-built program	Barnard et al. (2004)	Wellness/African Americans	United States http://1.usa. gov/1VusnkD
Volunteerism as an occupation and its relationship to health and wellbeing	Black & Living (2004)	Health and well-being/volunteers	United Kingdom http://bit.ly/ 1PDA2c3
Investigation of health perspectives of those with physical disabilities: The role of spirituality as a determinant of health	Faull et al. (2004)	Musculoskeletal disorders/patients	New Zealand http://bit.ly/ 1VusrRB
Spirituality in multicultural caregivers of persons with dementia	Farran (2003)	Dementia/ caregivers	United States http://bit.ly/ 2098S7W
The impact of an allotment group on mental health clients' health, wellbeing, and social networking	Fieldhouse (2003)	Mental health/ adults	United Kingdom http://bit.ly/ 1POChXw
No African renaissance without disabled women: A communal approach to human development in Cape Town, South Africa	Lorenzo (2003)	Occupational justice/women with disabilities	Africa http://bit.ly/ 1PlMYra
Occupational therapy intervention with children survivors of war	Simó-Algado, Mehta, Kronenberg, Cockburn, & Kirsh (2002)	Occupational justice/children	Kosovo http://bit.ly/ 20vMySX
Spirituality and psychological adaptation among women with HIV/AIDS: Implications for counseling	Simoni, Martone, & Kerwin (2002)	HIV and AIDS/ African American and Puerto Rican women	United States http://bit.ly/ 1PODfDd
Quality of life, life satisfaction, and spirituality: Comparing outcomes between rehabilitation and cancer patients	Tate & Forchheimer (2002)	Prostate cancer and disabilities/ patients	United States http://1.usa. gov/1Tqm0QQ
Disability and spirituality: A reciprocal relationship with implications for the rehabilitation process	Boswell, Knight, & Hamer (2001)	Long-standing disabilities/women	United States http://bit.ly/ 1PlObyL
Coping strategies that elicit psychological well-being and happiness among older Catholic nuns with physical impairments and disabilities	Brandthill et al. (2001)	Physical impairments/ Catholic nuns	United States
Conceptualizing quality of life for elderly people with stroke	Lau & McKenna (2001)	Cerebrovascular accident/elderly	Hong Kong http://1.usa. gov/1OSOdg8

(Continued)

Table 1.1. Evidence of the Value of Spirituality During Life Challenges and Transitions (*Cont.*)

Article Title	Author/Link	Focus/ Population	Country/Link
Spiritual issues associated with traumatic-onset disability	McColl et al. (2000)	Traumatic-onset disabilities/ patients	Canada http://bit.ly/ 1UtMhfs
Program planning for an assisted living community	McPhee & Johnson (2000) http://bit.ly/ 1oxBjvy	Assisted living/ older adults	United States
The occupation of gardening in life-threatening illness: A qualitative pilot project	Unruh, Smith, & Scammel (2000) http://bit.ly/ 23V3GEc	Breast cancer/ women	Canada
Occupational performance needs of a shelter population	Tryssenaar, Jones, & Lee (1999) http://bit.ly/ 1KfPYoW	Homelessness and occupational justice/adults in shelter	Canada
Ethnic differences in the wellness of elderly persons	White (1998) http://bit.ly/ 1oxC3ka	Health benefits/ elderly	United States

The engagement of spirituality or religious practices also provided a greater sense of *awareness,* or insight about life. Authors and participants linked spirituality with the recognition of a connection between self and others and the world (Faull et al., 2004; Schulz, 2005) and a general understanding of suffering (Holt et al., 2011; Walton, 2007). It also offered the possibility of gaining personal meaning out of chaos, loss, or suffering (Ojalehto & Wang, 2008; Simó-Algado et al., 2002; Schulz, 2005; Tzanidaki & Reynolds, 2011).

Initiating or reengaging spirituality often served as a catalyst for *spiritual awakening,* that is, a heightened connection to religious life (Gillen, 2005; Schulz, 2005; Tzanidaki & Reynolds, 2011). Spirituality was also linked with a process of transformation, shifting identity, and discovering oneself as a new being (Griffith et al., 2007; Lee & Kirsh, 2006; MacGillivray, Sumsion, & Wicks-Nicholls, 2006). Spirituality connected feelings and values (Simó-Algado et al., 2002) and gave people the ability to attend to and be present in the moment (Beauregard & Solomon, 2005; Tryssenaar et al., 1999; Unruh, Smith, & Scammel, 2000).

Spirituality and the engagement in religious practices were also described in the literature as they related to a perceived outcome or result. For example, in some of the articles reviewed, spirituality was associated with *coping,* or the ability to handle life's challenges, and at times, the ability to develop strategies for personal growth (Koenig, 2013). The literature shows that spirituality helped people cope in the following ways:

- Mediated the stress of caregiving (Farran, Paun, & Elliott, 2003; Pillay, Girdler, Collins, & Leonard, 2012; Watts & Teitelman, 2005)
- Enabled the ability to endure life events (Beauregard & Solomon, 2005; Constantine, Miville, Warren, Gainor, & Lewis-Coles, 2006; Lau & McKenna, 2001; Simoni, Martone, & Kerwin, 2002; Tzanidaki & Reynolds, 2011)
- Provided the perseverance to overcome racism and other issues of occupational justice (Beagan, Etowa, & Bernard, 2012; Constantine et al., 2006; Hattie & Beagan, 2013; Lorenzo, 2003; Ojalehto & Wang, 2008)

- Provided the strength to deal with the effects of long-term disabilities (Giaquinto, Sarno, Dall'Armi, & Spiridigliozzi, 2010; Glover-Graf et al., 2007; Lau & McKenna, 2001; Revheim et al., 2010; Specht, King, Willoughby, Brown, & Smith 2005; Webb & Emery, 2009).
- Provided general, overall health benefits (Holt et al., 2012)
- Supported wellness and quality of life with select populations (Barnard et al., 2004; Brandthill et al. 2001; Morris, Johnson, Losier, Pierce, & Sridhar, 2013; Tyszka & Farber, 2010; Wilding, 2007).

Spiritual engagement served as a mechanism to empower personal development and strengthen community relationships (Lorenzo, 2003). It also provided meaning in life (Glover-Graf et al., 2007; Lau & McKenna, 2001; MacGillivray et al., 2006; Selman et al., 2011; Schulz, 2005; Unruh et al., 2000; Wilding, 2007) and purpose in life (Black & Living, 2004; Constantine et al., 2006; Egan et al., 2011; Faull et al., 2004; Schwarz & Fleming Cottrell, 2007; Schulz, 2005).

Caution: Spirituality in Practice and Research

Although preliminary evidence suggests some perceived value of spirituality by clients, family members, and others, some studies and literature, within and outside the occupational therapy profession, caution whole-hearted acceptance of inclusion of spirituality in practice and research. Challenges include the process of developing resiliency, psychological variables, duration, development of spirituality, differing constructs, and spirituality compromising wellness.

Process of Resiliency

It has been suggested that developing *resiliency,* the ability to face ongoing and often mounting challenges, while dealing with long-term pain and disabilities requires a process of reflection, introspection, or contemplation. Spirituality may provide additional avenues to develop and enhance contemplation and offer alternative ways to consider life meaning and purpose (Faull et al., 2004; Schulz, 2004). Although some clients can understand

and undertake this process, it may not be accessible to or compatible with all clients (Johnstone et al., 2012).

Psychological Variables

Multiple psychological variables may play a role in clients' valuation of spirituality. For example, attributes of self-worth, insights into personal control over pain, and acceptance of the condition might need to be present, along with the use of spirituality, to promote progression to health. Clients' personal beliefs about themselves need to be compatible with those particular spiritual beliefs and practices being promoted for health and wellness (Faull et al., 2004; Johnstone et al., 2012).

Duration

Using and understanding spirituality may differ among people according to their personal life journeys, whether it relates to disability or justice issues (e.g., racism, sexism). How people make sense of and respond to particular circumstances evolves over time and is influenced by their spirituality (Boswell, Knight, & Hamer, 2001; Hattie & Beagan, 2013; Schulz, 2005). Therefore, it is important to appreciate spirituality as dynamic and often evolving as well as to understand a person's current beliefs, practices, and views of his or her life circumstance.

Development of Spirituality

Sinclair et al. (2006) reviewed spiritual literature on palliative care. Most of the literature relating to clients and caregivers focused on conceptual and attitudinal issues, with little insight on how spiritual experiences were developed and supported in practice. The studies frequently identified the value of spirituality by the client or family and, in some instances, articulated the activities used to support spirituality or the meaning of spirituality to the client. However, the process of selecting, developing, and using spiritual practices, in the short term and long-range response to the life event, was not determined or discussed.

Occupational therapy practitioners must remember that a client's religious or spiritual convictions may not correlate to improvement in functional recovery (Giaquinto et al., 2010; Jones et al., 2015). Therefore, further research to understand how spiritual or religious practices actually support people and assist them through crises and long-term challenges is needed.

Differing Constructs

Religious practices and spirituality have often been considered different constructs; however, the definition and use of these terms may have varying effects on or elicit varying responses from different people (Holt et al., 2012; Revheim et al., 2010). For research purposes, these differences need to be made clear but often are not. For example, when people who identify themselves as religious have difficulty conceiving spirituality outside the framework of religion (Egan et al., 2011), they may use these terms interchangeably. Even with good intentions, great challenges exist when the constructs of spirituality and religion are either integrated or separated in life or in practice (Egan et al., 2011).

Clients may also have challenges separating and relating constructs of culture and spirituality and may not be able to clearly articulate how their spiritual practices or culture affects their approach to disease or disability or dealing with life events (Cobb, Puchalski, & Rumbold, 2012). For example, a person may be asked whether he or she has any particular spiritual practices, and the response is to pray. Is prayer then considered a religious expression, a spiritual one, or both? What is the essence of the prayer that provides meaning? What is important to the person: the words, the act of praying, or the place where he or she prays? How does prayer assist the person in dealing with life events?

Spirituality Compromising Wellness

Despite a general, and sometimes high, value by practitioners, clients, and families given to spirituality related to coping and wellness, some authors have noted potential negative ramifications of spirituality or religious practices on health and well-being. For example, *negative religious coping* (sometimes referred to as *spiritual distress*) occurs when a person's beliefs or practices bring additional confusion, dissatisfaction, or increased angst about his or her life situation. Religious struggles between beliefs and practices can compromise health and wellness. Diverse, and perhaps conflicting, ideas related to goodness, punishment, benevolence, and personal control may affect how clients perceive a health-related or life crisis and how they should respond (Hattie & Beagan, 2013; Holt et al., 2011; Jones et al., 2015; Koenig, McCullough, & Larson, 2001; Schulz, 2004).

First, attending to spiritual issues may raise challenges, such as loss, a sense of emptiness, despair, and difficult relationships (Hattie & Beagan, 2013; Tryssenaar et al., 1999). Questions about personal meaning and desires (e.g., What is next for you in this life? What brings you hope? How do you move on from this devastating injury?) may produce great anxiety of the unknown or questioning of long-held beliefs.

Second, religious beliefs may present serious ramifications to health care decision making about what procedures and health practices will be consented to and engaged in (Holt et al., 2011; Koenig et al., 2001).

Third, the practitioner–client relationship may be compromised if the practitioner or client has difficulty relating to the other when spiritual and religious values are not consistent or compatible (Bray et al., 2012; Schulz, 2004).

Client-Centered Care

Occupational therapy is a client-centered profession. Therefore, regarding the topic of this text, *client-centered care* means practitioners must appreciate how clients and families view and value spirituality. Becoming culturally effective practitioners includes understanding spirituality as it pertains to clients and their families. Practitioners are asked to appreciate the dynamic cultural experiences that clients and families bring with them as they relate to the therapy process and when making health care decisions (Johnstone et al., 2012; Keightley, 2011; Kwok, 2014; Salvatori, Berry, & Eva, 2007; Tafur, Crowe, & Torres, 2009; Wells, Black, & Gupta, in press). Having a greater sensitivity to diverse cultural perspectives allows practitioners to better support clients in crisis and when life, therapeutic, and health care decisions need to be made (Chiang & Carlson, 2003; Cobb et al., 2012; Keightley, 2011; Wells et al., in press).

Cultural Differences

Culture, people's beliefs about and perspectives of the world, along with their lived experiences, is complex and dynamic. This intricate mix of beliefs and experiences affects a person's occupational engagement and how he or she might respond within the therapeutic context. Expanding occupational therapy practitioners' sensitivity and responsiveness to this dynamic mix and supporting cultural pluralism further promote client-centered care.

The literature contains some evidence that the clients' or families' responses to therapy depend on their perspectives on spirituality. Whereas one client may readily accept a suggested course of action, another may be dramatically opposed to it because it conflicts (or appears to conflict) with spiritual beliefs.

For example, a client dealing with the aftermath of a severe stroke may be reluctant to fully engage in rehabilitation efforts. Instead, he or she may rely on personal beliefs about the possibility of recovery or physical healing through engaging in spiritual or religious practices. The client may prefer to spend time and energy pursuing those efforts. Occupational therapy practitioners should not expect that they can fully anticipate how clients and families will respond to their requests or suggestions because practitioners often have limited understanding of their cultural beliefs, especially if those beliefs are highly influenced by spiritual or religious beliefs (Johnstone et al., 2012; Keightley, 2011; Kwok, 2014; Tafur et al., 2009).

A study conducted by Sage and Jegatheesan (2010) explored cultural differences between two families who had children with autism spectrum disorder (ASD) and other siblings in the family. The authors suggested that the parents' spiritual and religious beliefs greatly influenced the family's responses to the children, which ultimately influenced the siblings' relationships. One family believed genetics contributed to ASD, and the other believed that "karma and retribution for past evil deeds" was the reason they had a child with ASD. Beliefs associated with the reasons for the disability, the nature of the disability, and how others should respond to a person with a disability could provide a context of care and compassion or indifference.

Sage and Jegatheesan (2010) also suggested that cultural and spiritual or religious beliefs influenced perspectives on the personal responsibility within the family and the community of the child with disabilities. A family's beliefs about disability, healing, individual worth and value, and ability to contribute to the larger good may affect what is expected of a child with disabilities. In the study, shame of having a child with a disability prevented the family from talking about ASD with their other child, seeking early intervention services, and encouraging sibling interaction and play. The family also communicated to their son that it was his ultimate responsibility to provide ongoing, life-long care to his sibling. Having greater understanding of clients' and families' cultural and spiritual beliefs better prepares occupational therapy practitioners to effectively conduct therapy with them.

Despite occupational therapy's goal to provide client-centered care, that goal may not always be achieved in practice. Kirsh, Trentham, and Cole (2006) conducted a study with occupational therapy clients who identified themselves as minorities. Their poignant expressions of discrimination and misunderstanding point to a lack of cultural responsiveness during the therapy process. Therefore, the authors encouraged occupational therapy practitioners to challenge themselves about their own beliefs by further exploring occupational choices, experiences of oppression, and how their own culture affects the therapeutic process.

Iwama (2007) moved the conversation about culture even further in hopes that the profession of occupational therapy and those who articulate the values of the profession understand the full meaning of culture and make it an integral part of the profession. He stated,

> If we can broaden our conception of culture to mean also "shared spheres of experience and the ascription of meaning to objects and phenomena in the world," then occupational therapists ought to comprehend *culture* more fundamentally, taking it beyond individual embodiment and the mere markings of distinction that define therapist and client, to the very form, function, and meanings of occupational therapy itself. Matters of culture not only speak to issues of diversity and inclusion but also to the creation of knowledge, theories and the structures and contents of occupational therapy practices. In these ways, culture is at the core of occupational therapy

and should compel all occupational therapists to consider its integral nature and place within facets of this great profession. (p. 184)

Note. Copyright © 2007 by Wiley. Used with permission.

Rudman and Dennhardt (2008) also challenged the understanding of culture as a construct that includes only the individual, that is, going beyond the individual to also include extended groups, such as families and identified communities. They stated, "If we focus on the theoretical development of the concept of *occupational therapy* identity in terms of the individual's sense of self, we need to understand that not all individuals interpret the world in terms of themselves" (p. 159, italics added). Practitioners might aspire to understand what a client personally desires for his or her life, or what occupations are most meaningful for that person to determine applicable therapeutic goals, keeping in mind that his or her perceived roles, desires, and goals may be constructed and influence by the family group.

Conflicted Beliefs

Even when an occupational therapy practitioner has identified a client's particular cultural group and knows his or her religious beliefs and practices, misunderstandings can occur between practitioner and client. In addition, clients may struggle with conflicts between their long-held beliefs and therapeutic interventions sought as a result of mental or physical problems (Awaad, 2003a; Hattie & Beagan, 2013; Keightley, 2011).

For example, Awaad (2003b) shed light on the challenges of young Middle Eastern women who espoused traditional religious values as they were seeking psychiatric intervention, attempting to bridge the gap between their traditional values and a modern perspective. These women were eventually able to integrate some of their traditional practices into the therapy sessions while also dismissing some traditional aspects of mental health care.

Shifting Beliefs

Because spiritual beliefs shift and change over time, understanding another person's culture is complicated. Boswell et al. (2001) provided insights from

their phenomenological study that women with long-standing disabilities viewed their life and spirituality as evolving. The women "characterized the interaction of disability and spirituality as reciprocal. This reciprocal interaction often resulted in adjustments of their views of themselves, the world, and their disability" (p. 22).

Boswell et al. (2001) suggested that "professionals in the area of rehabilitation are encouraged to recognize that women may characterize their disabilities as dynamic and inextricably interrelated with their spirituality . . . and a basis for developing meaning and acceptance of disability in their lives" (p. 24). Depending on the personal and spiritual journey of each client, perspectives of self-identity, empowerment, and independence may vary and affect the client's goals for therapy. Therefore, practitioners should have an appreciation for and an understanding of clients' shifting perspectives of disability and personal and occupational goals and ensure that therapy is consistent with these changing ideals and goals.

Practitioner Beliefs

As part of culturally effective care, practitioners must be aware of their own cultural beliefs and how they may affect the way they perceive and respond to others (Chiang & Carlson, 2003; Muñoz, 2007; Wells et al., in press). Within the therapeutic context, practitioners may be asked to include particular spiritual or religious practices into clients' occupations and also appreciate the meanings behind those practices in interventions (Angelo & Wilson, 2014; Gullick & Stainton, 2008; Luboshitzky & Gaber, 2001; McKenna, Broome, & Liddle, 2007; Smith, 2008; Tafur et al., 2009). Moreover, if practitioners hold biases and stereotyped ideas about a client's valued practice or misunderstand the significance of an occupation to a client, they may not be able to deliver high-quality, effective occupational therapy services.

When practitioners' worldviews and ideas conflict with those of their clients, they need to further engage interactive and integrated clinical reasoning and seek supervision and conversations with other professionals (e.g., chaplains) to better understand and clarify any disagreement. Being able to recognize any underlying struggles and find ways to provide the necessary therapy while supporting client-centered care is expected of occupational therapy practitioners (Hess & Ramugondo, 2014; Unsworth, 2004).

Summary

Whatever practitioners and students think about spirituality having a direct role in occupational therapy practice (and how it may be implemented), they need to understand the information that is communicated and espoused in the occupational therapy literature about the topic. This conversation has been ongoing and in some contexts may even be pushed to the forefront of health care and wellness debates by the medical community (Koenig, 2013). If practitioners want to be part of the conversation, or embrace the cultural aspects of client-centered care, the profession must have language and constructs that support this conversation. Developing such language and constructs is the goal of this text.

References

American Occupational Therapy Association. (2014). Occupational therapy practice framework: Domain and process (3rd ed.). *American Journal of Occupational Therapy, 68*(Suppl. 1), S1–S48. http://dx.doi.org/10.5014/ajot.2014.682006

Angelo, J., & Wilson, L. (2014). Exploring occupation roles of hospice family caregivers from Maori, Chinese and Tongan ethnic backgrounds living in New Zealand. *Occupational Therapy International, 21,* 81–90. http://dx.doi.org/10.1002/oti.1367

Awaad, T. (2003a). Culture, cultural competency and occupational therapy: A review of the literature. *British Journal of Occupational Therapy 66,* 356–367.

Awaad, T. (2003b). Culture, cultural competency and psychosocial occupational therapy: A Middle Eastern perspective. *British Journal of Occupational Therapy 66,* 409–415.

Baldacchino, D. R., & Bonello, L. (2013). Anxiety and depression in care homes in Malta and Australia: Part 2. *British Journal of Nursing, 22,* 780–785. http://dx.doi.org/http://dx.doi.org/10.12968/bjon.2013.22.13.780

Barnard, S., Dunn, S., Reddic, E., Rhodes, K., Russell, J., Tuitte, T. S., . . . White, K. (2004). Wellness in Tillery: A community-built program. *Family and Community Health, 27,* 151–157.

Barry, E., & Gibbens, R. (2011). Spirituality in practice: Using personal reflection to prepare occupational therapy students. *British Journal of Occupational Therapy, 74,* 176–180.

Beagan, B., & Kumas-Tan, Z. (2005). Witnessing spirituality in practice. *British Journal of Occupational Therapy, 68,* 17–28. http://dx.doi.org/10.1080/13674676.2011.560145

Beagan, B. L., Etowa, J., & Bernard, W. T. (2012). "With God in our lives he gives us the strength to carry on": African Nova Scotian women, spirituality, and racism-related stress. *Mental Health, Religion and Culture, 15,* 103–120.

Beauregard, C., & Solomon, P. (2005). Understanding the experience of HIV/AIDS for women: Implications for occupational therapists. *Canadian Journal of Occupational Therapy, 72,* 113–120. http://dx.doi.org/10.1177/000841740507200206

Black, W., & Living, R. (2004). Volunteerism as an occupation and its relationship to health and well-being. *British Journal of Occupational Therapy, 67,* 526–537. http://dx.doi.org/10.1177/030802260406701202

Boswell, B. B., Knight, S., & Hamer, M. (2001). Disability and spirituality: A reciprocal relationship with implications for the rehabilitation process. *Journal of Rehabilitation, 67*(4), 20–25. http://dx.doi.org/10.1007/s10943-013-9676-3

Boswell, B., Hamer, M., Knight, S., Glacoff, M., & McChesney, J. (2007). Dance of disability and spirituality. *Journal of Rehabilitation, 73*(4), 33–40.

Brandthill, S. L., Duczeminiski, J. E., Surak, E. A., Erdly, A. M., Bayer, S. J., & Holm, M. B. (2001). Coping strategies that elicit psychological well-being and happiness among older Catholic nuns with physical impairments and disabilities. *Physical and Occupational Therapy in Geriatrics, 19,* 87–98.

Bray, K. E., Egan, M. Y., & Beagan, B. L. (2012). The practice experience of evangelical Christian occupational therapists. *Canadian Journal of Occupational Therapy, 79,* 285–292. http://dx.doi.org/10.2182/cjot.2012.79.5.4

Bursell, J. (2010). Spirituality within dementia care: Perceptions of health professionals. *British Journal of Occupational Therapy, 73,* 144–151.

Canadian Association of Occupational Therapists. (2007). *Enabling occupation II: Advancing an occupational therapy vision for health, well-being, and justice through occupation.* Ottowa, ON: CAOT Publications.

Chiang, M., & Carlson, G. (2003). Occupational therapy in multicultural contexts: Issues and strategies. *British Journal of Occupational Therapy, 66,* 559–567.

Christiansen, C. H. (2008). The dangers of thin air: A commentary on exploring prayer as a spiritual modality. *Canadian Journal of Occupational Therapy, 75,* 14–15. http://dx.doi.org/10.1177/000841740807500104

Cobb, M., Puchalski, C. M., & Rumbold, B. (2012). *Oxford textbook of spirituality in healthcare.* New York: Oxford University Press.

Collins, J. S., Paul, S., & West-Frasier, J. (2001). The utilization of spirituality in occupational therapy: Beliefs, practices, and perceived barriers. *Occupational Therapy in Health Care, 14*(3/4), 73–92.

Constantine, M. G., Miville, M. L., Warren, A. K., Gainor, K. A., & Lewis-Coles, M. E. T. (2006). Religion, spirituality, and career development in African-American college students: A qualitative inquiry. *Career Development Quarterly, 54,* 227–241.

Csontó, S. (2009). Occupational therapy students' consideration of clients' spirituality in practice placement education. *British Journal of Occupational Therapy, 72,* 442–449. http://dx.doi.org/10.1177/030802260907201005

Egan, M., & DeLaat, M. D. (1994). Considering spirituality in occupational practice. *Canadian Journal of Occupational Therapy, 61,* 95–101. http://dx.doi.org/10.1177/000841749406100205

Egan, R., MacLeod, R., Jaye, C., McGee, R., Baxter, J., & Herbison, P. (2011). What is spirituality? Evidence from a New Zealand hospice study. *Mortality: Promoting the Interdisciplinary Study of Death and Dying, 16,* 307–324. http://dx.doi.org/10.1080/13576275.2011.613267

Engquist, D. E., Short-DeGraff, M., Gliner, J., & Oltjenbruns, K. (1997). Occupational therapists' beliefs and practices with regard to spirituality and therapy. *American Journal of Occupational Therapy, 51,* 173–180. http://dx.doi.org/10.5014/ajot.51.3.173

Farran, C. J., Paun, C., & Elliott, M. H. (2003). Spirituality in multicultural caregivers of persons with dementia. *Dementia, 2,* 353–377. http://dx.doi.org/10.1177/14713012030023005

Farrar, J. E. (2001). Addressing spirituality and religious life in occupational therapy practice. *Physical and Occupational Therapy in Geriatrics, 18,* 65–85.

Faull, K., Hills, M. D., Cochrane, G., Gray, J., Hunt, M., McKenzie, C., & Winter, L. (2004). Investigation of health perspectives of those with physical disabilities: The role of spirituality as a determinant of health. *Disability and Rehabilitation, 26,* 129–144. http://dx.doi.org/10.1080/09638280500265946

Fearing, V. G., Law, M., & Clark, J. (1997). An occupational performance process model: Fostering client and therapist alliances. *Canadian Journal of Occupational Therapy, 64,* 7–15. http://dx.doi.org/10.1177/000841749706400103

Fieldhouse, J. (2003). The impact of an allotment group on mental health clients' health, wellbeing, and social networking. *British Journal of Occupational Therapy, 66,* 286–296. http://dx.doi.org/10.1177/030802260306600702

Giaquinto, S., Sarno, S., Dall'Armi, V., & Spiridigliozzi, C. (2010). Religious and spiritual beliefs in stroke rehabilitation. *Clinical and Experimental Hypertension, 32,* 329–334. http://dx.doi.org/10.3109/10641960903443566

Gillen, G. (2005). Positive consequences of surviving a stroke. *American Journal of Occupational Therapy, 59,* 346–350. http://dx.doi.org/10.5014/ajot.59.3.346

Glover-Graf, N. M., Marini, I., Baker, J., & Buck, T. (2007). Religious and spiritual beliefs and practices of persons with chronic pain. *Rehabilitation Counseling Bulletin, 51,* 21–33. http://dx.doi.org/10.1177/00343552070510010501

Griffith, J., Caron, C. D., Desrosiers, J., & Thibeault, R. (2007). Defining spirituality and giving meaning to occupation: The perspective of community-dwelling older adults and autonomy loss. *Canadian Journal of Occupational Therapy, 74,* 78–90. http://dx.doi.org/10.2182/cjot.06.0016

Gullick, J., & Stainton, M. C. (2008). Living with chronic obstructive pulmonary disease: Developing conscious body management in a shrinking life-world. *Journal of Advanced Nursing, 64,* 605–614. http://dx.doi.org/10.1111/j.1365-2648.2008.04823.x

Hammel, K. W. (2001). Intrinsicality: Reconsidering spirituality, meaning(s), and mandates. *Canadian Journal of Occupational Therapy, 68,* 186–194. http://dx.doi.org/10.1177/000841740106800307

Hattie, B., & Beagan, B. L. (2013). Reconfiguring spirituality and sexual/gender identity: "It's a feeling of connection to something bigger, it's part of a wholeness." *Journal of Religion and Spirituality in Social Work: Social Thought, 32,* 244–268. http://dx.doi.org/10.1080/15426432.2013.801733

Hess, K. Y., & Ramugondo, E. (2014). Clinical reasoning used by occupational therapists to determine the nature of spiritual occupations in relation to psychiatric pathology. *British Journal of Occupational Therapy, 77,* 234–242. http://dx.doi.org/10.4276/030802214x13990455043449

Holt, C. L., Schulz, E., Williams, B., Clark, E. M., Wang, M. Q., & Southward, P. L. (2012). Assessment of religious and spiritual capital in African American communities. *Journal of Religious Health, 51,* 1061–1074. http://dx.doi.org/10.1007/s10943-012-9635-4

Holt, C. L., Wang, M. Q., Caplan, L., Schulz, E., Blake, V., & Southward, V. L. (2011). Role of religious involvement and spirituality in functioning among African Americans with cancer: Testing a mediational model. *Journal of Behavioral Medicine, 34,* 437–448. http://dx.doi.org/10.1007/s10865-010-9310-8

Humbert, T. K., Bess, J. L., & Mowery, A. M. (2013). Exploring women's perspectives of overcoming intimate partner violence: A phenomenological study. *Occupational Therapy in Mental Health, 29,* 246–265. http://dx.doi.org/10.1080/0164212x.2013.819465

Iwama, M. K. (2007). Culture and occupational therapy: Meeting the challenges of relevance in a global world. *Occupational Therapy International, 14,* 183–187.

Johnston, D., & Mayers, C. (2005). Spirituality: A review of how occupational therapists acknowledge, assess, and meet spiritual needs. *British Journal of Occupational Therapy, 68,* 386–392. http://dx.doi.org/10.1177/030802260506800902

Johnstone, B., Yoon, D. P., Cohen, D., Schopp, L. H., McCormick, G., Campbell, J., & Smith, M. (2012). Relationships and spirituality: Religious practices, personality factors, and health for five different faith traditions. *Journal of Religion and Health, 51,* 1017–1041. http://dx.doi.org/10.1007/s10943-012-9615-8

Jones, A., Cohen, D., Johnstone, B., Yoon, D. P., Schopp, L. H., McCormack, G., & Campbell, J. (2015). Relationships between negative spiritual beliefs and health outcomes for individuals with heterogeneous medical conditions. *Journal of Spirituality in Mental Health, 17,* 135–152. http://dx.doi.org/10.1080/19349637.2015.1023679

Kang, C. (2003). A psychospiritual integration frame of reference for occupational therapy. Part 1: Conceptual foundations. *Australian Occupational Therapy Journal, 50,* 92–103. http://dx.doi.org/10.1046/j.1440-1630.2003.00358.x

Keightley, M. L. (2011). Brain injury from a First-Nations' perspective: Teachings from elders and traditional healers. *Canadian Journal of Occupational Therapy, 78,* 237–245. http://dx.doi.org/10.2182/cjot.2011.78.4.5

Kirsh, B., Dawson, D., Antolikova, S., & Reynolds, L. (2001). Developing awareness of spirituality in occupational therapy students: Are our curricula up to the task? *Occupational Therapy International, 8,* 119–125.

Kirsh, B., Trentham, B., & Cole, S. (2006). Diversity in occupational therapy: Experiences of consumers who identify themselves as minority group members. *Australian Occupational Therapy Journal, 53,* 310–313. http://dx.doi.org/10.1111/j.1440-1630.2006.00576.x

Koenig, H. G. (2013). *Spirituality in patient care: Why, how, when and what* (3rd ed.). West Conshohocken, PA: Templeton Press.

Koenig, H. G., McCullough, M. F., & Larson, D. B. (Eds). (2001). *Handbook of religion and health.* New York: Oxford University Press.

Kwok, C. F. Y. (2014). Beyond the clinical model of recovery: Recovery of a Chinese immigrant woman with bipolar disorder. *East Asian Archives of Psychiatry, 24,* 129–133.

Lau, A., & McKenna, K. (2001). Conceptualizing quality of life for elderly people with stroke. *Occupational Therapy in Health Care, 23,* 227–238.

Lee, K., & Kirsh, B. (2006). An occupational journey: Narratives of two women who divorced a spouse with alcoholism. *Journal of Occupational Science, 13,* 134–144. http://dx.doi.org/10.1080/14427591.2006.9726506

Lloyd, C., Wong, S. R., & Petchkovsky, L. (2007). Art and recovery in mental health: A qualitative investigation. *British Journal of Occupational Therapy, 70,* 207–214. http://dx.doi.org/10.1177/030802260707000505

Lorenzo, T. (2003). No African renaissance without disabled women: A communal approach to human development in Cape Town, South Africa. *Disability and Society, 18,* 759–778. http://dx.doi.org/10.1080/0968759032000119505

Luboshitzky, D., & Gaber, L. B. (2001). Holidays and celebrations as a spiritual occupation. *Australian Occupational Therapy Journal, 48,* 66–74. http://dx.doi.org/10.1046/j.1440-1630.2001.00251.x

MacGillivray, P. S., Sumsion, T., & Wicks-Nicholls, J. (2006). Critical elements as identified by adolescent mental health clients. *Canadian Journal of Occupational Therapy 73,* 295–302. http://dx.doi.org/10.2182/cjot.06.006

Martins Silva, F. C., Sampaio, R. F., Mancini, M. C., Luz, M. T., & Alcántara, A. (2011). A qualitative study of workers with chronic pain in Brazil and its social consequences. *Occupational Therapy International, 18,* 85–95. http://dx.doi.org/10.1002/oti.302

Meredith, P. J. (2010). Has undergraduate education prepared occupational therapy students for possible practice in palliative care? *Australian Occupational Therapy Journal, 57,* 224–232. http://dx.doi.org/10.1111/j.1440-1630.2009.00836.x

McColl, M. A. (2011). *Spirituality and occupational therapy* (2nd ed.). Ottawa, ON: CAOT Publications.

McColl, M. A., Bickenbach, J., Johnston, J., Nishihama, S., Schumaker, M., Smith, K., . . . Yealand, B. (2000). Spiritual issues associated with traumatic-onset disability. *Disability and Rehabilitation, 22,* 555–564. http://dx.doi.org/10.1016/S0003-9993(00)90117-5

McKenna, K., Broome, K., & Liddle, J. (2007). What older people do: Time use and exploring the link between role participation and life satisfaction in people aged 65 years and over. *Australian Occupational Therapy Journal, 54,* 273–284. http://dx.doi.org/10.1111/j.1440-1630.2007.00642.x

McPhee, S. D., & Johnson, T. (2000). Program planning for an assisted living community. *Occupational Therapy in Health Care, 12*(2/3), 1–17. http://dx.doi.org/10.1080/J003v12n02_01

Mische Lawson, L., Glennon, C., Amos, M., Newberry, T., Pearce, J., Salzman, S., & Young, J. (2012). Patient perceptions of an art-making experience in an outpatient blood and marrow transplant clinic. *European Journal of Cancer Care, 21,* 403–411. http://dx.doi.org/10.1111/j.1365-2354.2011.01316.x

Mollineux, M. (Ed.). (2006). *Occupation for occupational therapists.* Oxford, England: Blackwell Publishing.

Moreira-Almeida, A., & Koenig, H. G. (2006). Retaining the meaning of the words religiousness and spirituality: A commentary on the WHOQOL SRPB group's "A cross-cultural study of spirituality, religion, and personal beliefs as components of quality of life." *Social Science and Medicine, 63,* 843–845.

Morris, D. N. (2013). Perceptions of spirituality and spiritual care in occupational therapy practice. *Occupational Therapy in Mental Health, 29,* 60–77. http://doi.dx.org/10.1080/0164212x.2013.761109

Morris, D. N., Johnson, A., Losier, A., Pierce, M., & Sridhar, V. (2013). Spirituality and substance abuse recovery. *Occupational Therapy in Mental Health, 29,* 78–84. http://dx.doi.org/10.1080/0164212X.2013.761112

Morris, D. N., Stecher, J., Briggs-Peppler, K. M., Chittenden, C. M., Rubira, J., & Wismer, L. K. (2014). Spirituality in occupational therapy: Do we practice what we teach? *Journal of Religious Health, 53,* 27–36. http://dx.doi.org/10.1007/s10943-012-9584-y

Muñoz, J. (2007). Culturally responsive caring in occupational therapy. *Occupational Therapy International, 14,* 256–280. http://dx.doi.org/10.1002/oti.238

Ojalehto, B., & Wang, Q. (2008). Children's spiritual development in forced displacement: A human rights perspective. *International Journal of Children's Spirituality, 13,* 129–143. http://dx.doi.org/10.1080/13644360801965933

Okon, S., Webb, D., Zehnder, E., Kobylski, M., Morrow, C., Reid, V., & Schultz-Keil, E. (2015). Health and wellness outcomes for members in a psychosocial rehabilitation clubhouse participating in a healthy lifestyle design program. *Occupational Therapy in Mental Health, 31,* 62–81. http://dx.doi.org/10.1080/0164212x.2014.1001012

Orellano, E. M., Mountain, G., Varas, N., & Labault, N. (2014). Occupational competence strategies in old age: A mixed-methods comparison between Hispanic women with different levels of daily participation. *OTJR: Occupation, Participation, and Health, 34,* 32–40.

Peloquin, S. M. (2008). Morality preempts modality: A commentary on exploring prayer as a spiritual modality. *Canadian Journal of Occupational Therapy, 75,* 15–16. http://dx.doi.org/10.1177/000841740807500105

Pillay, D., Girdler, S., Collins, M., & Leonard, H. (2012). "It's not what you were expecting, but it's still a beautiful journey": The experience of mothers of children with Down syndrome. *Disability and Rehabilitation, 34,* 1501–1510. http://dx.doi.org/10.3109/09638288.2011.650313

Revheim, N., Greenberg, W. M., & Citrome, L. (2010). Spirituality, schizophrenia and state hospitals: Program description and characteristics of self-selected attendees of a spirituality therapeutic group. *Psychiatric Quarterly, 81,* 285–292. http://dx.doi.org/10.1007/s11126-010-9137-z

Rose, A. (1999). Spirituality and palliative care: The attitudes of occupational therapists. *British Journal of Occupational Therapy, 62,* 307–312. http://dx.doi.org/10.1177/030802269906200707

Rudman, D. L., & Dennhardt, S. (2008). Shaping knowledge regarding occupation: Examining the cultural underpinnings of the evolving concept of occupational identity. *Australian Occupational Therapy Journal, 55,* 153–162. http://dx.doi.org/10.1111/j.1440-1630.2007.00715.x

Sage, K. D., & Jegatheesan, B. (2010). Perceptions of siblings with autism and relationships with them: European American and Asian American siblings draw and tell. *Journal of Intellectual and Development Disability, 35,* 92–103. http://dx.doi.org/10.3109/13668251003712788

Salvatori, P. S., Berry, S., & Eva, K. W. (2007). Implementation and evaluation of an interprofessional education initiative for students in the health professions. *Learning in Health and Social Care, 6,* 72–82.

Schulz, E. K. (2004). Spirituality and disability: An analysis of select themes. *Occupational Therapy in Health Care, 18,* 57–83. http://dx.doi.org/10.1080/J003v18n04_05

Schulz, E. K. (2005). The meaning of spirituality for individuals with disabilities. *Disability and Rehabilitation, 27,* 1283–1295. http://dx.doi.org/10.1080/09638280500076319

Schwarz, L., & Fleming Cottrell, R. P. (2007). The value of spirituality as perceived by elders in long-term care. *Physical and Occupational Therapy in Geriatrics, 26,* 43–61. http://dx.doi.org/10.1300/J148v26n01_04

Selman, L. E., Higginson, I. J., Agupio, G., Dinat, N., Downing, J., Gwyther, L., . . . Harding, R. (2011). Quality of life among patients receiving palliative care in South Africa and Uganda: A multi-centred study. *Health and Quality of Life Outcomes, 9*(21), 1–14. http://dx.doi.org/10.1186/1477-7525-9-21.

Simó-Algado, S., Mehta, N., Kronenberg, F., Cockburn, L., & Kirsh, B. (2002). Occupational therapy intervention with children survivors of war. *Canadian Journal of Occupational Therapy, 69,* 205–218. http://dx.doi.org/10.1177/000841740206900405

Simoni, J. M., Martone, M. G., & Kerwin, J. F. (2002). Spirituality and psychological adaptation among women with HIV/AIDS: Implications for counseling. *Journal of Counseling Psychology, 49,* 139–147. http://dx.doi.org/10.1037//0022-0167.49.2.139

Sinclair, S., Pereira, J., & Raffin, S. (2006). A thematic review of spirituality literature within palliative care. *Journal of Palliative Medicine, 9,* 464–479.

Smith, S. (2008). Considering ideology, context and client-centered language: A commentary on exploring prayer as a spiritual modality. *Canadian Journal of Occupational Therapy, 75,* 16–17. http://dx.doi.org/10.1177/000841740807500106

Smith, S., & Suto, M. (2012). Religious and/or spiritual practices: Extending spiritual freedom to people with schizophrenia. *Canadian Journal of Occupational Therapy, 79,* 77–85. http://dx.doi.org/10.2182/cjot.2012.79.2.3

Specht, J. A., King, G. A., Willoughby, C., Brown, E. G., & Smith L. (2005). Spirituality: A coping mechanism in the lives of adults with congenital disabilities. *Counseling and Values, 50,* 51–62. http://dx.doi.org/10.1002/j.2161-007X.2005.tb00040.x

Tafur, M. M., Crowe, T. K., & Torres, E. (2009). A review of *curanderismo* and healing practices among Mexicans and Mexican Americans. *Occupational Therapy International, 16,* 82–88. http://dx.doi.org/10.1002/oti.265

Tate, D. G., & Forchheimer, M. (2002). Quality of life, life satisfaction, and spirituality: Comparing outcomes between rehabilitation and cancer patients. *American Journal of Physical Medicine and Rehabilitation, 81,* 400–410.

Tryssenaar, J., Jones, E. J., & Lee, D. (1999). Occupational performance needs of a shelter population. *Canadian Journal of Occupational Therapy, 66,* 188–196. http://dx.doi.org/10.1177/000841749906600406

Tyszka, A. C., & Farber, R. S. (2010). Exploring the relation of health-promoting behaviors to role participation and health-related quality of life in women with multiple sclerosis: A pilot study. *American Journal of Occupational Therapy, 64,* 650–659. http://dx.doi.org/10.5014/ajot.2010.07121

Tzanidaki, D., & Reynolds, F. (2011). Exploring the meaning of making traditional arts and crafts among older women in Crete, using interpretative phenomenological analysis. *British Journal of Occupational Therapy, 74,* 375–382. http://dx.doi.org/10.4276/030802211X13125646370852

Unruh, A. M., Smith, N., & Scammell, C. (2000). The occupation of gardening in life-threatening illness: A qualitative pilot project. *Canadian Journal of Occupational Therapy, 67,* 70–77. http://dx.doi.org/10.1177/000841740006700110

Unruh, A. M., Versnel, J., & Kerr, N. (2002). Spirituality unplugged: A review of commonalties and contentions, and a resolution. *Canadian Journal of Occupational Therapy, 69,* 5–20. http://dx.doi.org/10.1177/000841740206900101

Unsworth, C. A. (2004). Clinical reasoning: How do pragmatic reasoning, worldview, and client-centeredness fit? *British Journal of Occupational Therapy, 67,* 10–19. http://dx.doi.org/10.1177/030802260406700103

Walton, J. (2007). Prayer warriors: A grounded theory study of American Indians receiving hemodialysis. *Nephrology Nursing, 34,* 377–386.

Watts, J. H., & Teitelman, J. (2005). Achieving a restorative mental break for family caregivers of persons with Alzheimer's disease. *Australian Occupational Therapy Journal, 52,* 282–292. http://dx.doi.org/10.1111/j.1440-1630.2005.00524.x

Webb, M. A., & Emery, L. J. (2009). Self-identity in an adolescent a decade after spinal cord injury. *Occupational Therapy in Health Care, 23,* 267–287. http://dx.doi.org/10.3109/07380570903214796

Wells, S., Black, R., & Gupta, J. (Eds.). (in press). *Culture and occupation: Effectiveness for occupational therapy, practice, education, and research* (3rd ed.). Bethesda, MD: AOTA Press.

White, V. K. (1998). Ethnic differences in the wellness of elderly persons. *Occupational Therapy in Health Care, 11*(3), 1–15. http://dx.doi.org/10.1080/J003v11n03_01

Wilcock, A. (1998). Reflections on doing, being, and becoming. *Canadian Journal of Occupational Therapy, 65,* 248–256. http://dx.doi.org/10.1177/000841749806500501

Wilding, C. (2002). Where angels fear to tread: Is spirituality relevant to occupational therapy practice? *Australian Occupational Therapy Journal, 49,* 44–47. http://dx.doi.org/10.1046/j.0045-0766.2002.00292.x

Wilding, C. (2007). Spirituality as sustenance for mental health and meaningful doing: A case illustration. *Medical Journal of Australia, 186,* S67–S69.

Williams, B. J. (2008). An exploratory study of older adults' perspectives of spirituality. *Occupational Therapy in Health Care, 22,* 3–19. http://dx.doi.org/10.1080/J003v22n01_02

Wilson, L. (2010). Spirituality, occupation, and occupational therapy revisited: Ongoing consideration of the issues for occupational therapists. *British Journal of Occupational Therapy, 73,* 437–444. http://dx.doi.org/10.4276/0308022 10X12839367526219

Wong-McDonald, A. (2007). Spirituality and psychosocial rehabilitation: Empowering persons with serious psychiatric disabilities at an inner-city community program. *Psychiatric Rehabilitation Journal, 30,* 295–300. http://dx.doi.org/10.2975/30.4.2007.295.300

CHAPTER 2.

CONTEMPORARY HISTORY OF SPIRITUALITY AND OCCUPATIONAL THERAPY

Tamera Keiter Humbert, MA, DEd, OTR/L

Chapter Highlights

✧ AOTA and CAOT definitions and descriptions of *spirituality*
✧ Spirituality and religious practices as occupations in the literature
✧ Client-centered care
✧ Mary Ann McColl: Spirituality in occupational therapy
✧ Challenging spirituality
✧ Occupational science and spirituality
✧ Social justice
✧ Current changes and challenges.

Key Terms and Concepts

✧ Agency
✧ Canadian Model of Occupational Performance
✧ Canadian Model of Occupational Performance and Engagement
✧ Client factor
✧ Client narratives
✧ Client-centered care
✧ Cultural competence
✧ Doing, Being, Becoming, and Belonging approach
✧ Eudaimonic well-being
✧ Inclusiveness
✧ Interdisciplinary approaches
✧ Intrinsicality

✧ Model of Occupational Performance
✧ Occupational identity
✧ Occupational integrity
✧ Occupational rights for all people
✧ Occupational science
✧ *Occupational Therapy Practice Framework*
✧ Recovery
✧ Recovery Model
✧ Resiliency
✧ Roles
✧ Social justice
✧ Spirit
✧ Spiritual context
✧ Spirituality
✧ Transcendence

An historical perspective of spirituality and occupational therapy can help put the topic into present-day context. This chapter provides an overview of the contemporary history of the occupational therapy profession as it directly relates to or has indirectly supported the idea of spirituality. It discusses the perspectives of the American Occupational Therapy Association (AOTA) and the Canadian Association for Occupational Therapists (CAOT) and their official definitions and descriptions of spirituality to illustrate how this topic has evolved.

The chapter then examines the occupational therapy profession from a global perspective, which has prompted the profession to address the topic of spirituality. Major movements in occupational therapy, such as client-centered care, occupational justice, recovery and health and wellness models, and the emergence of occupational science, have contributed to discussions of spirituality in the profession. These movements, initiated and promoted by occupational therapy practitioners and groups, either directly or through the influence of others outside the field, have endorsed and incorporated, but also have questioned, the ideals and constructs of spirituality within the occupational therapy profession.

The chapter provides an overview of contemporary perspectives and historical markers of spirituality in occupational therapy. It also highlights references to and varying constructs of spirituality espoused by select authors, recognizing that many of these ideas occurred simultaneously and frequently influenced one other.

AOTA and CAOT Definitions and Descriptions of *Spirituality*

AOTA and CAOT have articulated the value and importance of spirituality in occupational therapy through their publications on the topic, including formal association documents (e.g., AOTA, 2014; CAOT, 2007) and published articles and texts. Their public recognition that spirituality has been and is part of occupational therapy practice is noteworthy. This section explores how these organizations have described and upheld this complex construct.

AOTA and Spirituality

AOTA's first public endorsement of spirituality in occupational therapy was in the first edition of the *Occupational Therapy Practice Framework: Domain and Process* (AOTA, 2002). In this document, *spirituality* was considered a context in which people engaged, and *spiritual context* was defined as "the fundamental orientation of a person's life; that which inspires and motivates that individual" (p. 623). Indirectly, this document linked spirituality to a client's meaning, values, and beliefs, such as in the area of contexts that might support spiritual engagement.

In the second edition of the *Framework* (AOTA, 2008), the understanding of spirituality shifted from a contextual to a client perspective. Spirituality was now considered a *client factor* under the subcategory of Values, Beliefs, and Spirituality to "[r]eflect the way in which occupational therapy practitioners view and analyze meaning, values and beliefs of a broad range of clients" (AOTA, 2008, p. 665). The rationale given for this change included the idea that spirituality resides within the client instead of being part of a context. The official definition for *spirituality* given in this edition of the *Framework* was "the personal quest for understanding answers to ultimate questions about life, about meaning and about the sacred or transcendent, which may (or may not) lead to or arise from the development of religious rituals and the formation of community (Moreira-Almeida & Koenig, 2006, p. 844)" (p. 634).

In the third edition of the *Framework* (AOTA, 2014), the construct of spirituality shifted again. The term *spirituality,* still considered a client factor, was now defined as "the aspect of humanity that refers to the way individuals seek and express meaning and purpose and the way they experience their connectedness to the moment, to self, to others, to nature, and to the significant or sacred" (p. S7). In this iteration, spirituality shifted from a philosophical approach to understanding the mysteries and questions of life to a rational approach of engaging in occupations to find meaning or purpose in life. Spirituality and ritual are also now more explicitly related to the instrumental activity of daily living of religious and spiritual activities and expressions.

The changes in how AOTA has considered spirituality within the profession over time is evident in the three editions of the *Framework* (AOTA, 2002, 2008, 2014; Table 2.1). In addition, many

Table 2.1. Changes in Understanding of Spirituality in the *Framework*

Area	Description
Framework (2002): Spiritual context	
Contexts: "[R]efers to a variety of interrelated conditions within and surrounding the client that influence performance" (p. 623). Contexts can be cultural, physical, social, personal, spiritual, temporal, and virtual. Some contexts are external to the client (e.g., physical, social, virtual); some are internal to the client (e.g., personal, spiritual); and one is external but is internalized by the client (i.e., cultural) through beliefs and values.	*Spiritual context:* "The fundamental orientation of a person's life; that which inspires and motivates that individual" (p. 633).
Framework (2nd edition, 2008): Religious observance and spirituality	
IADLs: "Activities to support daily life within the home and community that often require more complex interactions than self-care used in ADLs" (p. 631).	*Religious observance*: "Participating in *religion*, 'an organized system of beliefs, practices, rituals, and symbols designed to facilitate closeness to the sacred or transcendent' (Moreira-Almeida & Koenig, 2006, p. 844)" (p. 631).
Client factors—person: "[I]nclude (1) values, beliefs, and spirituality; (2) body functions; and (3) body structures that reside within the client and may affect performance in areas of occupation" (p. 634).	*"Values, beliefs, and spirituality* influence a client's motivation to engage in occupations and give his or her life meaning" (p. 633).
	Values: "[P]rinciples, standards, or qualities considered worthwhile by the client who holds them" (p. 633).
	Beliefs: "'[C]ognitive content held as true' (Moyers & Dale, 2007, p. 28)" (p. 633).
	Spirituality: "'[T]he personal quest for understanding answers to ultimate questions about life, about meaning and about relationship with the sacred or transcendent, which may (or may not) lead to or arise from the development of religious rituals and the formation of community' (Moreira-Almeida & Koenig, 2006, p. 844)" (p. 633).
Performance patterns—person and population: "Patterns of behavior related to an individual's or significant other's daily life activities (or related to a population) that are habitual or routine" (p. 643).	*Rituals—person:* "Symbolic actions with spiritual, cultural, or social meaning, contributing to the client's identity and reinforcing values and beliefs. Rituals have a strong affective component and represent a collection of events" (Fiese et al., 2002; Segal, 2004) (p. 643). "Habits, routines, roles, and rituals can support or hinder occupational performance" (p. 642).
	Rituals—population: "[S]hared social actions with traditional, emotional, purposive, and technological meaning, contributing to values and beliefs within the population" (p. 644).

(Continued)

Table 2.1. Changes in Understanding of Spirituality in the *Framework* (*Cont.*)

Area	Description
Framework (3rd edition, 2014): Religious observance and spirituality	
IADLs: Same definition as 2nd ed.	*Religious and spiritual activities and expression:* "Participating in *religion*, 'an organized system of beliefs, practices, rituals, and symbols designed to facilitate closeness to the sacred or transcendent' (Moreira-Almeida & Koenig, 2006, p. 844), and engaging in activities that allow a sense of connectedness to something larger than oneself or that are especially meaningful, such as taking time out to play with a child, engaging in activities in nature, and helping others in need (Spencer, Davidson, & White, 1997)" (p. S20).
Client factors—person: Same definition as 2nd ed.	*Values, beliefs, and spirituality:* "Clients' perceptions, motivations, and related meaning that influence or are influenced by engagement in occupations" (p. S22).
	Values: "Acquired beliefs and commitments, derived from culture, about what is good, right, and important to do (Kielhofner, 2008)" (p. S22).
	Beliefs: "Cognitive content held as true by or about the client" (p. S22).
	Spirituality: "'The aspect of humanity that refers to the way individuals seek and express meaning and purpose and the way they experience their connectedness to the moment, to self, to others, to nature, and to the significant or sacred' (Puchalski et al., 2009, p. 887)" (p. S22).
Performance patterns—person and population: "[T]he habits, routines, roles, and rituals used in the process of engaging in occupations or activities; these patterns can support or hinder occupational performance" (p. S27).	*Rituals—person:* "Symbolic actions with spiritual, cultural, or social meaning contributing to the client's identity and reinforcing values and beliefs. Rituals have a strong affective component and consist of a collection of events (Fiese, 2007; Fiese et al., 2002; Segal, 2004)" (p. S27).
	Rituals—population: "Shared social actions with traditional, emotional, purposive, and technological meaning contributing to values and beliefs within the group or population" (p. S27)

Note. ADLs = activities of daily living; IADLs = instrumental activities of daily living.

occupational therapy practitioners (from inside and outside the United States) had been writing about the topic well before the publication of the first edition of the *Framework* (AOTA, 2002), when AOTA first publicly endorsed the concepts of spirituality in the profession.

CAOT and Spirituality

Canadian occupational therapy practitioners point to 1919 as a landmark year because the integration of mind–body–spirit was conveyed in CAOT's emblem and badge worn by practitioners (CAOT, 2002).

Publically supported identification of spirituality has had a long history in Canadian occupational therapy and is also highlighted in contemporary literature. In 1997, CAOT unveiled the **Canadian Model of Occupational Performance** (**CMOP;** Fearing, Law, & Clark, 1997), which was then revised in 2002 (CAOT, 2002). Both the original and revised articles provided a practice model that endorsed spirituality as the central core of each person. *Spirituality* was defined as "a pervasive life force, manifestation of a higher self, source of will and self-determination, and a sense of meaning, purpose and connectedness that people experience in the context of their environment" (CAOT, 2002, p. 182).

In 2007, the CMOP was further revised and renamed the **Canadian Model of Occupational Performance and Engagement** (**CMOP–E;** CAOT, 2007). This most current revision of the model maintained the original definition of *spirituality* with the addition of the phrases "spirituality is sensitivity to the presence of spirit" and "spirituality resides in persons, is shaped by the environment, and gives meaning to occupations" (CAOT, 2007, p. 374).

Spirituality and Religious Practices as Occupations in the Literature

Articles specifically related to religious or spiritual practices as occupations began appearing in the 1990s in the *American Journal of Occupational Therapy*, the *Canadian Journal of Occupational Therapy*, and other journals (Exhibit 2.1 includes a sample of these articles as well as texts). The purpose of the articles ranged from describing spiritual and religious occupations from an analytical perspective to articulating the challenges of completing such tasks when clients have experienced particular illnesses or disabilities and describing how people with illnesses or disabilities attend to and accomplish such tasks. These articles started to point occupational therapy practitioners in the direction of considering spirituality as an occupation or as an aspect within a select occupation that might be addressed in the therapeutic process.

Client-Centered Care

The idea of **client-centered care,** or shifting the power dynamics in the therapeutic relationship from the practitioner to the client, espoused through

---

Exhibit 2.1. Sample of Articles and Texts Related to Spirituality and Occupations

- *Spirituality, Daily Practice, and the Occupational Performance Model* (Urbanowski & Vargo, 1994)
- *Jewish Spirituality Through Actions in Time: Daily Occupations of Young Orthodox Jewish Couples in Los Angeles* (Frank et al., 1997)
- *Reflections on . . . Spirituality and Occupation: Garden Musings and the Himalayan Blue Poppy* (Unruh, 1997)
- *Occupational Therapy and Spirituality: Reflecting on Quality of Experience in Therapeutic Interventions* (Collins, 1998)
- *The Art of Observation: Reflecting on a Spiritual Moment* (Toomey, 1999)
- *The Experience of Pet Ownership as a Meaningful Occupation* (Allen, Kellegrew, & Jaffe, 2000)
- *Spiritual Agent Modalities for Occupational Therapy Practice* (Rosenfeld, 2000)
- *The Occupation of Gardening in Life-Threatening Illness* (Unruh, Smith, & Scammel, 2000)
- *Holidays and Celebrations as a Spiritual Occupation* (Luboshitzky & Gaber, 2001)
- *Spirituality, Motivation and Performance* (Rosenfeld, 2001)
- *The Impact of an Allotment Group on Mental Health Clients' Health, Well-Being and Social Networking* (Fieldhouse, 2003)
- *The Presence of Child Spirituality* (Burgman & King, 2005)
- *Spirituality: A Review of How Occupational Therapists Acknowledge, Assess, and Meet Spiritual Needs* (Johnston & Mayers, 2005)
- *Exploring Prayer as a Spiritual Modality* (Farah & McColl, 2008)
- *Relationships Among Religiousness, Spirituality, and Health for Individuals With Spinal Cord Injury* (Franklin, Yoon, Acuff, & Johnstone, 2008)
- *The Meaning and Functions of Occupations Related to Spirituality for African Nova Scotian Women* (Beagan & Etowa, 2011)

---

the CMOP and then later expanded on through the CMOP–E, directed occupational therapy practitioners to consider the client's perspectives within the therapy process. It also helped practitioners shift their understanding of power and authority within the therapeutic relationship and process and begin to look at health and wellness from a perspective of hope (vs. limitations) and resiliency (vs. dependency). Some occupational therapy scholars and practitioners have suggested that some notion of spirituality is essential to these ideas about client-centered care. Although differences may exist in how spirituality has been conceptualized and upheld, client-centeredness centralizes honoring clients and families and their personal meaning of life, choice, hope, and resilience (Kirsh, Trentham, & Cole, 2006).

The following evidence-based literature within occupational therapy has highlighted a client-centered approach and implicitly or explicitly identified spirituality:

- Clients' perspectives of care, wellness, and quality of life (Pereira & Stagnitti, 2008; Schleinich, Warren, Nekolaichuk, Kaasa, & Watanabe, 2008; Thomas, Gray, McGinty, & Ebringer, 2011)
- Clients' perspectives and responses to rehabilitation and community-based programs (Haltiwanger & Brutus, 2012; Lloyd, Wong, & Petchkovsky, 2007; Peoples, Satink, & Steultjens, 2011; Schleinich et al., 2008; Thomas et al., 2011)
- Practice suggestions seeking to acknowledge and incorporate clients' sociocultural, spiritual, or religious practices and therapeutic activities (Feeney & Toth-Cohen, 2008; Liddle & McKenna, 2000; Lloyd & O'Connor, 2007).

Model of Occupational Performance

Guidelines for client-centered care had been developed in waves from 1979 through 1987. In 1990, Townsend, Brintnell, and Staisey published "Developing Guidelines for Client-Centered Occupational Therapy Practice," which outlined their *Model of Occupational Performance* to address client-centered care. The model promoted a way to make sense of practice from a personal, client perspective versus a fundamentally treatment or protocol approach.

Townsend et al. (1990) highlighted occupational therapy's interest and domain in health as "an individual's ability to integrate everyday activity/occupation into a holistic, developmentally appropriate way of life which that individual defines as purposeful" (p. 70). They furthered the concept of *intervention* to consider working directly with the client and with the people with whom the

client relates. According to Townsend et al., occupational therapy practitioners may be considered consultants or asked to provide therapy services indirectly to clients through caregivers, teachers, health care workers, members of the family, volunteers, and so forth.

Townsend et al. (1990) emphasized adaptation and activity as central to intervention, arguing that client-centered practice "promote[s] adaptation, not only of the self, but also of the environment where environmental change will enhance an individual's possibility for independence, a sense of internal control and a purposeful existence" (p. 72). Promoting purposeful existence started the conversation about considering spirituality as a core part of engagement in occupation.

Three volumes of guidelines (CAOT, 1991, 1997, 2002) were based on the Model of Occupational Performance, which involved integrating four performance components (i.e., physical, mental, sociocultural, and spiritual) for a person to engage in valued occupations. Townsend et al. (1990) explained *spirituality* as reflecting a

> mind–spirit paradigm . . . and [representing] the need to explore meaning in life and is central in assessment of and intervention in occupational performance. Spirituality provides a basis for motivation which represents one's intrinsic sense of purpose and energy. Motivation is the integration of spiritual, socio-cultural and mental components of occupational performance. (p. 72)

When implementing the guidelines, some practitioners accepted and integrated the concept of client-centered practice but still faced challenges in the workplace to fully engage in this paradigm.

A follow-up study by Blain and Townsend (1993) assessed the understanding of the Model of Occupational Performance and the use of the guidelines. The results showed that the the model's constructs were implemented in practice, particularly in acute care and rehabilitation settings, but that practitioners were uncertain about the use of spirituality in practice. Even though practitioners saw spirituality as "integral to occupational therapy's concern with meaning and purpose in people's lives" (Blain & Townsend, 1993, p. 277), they also perceived its use in practice as complex.

Adoption of Client-Centered Care

Client-centered care has been widely adopted in the occupational therapy community and has pushed the profession to reconsider how it conceptualizes practice (AOTA, 2014; Christiansen, Baum, & Bass-Haugen, 2005), conducts assessments (AOTA, 2014; Klein, Barlow, & Hollis, 2008), and implements therapy (AOTA, 2014; CAOT, 2007; Christiansen et al., 2005). Practitioners have been urged to consider the perspectives of clients with whom they work to inform their practice (McCormack & Collins, 2010).

Perspectives about who should make health care decisions or who should establish the priorities and goals for therapy shifted when practitioners who assumed primary authority over and expertise about the therapy process came to recognize the importance of client-centered practice. These practitioners recognized the importance of clients having authority and power over their life choices and health care needs, including how they understand spirituality, meaning and purpose, and end-of-life care. Client-centered care principles also affirmed the client by "respecting the client's personal definitions of *hope* and his or her perspective on his or her own wellness" (McCormack & Collins, 2010, p. 342, *italics added*).

To better appreciate and respect client perspectives, some authors have suggested the use of ***client narratives,*** which are personal stories of lived experiences, to explore clients' understanding of meaning, purpose, and spirituality (Kirsh, 1996). By listening deeply to how and what the client shares about these lived experiences, practitioners have an opportunity to expand their understanding of what is most important to the client. Narratives may enlighten the practitioner about the importance of spiritual practices and beliefs, the meaning of a newly faced health challenge, and how meaning and hope had been found during past hardships.

Recovery Model

Client-centered care spurred the ***Recovery Model*** espoused in contemporary mental health intervention (Bassett, Lloyd, & Tse, 2008). The model considers what constitutes health for people with physical, social, or cognitive disabilities (Faull & Kalliath, 2001); supports the promotion of community health and wellness (Trentham,

Cockburn, & Shin, 2007; Tse, Lloyd, Petchkovsky, & Manaia, 2005); and upholds the incorporation of recovery principles in occupational therapy practice (Gruhl, 2005; Lloyd et al., 2007).

In promoting concepts of the Recovery Model, Bassett et al. (2008) offered suggestions on how practitioners may become more sensitive to the needs of clients by including spirituality and hope in assessment and intervention. In a review of the literature and conceptualization of spirituality, Bassett et al. included the constructs of motivation; personal goals; the pursuit of meaning and purpose; and, when applicable to the client, client religious beliefs in making sense of the world. The review suggested that ***recovery*** "can be viewed as the process by which people affected by mental health problems reclaim their lives and rebuild their connectedness with themselves, others, and with their environment, while developing a new sense of meaning and purpose to life" (Bassett et al., 2008, p. 255).

Resiliency

Trentham et al. (2007) discussed resiliency as an important aspect of recovery and health promotion for those with long-term mental health and physical challenges. ***Resiliency*** is the "capability of individuals and systems (families, groups, and communities) to cope successfully with significant adversity or risk.... [It] develops over time and is enhanced by protective factors within the individual or system and the environment and contributes to the maintenance of health" (Trentham et al., 2007, p. 55). Trentham et al. argued that by developing and strengthening both supportive communities and environments and client performance skills, clients would be able to engage in valued occupations and subsequently build resiliency. Trentham et al. also highlighted the importance of mental health promotion, collaboration, community action, and development and a consumer- or survivor-driven perspective as the focus of occupational therapy programs. They listed various workshops that facilitate such programs, one of which was on "discovering your spirituality" (p. 61).

Spirituality and health and wellness

Faull and Kalliath (2001) specifically identified spirituality as a determinant of health and wellness in people dealing with physical, social, or cognitive loss. They described spirituality as consisting of relationships (within self, between self and others, and external spiritual forces and nature), relatedness and connectedness (relationships that are experienced and perceived as an essential component of self), meaning (purpose of own life), and beliefs and clarity of principles (a personal belief system that helps interpret life meaning and life experiences). They furthered the notion that spirituality was central to health promotion:

> If spirituality is viewed as the core and essence of life, indeed the only permanent dimensions of self, then health would be perceived and defined somewhat differently than just optimal functioning of the objective dimensions of self. Indeed, if overall health is dependent on the health of the spiritual dimension as we have argued here, then accessing the dimension ought to lead to positive effects on the health status of the cognitive, social, and physical dimensions. (p. 13)

Therefore, spirituality is at the heart of health and wellness, and attending to spiritual aspects is paramount to addressing a person's health problems, whether they are physical, social, or psychological. From this perspective, spirituality should be at the forefront of intervention when considering health and wellness practices.

Mary Ann McColl: Spirituality in Occupational Therapy

In the first published book entirely and specifically related to spirituality in occupational therapy, *Spirituality and Occupational Therapy*, Mary Ann McColl (2003) described the assumptions and motivations that guided the text. Along with the historical understanding and value of spirituality as described by CAOT (2002), McColl also acknowledged

- The natural human drive to understand what lies beyond the known realm of their earthly experience and senses
- Health care professionals' impetus, provided by work, to better understand existential questions about death, pain, and suffering

- Practitioners' understanding of the possible link between spirituality and disability and desire to understand their clients' experiences from a holistic perspective, including the spiritual perspective.

Transcendence

McColl (2003) described the concept of **spirit** through the notion of **transcendence,** or "an experience that goes beyond normal human experience" (p. 221), as a difficult construct to fully articulate. However, she stated that spirit allows people to recognize a power greater than themselves and provides awareness of the cosmos. It is responsible for the connection between people and is "the force that dissolves the boundaries between self and others, and helps us realize that other people and other parts of the world are real" (McColl, 2003, p. 222). Spirit is the source of meaning or the "opportunity to see universal truths in specific activities, to obtain a view of the whole cosmos in relation to a particular daily pattern of life, and to see one's life as a whole in relation to the grander scheme of things" (McColl, 2003, p. 222).

Occupation and Health

In the second edition of her book, McColl (2011b) defined *spirituality* as "the desire for, or sensitivity to, the presence of spirit" (p. 18) and *spirit* as "the force that animates living things" (p. 18). She, along with the book's contributors, provided chapters related to concepts and definitions of *spirituality* and then built on conceptual models related to occupation and health (McColl, 2011a), occupational therapy values (Thibeault, 2011b) and gifts (Thibeault, 2011a), resilience and maturity (Thibeault, 2011c), transformation and maturity (Forster, Fardella, & McColl, 2011), occupational choice (Pentland & McColl, 2011), and the spiritual path (Brémault-Phillips & Chivorsky, 2011b).

The text provided models of practice in which particular modalities were suggested to evoke spirituality. The description of direct interventions included assessing spirituality (McColl, 2011b), working with chaplains (Huth, 2011), engaging in traditional spiritual practices (Brémault-Phillips & Chirovsky, 2011a), and using direct spiritual intervention (Farah & McColl, 2008, 2011).

Indirect intervention included the use of or engagement with narratives (Egan & Vallée, 2011; Kirsh, 2011), ritual (Thibeault, 2011d), creativity (Toomey, 2011; Woodbridge, 2011), work (Baptiste, 2011), and nature (Unruh, 2011).

Application to Practice

The most prevalent areas in which spirituality is addressed in the field, as indicated in the literature, include mental health (Clarke, 2003; Csontó, 2009), hospice and palliative care (AOTA, 2011; Dawson & Barker, 1995; Pizzi & Briggs, 2004; Shu Shan Teo, 2009; Trump, 2001), home-based or community-based programs (Csontó, 2009; Griffith, Caron, Desrosiers, & Thibeault, 2007; McPhee & Johnson, 2000), and occupational justice programs (Kronenberg, Algado, & Pollard, 2005; Kronenberg, Pollard, & Sakellariou, 2011). There is also some recognition that attending to spiritual needs in adult rehabilitation is feasible within an appropriately supported work context (Feeney & Toth-Cohen, 2008) and applicable to traditionally based medical models of practice (Donica, 2008; Weskamp & Ramugondo, 2005).

McColl (2011b) provided rich descriptions of how to understand spirituality within occupational therapy and many examples of how occupational therapy researchers and practitioners apply these constructs to practice. She also discussed the following challenges in moving forward:

> Another thing that is the same 10 years later is the ambivalent approach that we still take as a profession toward spirituality. At the same time that we acknowledge its importance, we still resist attempts to define spirituality, and we cling to an intuitive approach to spirituality. Thus the gap persists between the rhetoric and the behavior of occupational therapists. The rhetoric embraces the concept; but educational programs still allocate a tiny percentage of student contact time to spirituality, relatively few therapists address it in their practice, and the research is sparse to help us understand the relationship between spirituality and occupation. (p. 271)

McColl identified barriers to a "more wholesome approach to spirituality in occupational therapy"

(p. 270). She acknowledged the absence of language and clear descriptions of particular aspects of spirituality, the commodification of spirituality related only to outcome studies, the personal and professional beliefs that do not permit acknowledging the unknown, the focus of doing therapy versus "being" (i.e., honoring personal existence and experience), the insistence of an intuitive approach instead of a scholarship of spirituality, and the limitations of maintaining a rigid understanding of personal–professional boundaries.

McColl (2011b) acknowledged that the use of (or interest or involvement in) spirituality within practice is not for all practitioners. However, she also provided suggestions to help "move the field of spirituality in occupational therapy forward" (p. 274). For example, she stated that occupational therapy practitioners need to further their understanding of the concept of *meaning* and its application to spirituality. They also need to think about spirituality not as a system or modality used in practice but as a journey or path. Moreover, the occupations used as metaphorical doorways or bridges in that spiritual journey or path need to be further investigated and understood.

Challenging Spirituality

Several authors have challenged the use of the term *spirituality* regarding occupational performance and suggested alternatives. For example, Hammel (2001) proposed the term *intrinsicality,* and Unruh, Versnel, and Kerr (2002) the term *occupational identity.*

Intrinsicality

The term **intrinsicality** was proposed by Hammell (2001) as a better way to describe the inherent and universal quality of motivation and hope compared with the term *spirituality* as used in the CMOP. Hammell argued, "Use of the word *spirituality* is problematic and potentially ambiguous" (p. 186, *italics added*). Hammell furthered her opinion by stating, "We need a new term ... to avoid ambiguity, to clarify our understanding of client-centered practice, avoid imposing beliefs informed by our own class, cultural and educational backgrounds and to make explicit our mandate in informing client-centered intervention" (p. 191). Although the term *intrinsicality* was never officially adopted by CAOT, Hammell's argument heightened awareness about the controversy in using the term *spirituality* in occupational performance.

Occupational Identity

Unruh et al. (2002) argued that the central core of occupational therapy is occupation, not spirituality, and suggested the use of **occupational identity** as a better term for understanding the reason to engage in occupations. They defined it as "the expression of the physical, affective, cognitive and spiritual aspects of human nature, in an interaction with the institutional, social, cultural and political dimensions of the environment, across time and space of a person's life span, through the occupations of self-care, productivity and leisure" (p. 14).

One problem with using the term *spirituality* in occupational therapy is lack of a standard definition. In an extensive review of the literature in occupational therapy and other health-related fields, Unruh et al. (2002) presented several difficulties related to acceptance of a universal definition of *spirituality,* including, but not limited to, acknowledging religious connotations with spirituality, including reference to a higher being, and supporting the notion of another worldly dimension or the concept of transcendence. They then provided four dimensions of spirituality that were portrayed in the literature (i.e., secular, sacred, theistic, religious), highlighting the challenges of choosing one succinct description or definition of *spirituality.* In addition, they cautioned that use of only one dimension or perspective to define spirituality in occupational therapy can undermine true spiritual examination:

> [T]ension between religious, sacred, and secular perspectives of spirituality occurs in the field of spirituality and within occupational therapy. The tensions can obfuscate the spiritual questioning which underlies these perspectives. Regardless of whether a secular, sacred or religious definition is preferred, spirituality implies a search for answers to fundamental spiritual questions such as: How was the world created? What is the origin of life? Is there life after death? How do we account

for the presence of good and evil? What are our obligations to each other and the world around us? Is there redemption or forgiveness for wrongs and omissions? What is the meaning and purpose of human life? Is there a supreme being or a higher intelligence over all life? Why do bad things happen to good people? (p. 12)

Focus of therapy

Although spirituality may be closely connected to a person's occupational identity, Unruh et al. (2002) stated that occupational performance (and how it affects occupational identity) needs to be the focus of therapeutic intervention. Illness, injury, and other challenging life circumstances restrict a person's occupational performance and subsequently affect occupational identity. It is in the reconstruction of new roles, rituals, and routines in response to such difficulties that occupational performance is enhanced and ultimately occupational identity restored and affirmed. Spirituality may or may not be a component of that process.

Occupational therapy practitioners may need to address a client's occupational identity before occupational performance. For example, when a client experiences grief and despair because of the loss of occupational performance, the practitioner and client may need to collaboratively attend to the "reformulation" (Unruh et al., 2002, p. 16) of occupational identity before the client is able to pursue goals directly related to or focused on occupational performance. In other words, although the ultimate goal of therapy might be improved or increased occupational performance, it may be premature to start therapeutic interventions that target this performance before the client is able to create a new identity, including considering new potentials and possibilities.

Acknowledging clients' spirituality

Unruh et al. (2002) clarified their idea about occupational identity versus spirituality by acknowledging that the personal search for answers to life's questions, particularly during crises and altered life circumstances, may be part of the rehabilitation and recovery journey. Therefore, occupational therapy practitioners should be sensitive to how clients make meaning of these difficult times and be respectful of how clients incorporate spirituality into this meaning making. Listening and caring should be part of the therapeutic relationship; however, addressing the spiritual needs of the client is not, and should not be, the focus of occupational therapy.

In later work, Unruh, Versnel, and Kerr (2004) acknowledged that spirituality in occupational therapy could be understood through working with clients during the occupational therapy process. They presented two case studies. One linked spirituality with assessing and understanding a client's story or narrative in which a 4-year-old child engaged in play therapy. Through play, the child began acting out the events of and current occupational challenges due to her mother's death. The loss of connectedness through death was articulated by the authors as a spiritual matter. The therapist did not address the spiritual concern but did refer the child and family for grief counseling.

The other case illustrated a therapist working collaboratively with a client to engage in a spiritual activity of planning a private and personal graveside funeral service as a way to deal with grief and create a new image of identity. The case study featured a 15-year-old adolescent dealing with family conflicts, an unplanned pregnancy, and resulting emotional distress of running away from home and being rejected by the family. As therapy services were provided to attend to the emotional issues, the mother of the adolescent client unexpectedly died, furthering emotional turmoil and also highlighting the spiritual loss.

As part of the therapy process, the occupational therapist provided the client with the opportunity to construct and plan a funeral service for her mother. In the latter case study, the authors acknowledged the level of comfort and collaboration needed by the therapist to engage in such an occupation in therapy. Unruh et al. (2004) made it clear that the profession does not have a good understanding of the link among spirituality, occupation, and occupational well-being.

Cultural competence and occupational identity

Cultural competence is the ability to recognize and identify cultural aspects of occupations and support applicable use within intervention (Bonder, Martin, & Miracle, 2002). Examining occupational identity,

Rudman and Dennhardt (2008) urged occupational therapy practitioners to consider how their cultural understandings may prevent them from being truly client-centered. They argued that practitioners may present new images of potential and possibility to clients, offering them some hope in the recovery process, but that these images of improvement and self-determination may be only the practitioner's view and not consistent with or applicable to the client. For example, a practitioner might encourage a client to be independent in completing self-care, whereas the client and family consider it an honor to be cared for by the family.

Cultural competence extends to appreciating the culture of communities and groups and recognizing the conflict that may arise between individual perspectives and familial and community perspectives. Phelan and Kinsella (2009) highlighted the tension between the individual perspective of self, agency, and the essential self and the different perspective of self embedded, but not fully recognizable, within the larger community. The ideas of *agency* (i.e., choice and control) and productivity and the social dimensions that current models of occupational therapy practice highly esteem may not be shared by other cultures. Cultural competence suggests that practitioners are not only attuned to the individual's cultural contexts but also able to appreciate and attend to the larger social constructs of culture.

Although Phelan and Kinsella did not specifically link spirituality and occupational identity, they highlighted the complexity of understanding how occupational identity might be facilitated within the therapy process and the ensuing conflict that may arise between the practitioner and the client or family over different perceptions of values, goals, the meaning of the life crisis, and the purpose of life. Rudman and Dennhardt (2008) also encouraged practitioners and students to engage in critical reflection and analysis of their assumptions about occupation-based concepts, models, and assessments and to further research related to occupational science.

Occupational Science and Spirituality

Occupational science is the study of human participation in occupations. According to Hocking (2000), "the central concept within occupational science is occupation itself" (p. 59). The emergence of occupational science has assisted the occupational therapy profession in challenging long-held fundamental beliefs and assumptions about particular occupations being universally valued and engaged.

Occupational science began by exploring the essential elements of occupation. It expanded by examining the elements of occupational processes and then the complex and dynamic nature of occupations within socio–cultural–political and gender contexts (Hocking, 2000). Because occupations and occupational identity continually evolve, clients' personal perspectives must be considered when occupations are interpreted or analyzed during therapy (Christiansen, 1999). In addition, integrating clients' occupations, rituals, and routines, including those with religious or spiritual meaning, into therapy relies on the practitioner to understand how a person engages in an occupation and when he or she desires to or must make a change to that engagement.

Perspectives of Occupations

Persson, Erlandsson, Eklund, and Iwarsson (2001) provided a framework to better comprehend the complexity of human occupations by assigning levels or perspectives of occupations: macro, meso, and micro. The *macro* level is an integrated repertoire of chosen and valued occupations in which meaning is discovered or created within one's life and over time; *meso* is a select sampling of occupations conducted within a select time frame (e.g., day, week); and *micro* is related to the components of select occupations. Persson et al. also elucidated how life crises and the therapeutic process may change the meaning of an occupation for a person. All levels of occupations are important to consider within the therapeutic process.

The macro level of occupation, such as returning to work, assists practitioners in understanding the value and importance of occupations to a client, whereas the micro level, such as typing on a keyboard, is used to restore a client's occupational performance. A single occupation at the micro level may ultimately contribute to rebuilding the macro level. Moreover, ongoing development and integration of single occupations move the client to the meso level, where he or she may further judge the importance and value of each occupation and

the desire or need to move these occupations to the macro level.

According to Persson et al. (2001), the process of therapy should consist of ongoing assessment and integration of these levels with the knowledge that at any time, the client can make meaning of an occupation in relationship to his or her life circumstance. Persson et al.'s framework encouraged occupational therapy practitioners to focus on the meaning and value of occupations for each client throughout the therapeutic process.

For example, a client who wants to return to her vocation as an administrative assistant after a stroke may work toward that goal in therapy by completing select occupational tasks, such as typing. How well the client progresses with typing and her perceived ability to do so effectively and efficiently may provide insights into her desire and willingness to continue to pursue the ultimate goal of returning to her job. Additionally, the practitioner and client may discuss what her vocation means to the client, including how it correlates to her purpose in life or intrinsic connection to others. Therefore, attending to the client's work occupation can expand her understanding of the spiritual constructs of meaning, purpose, and connection.

Doing, Being, Becoming, and Belonging

Occupational science has been instrumental in heightening awareness about occupations, including how people make sense of, or derive meaning from, an occupation and ultimately how that meaning gives perspective about life. Wilcock's (2007) *Doing, Being, Becoming, and Belonging approach* describes a multidimensional progression of engagement (*doing*) leading to enlightenment (*being* and *becoming*) and inclusion (*belonging*). The concept of being was linked with spirituality as an aspect of the self related to a person's unique interpretation or meaning making of doing that informs life choices and satisfaction. Belonging is also associated with spirituality as it relates to connectedness with others.

Engagement in occupation is not only doing tasks but also having an internal awareness and integration of the self through doing. In other words, as people engage, or not, in occupations, they develop a sense of who they are. All of the dimensions of doing, being, becoming, and belonging can be seriously tested by injury, illness, or disability. Wilcock (2007) emphasized the dynamic interplay among these four dimensions and proposed that being, becoming, and belonging evolved over time and place. The sense of self can be affected by the therapeutic process as new meaning is attributed to engagement in occupations.

Roles

The changing nature of occupations and roles can produce conflict within the self and the community. *Roles* are "sets of behaviors expected by society and shaped by culture and context that may be further conceptualized and defined by the client (AOTA, 2014, p. S45). Abrahams (2008) suggested that engagement in multiple roles and their inherent cultural constructs could create tension, which ultimately needs to be resolved, at some level, for health and wellness. Abrahams stated that "a problem arises when cultural values and beliefs are in tension, such that conflict arises between equally meaningful occupations and in [the] way they are pursued. In my experience, it was the decision to resign from full-time employment to assume the role of mother and primary caregiver that was in conflict with the desire to be successful in my role as a health professional" (p. 187).

One example of the tension between self and community is coming of age in young adulthood to establish independent roles away from family and community. For example, Awaad (2003) discussed the conflict between being a young, devout conservative Muslim woman while also living and working in communities that upheld values of independence, self-determination, and assertiveness. This potential conflict between roles often compels people to deliberate about the meaning and integration of their roles or the need to change them. Spiritual engagement encourages people to work through and make sense of these struggles and helps affirm their core beliefs and ideals.

Eudaimonic Well-Being

The field of occupational science has expanded to embrace *interdisciplinary approaches* for examining occupations by drawing from related disciplines (Wilcock, 2007). For example, researchers have studied the interconnection and confluence among occupation, spirituality, and health and well-being, called eudaimonic well-being, by drawing on psychology, occupational therapy, and theology (Powell, Shahabi, & Thorensen, 2003; Seeman, Dubin, & Seeman, 2003). Eudaimonic well-being may develop on a personal or collective level, and spirituality supports and sustains that well-being.

In *eudaimonic well-being,* engaging in activities or occupations that hold deep value for a person can produce a sense of well-being, even if the activities or occupations are challenging. These deep values can be viewed as a form of spirituality, or the inner resource to engage in challenging but meaningful occupations (Hayward & Taylor, 2011). Examples of eudaimonic well-being include an athlete who trains for and then runs a triathlon or a working parent who enrolls in and completes an educational program.

The idea of eudaimonic well-being has been expanded to include the lived experience of *occupational integrity,* which involves a person living out his or her meaningful roles and occupations while considering the well-being of others and, at times, all humanity (Hayward & Taylor, 2011). Eudaimonic well-being, and the underlying spirituality to endure and embrace substantial challenges, is understood not by the amount of financial and material resources people have but by their inherent and universal capacity for hope, individually and collectively. Elelwani Ramugondo (2005), a South African occupational therapist and researcher, added to this conversation when she spoke about her experiences in South Africa:

Is it possible for people to live in hope and to achieve the meaning and purpose that spirituality brings while living in poverty and exposed to acute suffering? Do such people ever hope? Can one find even a glimmer of human potential, alive and active under such circumstances? These are important questions for any occupational therapist to ask. The question becomes even more relevant when one is working with any community groups of people, or individuals, and particularly when they come from impoverished sectors, as is often the case in South Africa. This takes on an even greater importance if the occupational therapist's work is community development. (p. 160)

Ramugondo (2005) suggested that spirituality, which is inherent in each person, may not be sufficient to attend to personal roles and occupations challenged under the extreme and constant circumstances of poverty, war, famine, and death. Working alongside mothers and their children who had been diagnosed with HIV/AIDS, Ramugondo realized that she would first need to form relationships with the mothers and children and then offer opportunities for them to come together as a group to attend to their own personal spirituality and roles and occupations. She discussed the power of this collectivism to develop personal inner strength in the women: "[T]he need to be acknowledged[,] allowed to inform . . . intervention strategies[, and be] part of a supportive family or group, without any tangible outputs, may sometimes be sufficient to fulfill the needs of an individual" (p. 163).

Hayward and Taylor (2011) suggested that multiple perspectives and influences should be considered within the concept of eudaimonic well-being because one person's or community's values may conflict with or negatively affect another person's or community's values and well-being. Therefore, it is important for occupational therapy practitioners to understand the occupations that enhance well-being for an individual and their impact on the wider community. "In other words, it is important to consider the macro level of well-being and to engage the 'being' before the 'doing' (Howard & Taylor, 2011, p. 139)...and [give] recognition to the importance of considering the sustainability of our social and natural environments" (Howard & Taylor, 2011, p. 142).

Social Justice

Townsend (1993) articulated that practitioners should consider their own spirituality, attitudes of inclusiveness, and collaborative meaning-making and consider how spirituality may be demonstrated within the therapeutic relationship and process. She challenged the occupational therapy community to consider the social nature of the profession and promote *social justice,* that is, addressing the inequalities and disparities within the larger community context. She suggested that individual practitioners and the collective profession do so by "enabling development of occupational potential"

to ensure social equality (p. 176). She linked her social vision to a "spiritual concept and vision" in which all people have equal worth and a commitment is made to a spirit of inclusiveness (p. 177).

Promoting a perspective of *inclusiveness* that "demands unconditional respect, caring, love, trust, and value, regardless of a person's characteristics and contributions to everyday life" (p. 177), Townsend encouraged clinicians to elicit people's own definition and understanding of meaningful occupations and to embrace the concept that it is "an essential need for humans to experience meaning and power as worthy persons included within and important in the universe" (p. 181).

Townsend (1997) used the construct of spirituality, as it is depicted in the CMOP, to highlight a person's desire for meaning and occupations. Her goal in emphasizing a social agenda was to show practitioners how a collaborative, sharing, and respectful approach to occupational therapy was needed because "communities [that] extend equal respect and opportunities to people of differing abilities and characteristics create an energizing interconnectedness based on a community spirituality of inclusiveness" (p. 146). She encouraged practitioners to consider ways to challenge injustice when people and communities did not engender inclusiveness or the right for all people to engage in meaningful occupations.

Occupational Rights for All People

Occupational therapy scholars have espoused the ideal of *occupational rights for all people* (Hammell, 2008), which is the belief that everyone, with or without disabilities, has the right to engage in meaningful occupations that contribute positively to personal and communal well-being. Some scholars have supported this principle of dignity and inclusion by providing examples of occupational rights for all people throughout the world through injustices realized and then addressed (Kronenberg et al., 2005), such as

- Children survivors of war engaging in new life experiences and developing resilience and spiritual awareness and clarity,
- Children in poverty discovering the value of and engaging in art and creative expression and

building community solidarity together through that participation,

• People experiencing significant learning abilities by developing and using writing communities and publication outlets.

In the foreword for *Occupational Therapy Without Borders* (Kronenberg et al., 2005), David Werner (2005), director of HealthWrights (Workgroup for People's Health and Rights), linked spirituality to occupational rights and justice:

> This book is subtitled *Learning From the Spirit of Survivors.* Indeed, it emphasizes the importance of spirituality in the pursuit of personal and societal transformation. But "spirituality" is used in its broadest (least doctrinaire) sense to imply "the discovery of meaning in our day-to-day lives." Meaning in its existential sense involves actively realizing the link between our personal health, our collective [well-being], and our small but vital place in the universe. (p. xi–xii)

In other examples that promote the importance of engagement in meaningful occupations, authors have identified occupations that have been deemed challenging to discuss (e.g., sexuality, death and dying) and brought them to the forefront, highlighting the personal and collective injustices that occur when practitioners negate or disregard the meaningfulness of such occupations (Pollard, 2006; Sakellariou & Algado, 2006; Shamberg & Barr, 2006). Occupational rights sends a powerful message: If occupations have the ability to bring meaning to people and communities, then all occupations need to be considered able to do so. It is not only spiritual and religious activities that bring meaning; any occupation—the mundane as well as the profound—that holds meaning for a person or community can evoke a sense of spirituality.

Current Changes and Challenges

Spirituality has been, and continues to be, promoted within the field of occupational therapy. Accordingly, several concerns and considerations have been discussed and debated, including the ability of the practitioner

to skillfully and appropriately address spirituality in practice, the extent of the use of spirituality in practice, inadequate preparation of students and practitioners to conceptualize and use spirituality in practice, limited evidence to support spirituality in practice, and overlap of services.

Practitioner Ability

Several authors have expressed concern about whether occupational therapy practitioners have the ability to "encompass [the] diverse, strongly held opinions and also be tolerant of conflicting views" about spirituality (Wilson, 2010, p. 439). Occupational therapy intervention includes the client or group, significant others, and the practitioner. Each of these entities may come to the intervention process with differing perspectives of spirituality or with perspectives and goals that may not directly relate to spirituality.

Practitioners' background, experience, and comfort level in addressing spiritual needs and their willingness to do so are variable (Belcham, 2004; Dawson & Barker, 1995; Meredith, 2010; Morris et al., 2012; Udell & Chandler, 2000). Moreover, several authors have questioned practitioners' ability to recognize whether it is appropriate to explicitly use spiritual dimensions of occupation (Christiansen, 2008; Farah & McColl, 2008, 2011; Peloquin, 2008; Wilding 2002; Wilson, 2010).

Extent of the Use of Spirituality in Practice

The extent of the use of spirituality in practice has been an ongoing consideration. For example, Wilson (2010) questioned whether spirituality can or should be considered a part of the concept of occupation or only an inherent quality of being human. Although spirituality is important in many people's lives, particularly when they experience crisis, loss, or death, the practitioner's ability to respect clients' beliefs while providing intervention might be all they expect or desire (Wilson, 2010).

However, occupations considered meaningful to the client or those that provide hope, wellness, resiliency, and strength to rise above life challenges, including resisting injustices, are powerful and should be understood through the perspective of the client and collaboratively and intentionally incorporated into therapy (MacGillivray, Sumsion,

& Wicks-Nicholls, 2006; McPhee & Johnson, 2000). Therefore, is it sufficient to just understand what occupations are meaningful for the person and incorporate those into therapy, or is there benefit in understanding the spiritual aspects of an occupation and intentionally using those occupations to further develop or enhance personal growth?

Educational Programs

Educational programs that advocate and address the concepts of client-centered care may lack credibility or conviction in fully embracing the topic of spirituality. Although holism is espoused and client-centered care promoted within many curriculums, the actual application of spirituality in practice is still limited (Belcham, 2004; Csontó, 2009; Kirsh, Dawson, Antolikova, & Reynolds, 2001; Udell & Chandler, 2000). Additionally, fieldwork placements often have differing views of the use of spirituality in practice and use varying degrees of spiritual elements, including references to spirituality within assessments (Belcham, 2004; Csontó, 2009).

Lack of Empirical Research

Occupational therapy lacks empirical research that clearly identifies links between particular occupations, or modalities, and spirituality; provides outcomes on the use of select modalities in the way they affect spirituality (Wells, 2009; Wilding, 2002); or provides insights into the spiritual journey or path (McColl, 2011b).

For example, one modality historically used in occupational therapy and frequently associated with occupation and spirituality or meaning making is art and creative expression (Atkinson & Wells, 2000; Eklund, 2013; Hasselkus, 2002; Sadlo, 2004; Schmid, 2004; Toomey, 1999, 2011; Woodbridge, 2011). Yet, only one article has been found in the professional literature that has focused on the use of art and its implications for spirituality (Lloyd et al., 2007).

Another frequently used modality associated with spirituality is reflection and life writing (Denshire, 2002) and narrative exploration (Egan & Vallée, 2011; Kirsh, 1996, 2011). However, the scarce research related to this modality, although important to the profession, has been limited to autoethnographic insights (Forhan, 2010).

Overlap of Services

Questions have arisen about overlapping of services (i.e., addressing spirituality in relation to health care and wellness practices) and blurring of disciplinary lines with chaplaincy, nursing, social work, and psychology when occupational therapy practitioners use aspects of spirituality in care (Beagan & Kumas-Tan, 2005; Chochinov & Cann, 2005; Hummel, Galek, Murphy, Tannenbaum, & Flannelly, 2008; St. James O'Connor et al., 2012). In addition, use of spirituality in occupational therapy services may cause other health care professionals to perceive occupational therapy as lacking in value (Egan & Swedersky, 2003). Egan and Swedersky (2003) interviewed 8 occupational therapists who acknowledged that they considered spirituality while working with clients. In addition, these therapists assisted clients in dealing with suffering as it related to their current situation and were attentive to clients' expression of religious concerns. However, this approach used by the therapists sometimes caused conflict within the health care team about the exact nature and role of occupational therapy.

Summary

Despite the problems of theoretical models with limited empirical evidence to support spirituality in occupational therapy, insufficient preparation of students and practitioners for using spirituality in practice, and unclear practice roles regarding spirituality for practitioners in real-world contexts, there is some documented historical precedent for the use of spirituality in occupational therapy.

At the most basic level, spirituality is understood within the profession as an important aspect of life. It is valued and used by many clients in dealing with major life events and transitions, and respect and care about clients' and community's religious and spiritual practices needs to be offered for client-centered care. Some scholars and practitioners have furthered this basic appreciation and understanding to promote the use of spirituality within practice and intentionally address issues of spirituality with clients. The profession must continue the dialogue about the challenges of using spirituality in practice and promote research related to spirituality and occupation.

References

Abrahams, T. (2008). Occupation, identity and choice: A dynamic interaction. *Journal of Occupational Science, 15,* 186–189. http://dx.doi.org/10.1080/14427591.2008.9686629

Allen, J. M., Kellegrew, D. H., & Jaffe, D. (2000). The experience of pet ownership as a meaningful occupation. *Canadian Journal of Occupational Therapy, 67,* 271–278. http://dx.doi.org/10.1177/000841740006700409

American Occupational Therapy Association. (2002). Occupational therapy practice framework: Domain and process. *American Journal of Occupational Therapy, 56,* 609–639. http://dx.doi.org/10.5014/ajot.56.6.609

American Occupational Therapy Association. (2008). Occupational therapy practice framework: Domain and process (2nd ed.). *American Journal of Occupational Therapy, 62,* 625–683. http://dx.doi.org/10.5014/ajot.62.6.625

American Occupational Therapy Association. (2011). The role of occupational therapy in end-of-life care. *American Journal of Occupational Therapy, 65*(Suppl.), S66–S75. http://dx.doi.org/10.5014/ajot.2011.65S66

American Occupational Therapy Association. (2014). Occupational therapy practice framework: Domain and process (3rd ed.). *American Journal of Occupational Therapy, 68*(Suppl. 1), S1–S48. http://dx.doi.org/10.5014/ajot.2014.682006

Atkinson, K., & Wells, C. (2000). *Creative therapies: A psychodynamic approach within occupational therapy.* Cheltenham, UK: Stanley Thornes.

Awaad, J. (2003). Culture, cultural competency, and psychosocial occupational therapy: A Middle Eastern perspective. *British Journal of Occupational Therapy 66,* 409–415. http://dx.doi.org/10.1177/030802260306600804

Baptiste, S. (2011). Work: Understanding spirituality and work. In M. A. McColl (Ed.), *Spirituality and occupational therapy* (2nd ed., pp. 241–248). Ottawa, ON: CAOT Publications.

Bassett, H., Lloyd, C., & Tse, S. (2008). Approaching in the right spirit: Spirituality and hope in recovery from mental health problems. *International Journal of Therapy and Rehabilitation, 15,* 254–261. http://dx.doi.org/10.12968/ijtr.2008.15.6.29444

Beagan, B. L., & Etowa, J. B. (2011). The meaning and functions of occupations related to spirituality for African Nova Scotian women. *Journal of Occupational Science 18,* 277–290. http://dx.doi.org/10.1080/14427591.2011.594548

Beagan, B., & Kumas-Tan, Z. (2005). Witnessing spirituality in practice. *British Journal of Occupational Therapy, 68,* 17–28. http://dx.doi.org/10.1177/030802260506800104

Belcham, C. (2004). Spirituality in occupational therapy: Theory in practice? *British Journal of Occupational Therapy, 67,* 39–46. http://dx.doi.org/10.1177/030802260406700106

Blain, J., & Townsend, E. (1993). Occupational therapy guidelines for client-centered practice: Impact study findings. *Canadian Journal of Occupational Therapy, 60,* 271–285. http://dx.doi.org/10.1177/000841749306000508

Bonder, B. R., Martin, L., & Miracle, A. (2002). *Cultural threads in clinical contexts.* Thorofare, NJ: Slack.

Brémault-Phillips, S., & Chirovsky, A. (2011a). Spiritual practices. In M. A. McColl (Ed.), *Spirituality and occupational therapy* (2nd ed., pp. 183:192). Ottawa, ON: CAOT Publications.

Brémault-Phillips, S., & Chirovsky, A. (2011b). The spiritual path. In M. A. McColl (Ed.), *Spirituality and occupational therapy* (2nd ed., pp. 151:158). Ottawa, ON: CAOT Publications.

Burgman, I., & King, A. (2005). The presence of child spirituality. In F. Kronenberg, S. A. Algado, & N. Pollard (Eds.), *Occupational therapy without borders: Learning from the spirit of survivors* (pp. 153–165). New York: Elsevier/Churchill Livingstone.

Canadian Association of Occupational Therapists. (1991). *Occupational therapy guidelines for client-centered practice.* Toronto, ON: CAOT Publications.

Canadian Association of Occupational Therapists. (1997). *Enabling occupation: An occupational therapy perspective.* Ottawa, ON: CAOT Publications.

Canadian Association of Occupational Therapists. (2002). *Enabling occupation: An occupational therapy perspective* (2nd ed). Ottawa, ON: CAOT Publications.

Canadian Association of Occupational Therapists. (2007). *Enabling occupation II: Advancing an occupational therapy vision for health, well-being and justice through occupation.* Ottawa, ON: CAOT Publications.

Chochinov, H. M., & Cann, B. J. (2005). Interventions to enhance the spiritual aspects of dying. *Journal of Palliative Medicine, 8,* S103–S115. http://dx.doi.org/10.1089/jpm.2005.8.s-103

Christiansen, C. H. (1999). Defining lives: Occupation as identity: An essay on competence, coherence, and the creation of meaning [Eleanor Clarke Slagle Lecture]. *American Journal of Occupational Therapy, 53,* 544–558. http://dx.doi.org/10.5014/ajot.53.6.547

Christiansen, C. H. (2008). The dangers of thin air: A commentary on exploring prayer as a spiritual modality. *Canadian Journal of Occupational Therapy, 75,* 14–15. http://dx.doi.org/10.1177/000841740807500104

Christiansen, C. H., Baum, M. C., & Bass-Haugen, J. (Eds). (2005). *Occupational therapy: Performance, participation, and well-being.* Thorofare, NJ: Slack.

Clarke, C. (2003). Clinical application of the Canadian Model of Occupational Performance in a forensic rehabilitation hostel. *British Journal of Occupational Therapy, 66,* 171–174. http://dx.doi.org/10.1177/030802260306600407

Collins, M. (1998). Occupational therapy and spirituality: Reflecting on quality of experience in therapeutic interventions.

British Journal of Occupational Therapy, 61, 280–284. http://dx.doi.org/10.1177/030802269806100614

Csontó, S. (2009). Occupational therapy students' consideration of clients' spirituality in practice placement education. *British Journal of Occupational Therapy, 72,* 442–449. http://dx.doi.org/10.1177/030802260907201005

Dawson, S., & Barker, J. (1995). Hospice and palliative care: A Delphi survey of occupational therapists' roles and training needs. *Australian Occupational Therapy Journal, 42,* 119–127. http://dx.doi.org/10.1111/j.1440-1630.1995.tb01323.x

Denshire, S. (2002). Reflections on the confluence of personal and professional. *Australian Occupational Therapy Journal, 49,* 212–216. http://dx.doi.org/10.1046/j.1440-1630.2002.00338.x

Donica, D. K. (2008). Spirituality and occupational therapy: The application of the pyschospiritual integration frame of reference. *Physical and Occupational Therapy in Geriatrics, 27,* 107–121. http://dx.doi.org/10.1080/02703180802206082

Egan, M., & Swedersky, J. (2003). Spirituality as experienced by occupational therapists in practice. *American Journal of Occupational Therapy, 57,* 525–533. http://dx.doi.org/10.5014/ajot.57.5.525

Egan, M., & Vallée, C. (2011). Narrative: Reflections for good ghostwriting. In M. A. McColl (Ed.), *Spirituality and occupational therapy* (2nd ed., pp. 209–216). Ottawa, ON: CAOT Publications.

Eklund, M. (2013). Applying object relations theory to psychosocial occupational therapy. *Occupational Therapy in Mental Health 15,* 1–26. http://dx.doi.org/10.1300/J004v15n01_01

Farah, J., & McColl, M. A. (2008). Exploring prayer as a spiritual modality. *Canadian Journal of Occupational Therapy, 75,* 5–13. http://dx.doi.org/10.1177/000841740807500103

Farah, J., & McColl, M. A. (2011). In M. A. McColl (Ed.), *Spirituality and occupational therapy* (2nd ed., pp. 193–200). Ottawa, ON: CAOT Publications. http://dx.doi.org/10.1177/000841740807500103

Faull, K., & Kalliath, T. J. (2001). *Spirituality as a determinant of health for those with disabilities.* The Australian Journal of Rehabilitation Counselling, 7, 43–51. http://dx.doi.org/10.1017/S1323892200000843

Fearing, V. G., Law, M., & Clark, J. (1997). An occupational performance process model: Fostering client and therapist alliances. *Canadian Journal of Occupational Therapy, 64,* 7–15. http://dx.doi.org/10.1177/000841749706400103

Feeney, L., & Cohen, S. (2008). *Addressing spirituality for clients with physical disabilities.* Retrieved from bit.ly/1QfijZ8

Fieldhouse, J. (2003). The impact of an allotment group on mental health clients' health, well-being, and social networking. *British Journal of Occupational Therapy, 66,* 286–296. http://dx.doi.org/10.1177/030802260306600702

Fiese, B. H. (2007). Routines and rituals: Opportunities for participation in family health. *OTJR: Occupation, Participation and Health, 27,* 41S–49S. http://dx.doi.org/10.1177/15394492070270S106

Fiese, B. H., Tomcho, T. J., Douglas, M., Josephs, K., Poltrock, S., & Baker, T. (2002). A review of 50 years of research on naturally occurring family routines and rituals: Cause for celebration? *Journal of Family Psychology, 16,* 381–390. http://dx.doi.org/10.1037//0893-3200.16.4.381

Forhan, M. (2010). Doing, being, and becoming: A family's journey through perinatal loss. *American Journal of Occupational Therapy, 64,* 142–151. http://dx.doi.org/10.5014/ajot.64.1.142

Forster, D., Fardella, J., & McColl, M.A. (2011). Transformation and maturity. In M. A. McColl (Ed.), *Spirituality and occupational therapy* (2nd ed., pp. 131–140). Ottawa, ON: CAOT Publications.

Frank, G., Bernardo, C. S., Tropper, S., Noguchi, F., Lipman, C., Maulhardt, B., & Weitze, L. (1997). Jewish spirituality through actions in time: Daily occupations of young Orthodox Jewish couples in Los Angeles. *American Journal of Occupational Therapy, 57,* 199–206. http://dx.doi.org/10.5014/ajot.51.3.199

Franklin, K. L., Yoon, D. P., Acuff, M., & Johnstone, B. (2008). Relationships among religiousness, spirituality, and health for individuals with spinal cord injury. *Topics in Spinal Cord Injury Rehabilitation, 14,* 76–81. http://dx.doi.org/10.1310/sci1402-76

Griffith, J., Caron, C. D., Desrosiers, J., & Thibeault, R. (2007). Defining spirituality and giving meaning to occupation: The perspective of community-dwelling older adults and autonomy loss. *Canadian Journal of Occupational Therapy, 74,* 78–90. http://dx.doi.org/10.2182/cjot.06.0016

Gruhl, K. L. R. (2005). The recovery paradigm: Should occupational therapists be interested? *Canadian Journal of Occupational Therapy, 72,* 96–102. http://dx.doi.org/10.1177/000841740507200204

Haltiwanger, E., P., & Brutus, H. (2012). A culturally sensitive diabetes peer support for older Mexican-Americans. *Occupational Therapy International, 19,* 67–75. http://dx.doi.org/10.1002/oti.320

Hammell, K. W. (2001). Intrinsicality: Reconsidering spirituality, meaning(s), and mandates. *Canadian Journal of*

Occupational Therapy, 68, 186–194. http://dx.doi.org/10.1177/000841740106800307

Hammell, K. W. (2008). Reflections on . . . well-being and occupational rights. *Canadian Journal of Occupational Therapy, 75,* 61–64. http://dx.doi.org/10.2182/cjot.07.007

Hasselkus, B. R. (2002). *The meaning of everyday occupation.* Thorofare, NJ: Slack Incorporated.

Hayward, C., & Taylor, J. (2011). Eudaimonic well-being: Its importance and relevance to occupational therapy for humanity. *Occupational Therapy International, 18,* 133–141. http://dx.doi.org/10.1002/oti.316

Hocking, C. (2000). Occupational science: A stock take of accumulated insights. *Journal of Occupational Science, 7,* 58–67. http://dx.doi.org/10.1080/14427591.2000.9686466

Hummel, L., Galek, K., Murphy, K., Tannenbaum, H. P., & Flannelly, L. T. (2008). Defining spiritual care: An exploratory study. *Journal of Health Care Chaplaincy, 15,* 40–51. http://dx.doi.org/10.1080/08854720802698509

Huth, J. (2011). Working with chaplains. In M. A. McColl (Ed.), *Spirituality and occupational therapy* (2nd ed., pp. 175–182). Ottawa, ON: CAOT Publications.

Johnston, D., & Mayers, C. (2005). Spirituality: A review of how occupational therapists acknowledge, assess, and meet spiritual needs. *British Journal of Occupational Therapy, 68,* 386–392. http://dx.doi.org/10.1177/030802260506800902

Kielhofner, G. (2008). *The Model of Human Occupation: Theory and application* (4th ed.). Philadelphia: Lippincott Williams & Wilkins.

Kirsh, B. (1996). A narrative approach to addressing spirituality in occupational therapy: Exploring personal meaning and purpose. *Canadian Journal of Occupational Therapy, 63,* 55–61. http://dx.doi.org/10.1177/000841749606300107

Kirsh, B. (2011). Narrative: What makes narratives spiritual and how can we use them in OT? In M. A. McColl (Ed.), *Spirituality and occupational therapy* (2nd ed., pp. 201–208). Ottawa, ON: CAOT Publications.

Kirsh, B., Dawson, D., Antolikova, S., & Reynolds, L. (2001). Developing awareness of spirituality in occupational therapy students: Are our curricula up to the task? *Occupational Therapy International, 8,* 119–125. http://dx.doi.org/10.1002/oti.138

Kirsh, B., Trentham, B., & Cole, S. (2006). Diversity in occupational therapy: Experiences of consumers who identify themselves as minority group members. *Australian Occupational Therapy Journal, 53,* 310–313. http://dx.doi.org/10.1111/j.1440-1630.2006.00576.x

Klein, S., Barlow, I., & Hollis, V. (2008). Evaluating ADL measures from an occupational therapy perspective. *Canadian*

Journal of Occupational Therapy, 75, 69–81. http://dx.doi.org/10.1177/000841740807500203

Kronenberg, F., Algado, S. A., & Pollard, N. (2005). *Occupational therapy without borders: Learning from the spirit of survivors.* London: Elsevier/Churchill Livingstone.

Kronenberg, F., Pollard, N., & Sakellariou, D. (2011). *Occupational therapies without borders: Towards an ecology of occupation-based practices* (Vol. 2). London: Elsevier/Churchill Livingstone.

Liddle, J., & McKenna, K. (2000). Quality of life: An overview of issues for use in occupational therapy outcome measures. *Australian Occupational Therapy Journal, 47,* 77–85. http://dx.doi.org/10.1046/j.1440-1630.2000.00217.x

Lloyd, C., & O'Connor, C. (2007). Integrating spirituality into mental health rehabilitation. *International Journal of Therapy and Rehabilitation, 14,* 168–172. http://www98.griffith.edu.au/dspace/bitstream/handle/10072/40514/72248_1.pdf?sequence=1

Lloyd, C., Wong, S. R., & Petchkovsky, L. (2007). Art and recovery in mental health: A qualitative investigation. *British Journal of Occupational Therapy, 70,* 207–214. http://dx.doi.org/10.1177/030802260707000505

Luboshitzky, D., & Gaber, L. B. (2001). Holidays and celebrations as a spiritual occupation. *Australian Occupational Therapy Journal, 48,* 66–74. http://dx.doi.org/10.1046/j.1440-1630.2001.00251.x

MacGillivray, P. S., Sumsion, T., & Wicks-Nicholls, J. (2006). Critical elements as identified by adolescent mental health clients. *Canadian Journal of Occupational Therapy, 73,* 295–302. http://dx.doi.org/10.2182/cjot.06.006

McColl, M. A. (Ed.). (2003). *Spirituality and occupational therapy.* Ottawa, ON: CAOT Publications.

McColl, M. A. (2011a). Models of spirituality, occupation and health. In M. A. McColl (Ed.), *Spirituality and occupational therapy* (2nd ed.). Ottawa, ON: CAOT Publications.

McColl, M. A. (Ed.). (2011b). *Spirituality and occupational therapy* (2nd ed.). Ottawa, ON: CAOT Publications.

McCormack, C., & Collins, B. (2010). Can disability studies contribute to client-centred occupational therapy practice? *British Journal of Occupational Therapy, 73,* 339–342. http://dx.doi.org/10.4276/030802210X12785840213328

McPhee, S. D., & Johnson, T. (2000). Program planning for an assisted living community. *Occupational Therapy in Health Care, 12*(2/3), 1–17. http://dx.doi.org/10.1080/J003v12n02_01

Meredith, P. J. (2010). Has undergraduate education prepared occupational therapy students for possible practice in palliative care? *Australian Occupational Therapy Journal, 57,* 224–232. http://dx.doi.org/10.1111/j.1440-1630.2009.00836.x

Moreira-Almeida, A., & Koenig, H. G. (2006). Retaining the meaning of the words religiousness and spirituality: A commentary on the WHOQOL SRPB group's "A cross-cultural study of spirituality, religion, and personal beliefs as components of quality of life." *Social Science and Medicine, 63,* 843–845. http://dx.doi.org/10.1016/j.socscimed. 2006.03.001

Moyers, P. A., & Dale, L. M. (2007). *The guide to occupational therapy practice* (2nd ed.). Bethesda, MD: AOTA Press.

Morris, D. N., Stetcher, J., Briggs-Peppler, K. M., Chittenden, C. M., Rubira, J., & Wismer, L. K. (2012). Spirituality in occupational therapy: Do we practice what we teach? *Journal of Religious Health, 53,* 27–36. http://dx.doi.org/10.1007/s10943-012-9584-y

Peloquin, S. M. (2008). Morality preempts modality: A commentary on exploring prayer as a spiritual modality. *Canadian Journal of Occupational Therapy, 75,* 15–16. http://dx.doi.org/10.1177/000841740807500105

Pentland, W., & McColl, M. A. (2011). Occupational choice. In M. A. McColl (Ed.), *Spirituality and occupational therapy* (2nd ed., pp. 141–149). Ottawa, ON: CAOT Publications.

Peoples, H., Satink, T., & Steultjens, E. (2011). Stroke survivors' experiences of rehabilitation: A systematic review of qualitative studies. *Scandinavian Journal of Occupational Therapy, 18,* 163–171. http://dx.doi.org/10.3109/11038128.2010.509887

Pereira, R. B., & Stagnitti, K. (2008). The meaning of leisure for well elderly Italians in the Australian community: Implications for occupational therapy. *Australian Occupational Therapy Journal, 55,* 39–46. http://dx.doi.org/10.1111/j.1440-1630.2006.00653.x

Persson, D., Erlandsson, L., Eklund, M., & Iwarsson, S. (2001). Value dimensions, meaning, and complexity in human occupation—a tentative structure for analysis. *Scandinavian Journal of Occupational Therapy, 8,* 7–18. http://dx.doi.org/10.1080/11038120119727

Phelan, S., & Kinsella, E. A., (2009). Occupational identity: Engaging socio-cultural perspectives. *Journal of Occupational Science, 16,* 85–91. http://dx.doi.org/10.1080/14427591.2009.9686647

Pizzi, M. A., & Briggs, R. (2004). Occupational and physical therapy in hospice: The facilitation of meaning, quality of life, and well-being. *Topics in Geriatric Rehabilitation, 20,* 120–130. http://dx.doi.org/10.1097/00013614-200404000-00007

Pollard, N. (2006). Is dying an occupation? *Journal of Occupational Science, 13,* 149–152. http://dx.doi.org/10.1080/14427591.2006.9726508

Powell, L. H., Shahabi, L., & Thorensen, C. E. (2003). Religion and spirituality: Linkages to physical health. *American Psychologist, 58,* 36–52. http://dx.doi.org/10.1037/0003-066X.58.1.36

Puchalski, C., Ferrell, B., Virani, R., Otis-Green, S., Baird, P., Bull, J.,...Sulmasy, D. (2009). Improving the quality of spiritual care as a dimension of palliative care: The report of the Consensus Conference. *Journal of Palliative Medicine, 12,* 885–904. http://dx.doi.org/10.1089/jpm.2009.0142

Ramugondo, E. L. (2005). Unlocking spirituality: Play as a health-promoting occupation in the context of HIV/AIDS. In F. Kronenberg, S. A. Algado, & N. Pollard (Eds.), *Occupational therapy without borders: Learning from the spirit of survivors* (pp. 313–325). New York: Elsevier/Churchill Livingstone.

Rosenfeld, M. S. (2000, January). Spiritual agent modalities for occupational therapy practice. *OT Practice, 5,* 17–21. https://www.caot.ca/otnow/nov01-eng/nov01-SPM.htm

Rosenfeld, M. S. (2001). Spirituality, motivation and performance. *Canadian Journal of Occupational Therapy, 3,* 5–9. https://www.caot.ca/otnow/nov01-eng/nov01-SPM.htm

Rudman, D. L., & Dennhardt, S. (2008). Shaping knowledge regarding occupation: Examining the cultural underpinnings of the evolving concept of occupational identity. *Australian Occupational Therapy Journal, 55,* 153–162. http://dx.doi.org/10.1111/j.1440-1630.2007.00715.x

Sadlo, G. (2004). Creativity and occupation. In M. Molineux (Ed.), *Occupation for occupational therapists* (pp. 90–100). Malden, MA: Blackwell Publishing.

Sakellariou, D., & Algado, S. S. (2006). Sexuality and occupational therapy: Exploring the link. *British Journal of Occupational Therapy, 69,* 350–356. http://dx.doi.org/10.1177/030802260606900802

Schleinich, M. A., Warren, S., Nekolaichuk, C., Kaasa, T., & Watanabe, S. (2008). Palliative care rehabilitation survey: A pilot study of patients' priorities for rehabilitation goals. *Palliative Medicine, 22,* 822–830. http://dx.doi.org/10.1177/0269216308096526

Schmid, T. (2004). Meanings of creativity within occupational therapy. *Australian Occupational Therapy Journal, 51,* 80–88. http://dx.doi.org/10.1111/j.1440-1630.2004.00434.x

Seeman, T. E., Dubin, L. F., & Seeman, M. (2003). Religiosity/spirituality and health: A critical review of the evidence for biological pathways. *American Psychologists, 58,* 53–63. http://dx.doi.org/10.1037/0003-066X.58.1.53

Segal, R. (2004). Family routines and rituals: A context for occupational therapy interventions. *American Journal of Occupational Therapy, 58,* 499–508. http://dx.doi.org/10.5014/ajot.58.5.499

Shamberg, S., & Barr, A. (2006). Access for all—access to prayer and ritual. *Israeli Journal of Occupational Therapy, 15,* E69–E87. Retrieved from http://www.jstor.org/stable/23468979

Shu Shan Teo, S. (2009). An occupational therapist's contribution to spiritual care within a palliative care setting: A student's perspective. *Australian Journal of Pastoral Care and Health, 3*(1). Retrieved from http://pandora.nla.gov.au/pan/98927/20100623-0144/www.pastoraljournal.findaus.com/pdfs/Occupational.pdf

Spencer, J., Davidson, H., & White, V. (1997). Help clients develop hopes for the future. *American Journal of Occupational Therapy, 51,* 191–198. http://dx.doi.org/10.5014/ajot.51.3.191

St. James O'Connor, T., Chow, M., Meakes, E., Young, J., Payne, G., Rivera, M.,...Howitt, J. (2012). Three doors to spiritual reflection: Ethnographic research on the role of emotion, images and sacred texts in spiritual reflection done by non-chaplaincy health care professionals. *Journal of Health Care Chaplaincy, 18,* 43–56. http://dx.doi.org/10.10 80/08854726.2011.616171

Thibeault, R. (2011a). Occupational gifts. In M. A. McColl (Ed.), *Spirituality and occupational therapy* (2nd ed., pp. 111–120). Ottawa, ON: CAOT Publications.

Thibeault, R. (2011b). Occupational therapy values. In M. A. McColl (Ed.), *Spirituality and occupational therapy* (2nd ed., pp. 103–110). Ottawa, ON: CAOT Publications.

Thibeault, R. (2011c). Resilience and maturity. In M. A. McColl (Ed.), *Spirituality and occupational therapy* (2nd ed., pp. 121–130). Ottawa, ON: CAOT Publications.

Thibeault, R. (2011d). Ritual: Ceremonies of life. In M. A. McColl (Ed.), *Spirituality and occupational therapy* (2nd ed., pp. 217– 222). Ottawa, ON: CAOT Publications.

Thomas, Y., Gray, M., McGinty, S., & Ebringer, S. (2011). Homeless adults engagement in art: First steps towards identity, recovery and social inclusion. *Australian Occupational Therapy Journal, 58,* 429–436. http://dx.doi.org/10.1111/j.1440-1630.2011.00977.x

Toomey, M. A. (1999). The art of observation: Reflecting on a spiritual moment. *Canadian Journal of Occupational Therapy, 66,* 197–199. http://dx.doi.org/10.1177/000841749906600407

Toomey, M. (2011). Creativity: Spirituality through the visual arts. In M. A. McColl (Ed.), *Spirituality and occupational therapy* (2nd ed., pp. 233–240). Ottawa, ON: CAOT Publications.

Townsend, E. (1993). Occupational therapy's social vision. *Canadian Journal of Occupational Therapy, 60,* 174–184. http://dx.doi.org/10.1177/000841749306000403

Townsend, E. (1997). Inclusiveness: A community dimension of spirituality. *Canadian Journal of Occupational Therapy, 64,* 146–155. http://dx.doi.org/10.1177/000841749706400111

Townsend, E., Brintnell, S., & Staisey, N. (1990). Developing guidelines for client-centered occupational therapy practice. *Canadian Journal of Occupational Therapy, 57,* 69–76. http://dx.doi.org/10.1177/000841749005700205

Trentham, B., Cockburn, L., & Shin (2007). Health promotion and community development: An application of occupational therapy in primary health care. *Canadian Journal of Community Mental Health, 26,* 53–70. http://dx.doi.org/10.7870/cjcmh-2007-0028

Trump, S. M., (2001). Occupational therapy and hospice: A natural fit. *OT Practice, 6*(20), 7–8, 10–11.

Tse, S., Lloyd, C., Petchkovsky, O., & Manaia, W. (2005). Exploration of Australian and New Zealand indigenous people's spirituality and mental health. *Australian Occupational Therapy Journal, 52,* 181–187. http://dx.doi.org/10.1111/j.1440-1630.2005.00507.x

Udell, L., & Chandler, C. (2000). The role of occupational therapists in addressing the spiritual needs of clients. *British Journal of Occupational Therapy, 63,* 489–495. http://dx.doi.org/10.1177/030802260006301006

Unruh, A. M. (1997). Reflections on...Spirituality and occupation: Garden musings and the Himalayan Blue Poppy. *Canadian Journal of Occupational Therapy, 64,* 156–160. http://dx.doi.org/10.1177/000841749706400112

Unruh, A. (2011). Appreciation of nature: Restorative occupations. In M. A. McColl (Ed.), *Spirituality and occupational therapy* (2nd ed., pp. 249–256). Ottawa, ON: CAOT Publications.

Unruh, A. M., Smith, N., & Scammel, C. (2000). The occupation of gardening in life-threatening illness. *Canadian Journal of Occupational Therapy, 67,* 70–77. http://dx.doi.org/10.1177/000841740006700110

Unruh, A. M., Versnel, J., & Kerr, N. (2002). Spirituality unplugged: A review of commonalties and contentions, and a resolution. *Canadian Journal of Occupational Therapy, 69,* 5–20. http://dx.doi.org/10.1177/000841740206900101

Unruh, A. M., Versnel, J., & Kerr, N. (2004). In M. Molineux (Ed.). *Occupation for occupational therapists* (pp. 32–45). Malden, MA: Blackwell Publishing.

Urbanowski, R., & Vargo, J. (1994). Spirituality, daily practice, and the Occupational Performance Model. *Canadian Journal of Occupational Therapy, 61,* 88–94. http://dx.doi.org/10.1177/000841749406100204

Wells, K. (2009). *There is limited evidence to support inclusion of spirituality in occupational therapy intervention in older adult populations with physical disabilities* (Physical Function CATs Paper 18). Forest Grove, OR: Pacific University. Retrieved from http://commons.pacificu.edu/cgi/viewcontent.cgi?article=1017&context=otpf

Werner, D. (2005). Foreword. In F. Kronenberg, S. A. Algado, & N. Pollard (Eds.), *Occupational therapy without borders: Learning from the spirit of survivors* (pp. xi–xii). London: Elsevier/Churchill Livingstone.

Weskamp, K., & Ramugondo, E. L. (2005). Taking account of spirituality. In R. Watson & L. Swartz (Eds.), *Transformation through occupation* (pp. 155–167). London: Whur.

Wilcock, A. (2007). Occupation and health: Are they one and the same? *Journal of Occupational Science, 14,* 3–8. http://dx.doi.org/10.1080/14427591.2007.9686577

Wilding, C. (2002). Where angels fear to tread: Is spirituality relevant to occupational therapy practice? *Australian Occupational Therapy Journal, 49,* 44–47. http://dx.doi.org/10.1046/j.0045-0766.2002.00292.x

Wilson, L. (2010). Spirituality, occupation, and occupational therapy revisited: Ongoing consideration of the issues for occupational therapists. *British Journal of Occupational Therapy, 73,* 437–444. http://dx.doi.org/10.4276/030802210X12839367526219

Woodbridge, M. (2011). Creativity: Soul sessions. In M. A. McColl (Ed.), *Spirituality and occupational therapy* (2nd ed., pp. 223–232). Ottawa, ON: CAOT Publications.

CHAPTER 3.

DEFINITIONS AND DESCRIPTIONS OF SPIRITUALITY IN OCCUPATIONAL THERAPY LITERATURE

Tamera Keiter Humbert, MA, DEd, OTR/L

Chapter Highlights

✧ Definition vs. description
✧ Historical overview of definitions and descriptions
✧ General conceptualizations of spirituality in occupational therapy
✧ Aspects of spirituality in the occupational therapy literature
✧ Therapy as spiritual practice
✧ Discourse analysis.

Key Terms and Concepts

✧ Anthroposophy
✧ Aspects of spirituality
✧ Becoming
✧ Being
✧ Centeredness
✧ Conceptualizations
✧ Connectedness
✧ Coping
✧ Definition
✧ Description
✧ Discourse analysis
✧ Expanse of life
✧ Hope
✧ Internal aspects
✧ Internal–external aspects

✧ Kawa Model
✧ Meaning
✧ Occupational identity
✧ Psychospiritual integration
✧ Religious
✧ Resilience
✧ Sacred
✧ Secular
✧ Spiritual disorder
✧ Spiritual emergence
✧ Spiritual emergency
✧ Spirituality
✧ Theistic
✧ Transcendence
✧ Transpersonal perspective

A statement that frequently precedes most definitions or descriptions of *spirituality* often goes like this: "Spirituality is difficult to describe." This brief, poignant disclaimer is given by authors to prepare readers to be cautious in embracing ultimate or singular ideas about spirituality and to acknowledge its complexity. Although caution is wise, it is not particularly conducive to moving along conversations with colleagues and others interested in learning more about this subject.

In occupational therapy, practitioners need to be able to talk about spirituality and express concepts related to the topic clearly and explicitly to engage in and promote occupational therapy practice (McColl, 2003, 2011). The following two questions can be asked to begin the discussion: (1) How do occupational therapy practitioners define or describe *spirituality* within the literature? and (2) How is spirituality understood within occupational therapy? This chapter provides an overview of spirituality's multiple definitions and descriptions in the occupational therapy literature, foundational constructs that link spirituality to occupations, and how authors have conceptualized spirituality within the profession.

Definition vs. Description

Both definitions and descriptions of spirituality are prevalent and diverse within the occupational therapy literature. For the sake of clarity, in this chapter, **definition** refers to the explicit explanation that authors give to the term *spirituality.* Definitions tend to be conclusive and exact, such as Phillips' (2003) definition of *spirituality:* "Spirituality is intrinsic personal beliefs and practices that can be experienced within and without formal religion" (p. 249). A definition such as this one provides clarity and exactness for discussing spirituality.

Unlike definition, **description** tends to be more expressive or elaborative in providing insights about the topic. A description often evokes the reader's interpretations or application to personal experience, such as Egan and DeLaat's (1994) description of spirituality:

> Attention to spirituality requires acknowledgement of the spirit. This is an aspect of the person which underlies the physical self. It is the truest self, which we attempt to express in all our actions. Our spirit motivates us to

connect with others and attempt to make meaning in our daily lives. (p. 116)

Many of spirituality's definitions and descriptions in occupational therapy literature can be classified as original, borrowed, or summations:

- *Original definitions:* Authors provide their own understanding of the concept through a reflection of the literature and then expand on and elaborate their conclusions, such as Townsend and Polatajko's (2007) definition of *spirituality* as the "essence of the person" (p. 30).
- *Borrowed definitions:* Authors give credit to another author's definition or description, inside or outside the field of occupational therapy. The *Occupational Therapy Practice Framework: Domain and Process* (3rd ed.; American Occupational Therapy Association [AOTA], 2014) includes a definition of *spirituality* as "The aspect of humanity that refers to the way individuals seek and express meaning and purpose and the way they experience their connectedness to the moment, to self, to others, to nature, and to the significant or sacred" (Puchalski et al., 2009, p. 887). This definition came from an interdisciplinary group of health care providers addressing spirituality within palliative care.
- *Summation of multiple authors' work:* Authors synthesize multiple definitions within the field. Johnston and Mayers (2005) gave credence to previous authors' views within occupational therapy in their description of spirituality as they attempted to acknowledge multiple understandings of the subject:

> *Spirituality* can be defined as the search for meaning and purpose in life, which may or may not be related to a belief in God or some form of higher power. For those with no conception of supernatural belief, spirituality may relate to the notion of a motivating force, which involves an integration of the dimensions of mind, body, and spirit. This personal belief or faith also shapes an individual's perspective on the world and is expressed in the way that he or she lives life. Therefore, spirituality is experienced through connectedness to God/a higher being and/or by one's relationship with self, others or nature. (p. 386, *italics added*)

- *Summation of research data:* Authors summarize participant descriptions or synthesize literature review definitions. Williams (2008) provided a description of spirituality as a result of completing a focused research study with older adults on the topic:

  > *Spirituality* is viewed as that which brings an individual a sense of peace and well-being while providing purpose and value. Spirituality as a source of personal power, vitality, and influence is a concept unique to each person, as it is perceived as an intrinsic source that provides personal meaning. (p. 8, *italics added*)

Whatever approach is taken by scholars who study spirituality in occupational therapy to define or describe the term, their goal is to ground their work and provide a basis in understanding and a starting point for conversation about the subject.

Historical Overview of Definitions and Descriptions

One way to make sense of the definitions and descriptions of spirituality within the occupational therapy literature is to provide a historical overview of the term's use. Table 3.1 provides definitions and descriptions in chronological order.

Two early references are directly associated with spirituality and explicitly use the term *spirituality*

Table 3.1. Definitions and Descriptions of Spirituality in Occupational Therapy Literature

Author/Year/Link	Definition/Description
Townsend (1993) http://bit.ly/1PxDFV8	"[O]ccupational therapy's reference to spirituality suggests a belief in the inclusiveness basic to social justice. Therapists attend to the spirit when people are approached with respect as holistic and worthy individuals. Therapists who elicit people's own definition of meaningful occupations in real life are demonstrating an inclusive spirituality" (p. 178).
Egan & DeLaat (1994) http://bit.ly/1nLfA2U	"[T]he spirit is not merely viewed as a component of the individual. Rather, the spirit is seen as the essence of the person. In this way the spirit cannot be made more healthy. It can only be allowed more freedom through a strengthening or adjustment to the tools which it uses to express itself" (p. 101).
Urbanowski & Vargo (1994) http://bit.ly/20nR60V	"Spirituality may be defined as the experience of meaning in everyday life" (p. 89).
Chapparo & Ranka (1997)	"A sense of harmony within self, nature, others and in some cases, an ultimate other . . . [and that which] seeks an existing mystery to life: inner conviction; hope and meaning" (pp. 13–14).
Christiansen (1997) http://bit.ly/1P16t6U	"Spirituality is a metaphysical phenomenon" (p. 169).
Egan & DeLaat (1997) http://bit.ly/1QazN8W	"Spirituality relates to our thoughts, feelings and actions concerning the meaning that we make of our daily lives. Meaning is constructed through our relationships with ourselves, other humans, other inhabitants of the earth itself and for many individuals, a higher power or Creator. We live this meaning and our relationships through doing or occupation.[a] Attention to spirituality requires acknowledgement of the spirit. This is an aspect of the person which underlies the physical self. It is the truest self, which we attempt to express in all our actions. Our spirit motivates us to connect with others and attempt to make meaning in our daily lives" (p. 116).

(Continued)

Table 3.1. Definitions and Descriptions of Spirituality in Occupational Therapy Literature (*Cont.*)

Author/Year/ Link	Definition/Description
Engquist, Short-DeGraff, Gliner, & Oltjenbruns (1997) http://bit.ly/ 1Pbk5uc	"[T]he client's spirituality, as a source of inspiration, plays an influential role in directing what purposeful activities are identified as meaningful" (p. 174).
Howard & Howard (1997) http://bit.ly/ 20nRqNi	"Spirituality stresses the person's subjective perception and experience of something or someone greater than himself or herself" (p. 181).
Law, Polatajko, Baptiste, & Townsend (1997)	"A pervasive life force, manifestation of a higher self, source of will and self-determination, and a sense of meaning, purpose and connectedness that people experience in the context of their environment" (p. 43).[a]
Peloquin (1997) http://bit.ly/ 1QFGPFm	"To see occupation as the *making* of lives and worlds is a deeper—and more spiritual—perspective than to see it as doing or performing.... The difference between doing and making is one of substance rather than semantic. *Making* suggests a creation" (pp. 167–168).
Simo-Algado, Gregori, & Egan (1997) http://bit.ly/ 1KVs7FL	"Spirituality can be viewed as a way of living which demonstrates essential values regarding the role of the individual in the world" (p. 139).[b]
Thibault (1997) http://bit.ly/ 20nRQ6f	"[Spirituality is] an experience of connectedness to a universal order and even, at times, to a benevolent Will" (p. 112).
Townsend (1997b) http://bit.ly/ 23HLihR	"Spirituality is not merely a concept; it involves reflection and action in occupations that generate meaningful experiences" (p. 21).
Unruh (1997) http://bit. ly/1PTd0UJ	"Spirituality is a subjective, intimate, and private construct" (p. 157).
Urbanowski (1997)	"Spirituality is simply the experience of meaning" (p. 23).
McColl (2000) http://bit.ly/ 1nLgxs3	"Spirituality is sensitivity to the presence of spirit. According to this definition, spirituality is a quality that human beings possess to a greater or lesser degree, that allows them to be aware of the presence of spirit" (p. 217).
	"That spirituality entails an innate knowledge of the essence of self; that it is the source of our will, intention, self-determination; that it is responsible for the connection between people; that it invests our daily occupations with meaning" (p. 220).
Vrkljan (2000)	"It is imperative that occupational therapists consider the spirituality of their clients, as it may provide the link to engaging them in meaningful occupations" (p. 7).
Baptiste (2003)	"Spirituality as one's inner culture" (p. 83).

(*Continued*)

Table 3.1. Definitions and Descriptions of Spirituality in Occupational Therapy Literature (*Cont.*)

Author/Year/ Link	Definition/Description
Kang (2003) http://bit.ly/ 1UHxD4o	"Spirituality is viewed as a quality that ultimately makes us who we are and our universe what it becomes. It has six interconnected but distinct dimensions: becoming, meaning, being, centeredness, connectedness, transcendence" (p. 95).
McColl (2003)	"...the opportunity to see universal truths in specific activities, to obtain a view of the whole cosmos in relation to a particular daily pattern of life, and to see one's life as a whole in relation to the grander scheme of things" (p. 222).
Phillips (2003) http://bit.ly/ 1PeGk2v	"Spirituality is intrinsic personal beliefs and practices that can be experienced within and without formal religion" (p. 249).[b]
Schulz (2004) http://bit.ly/ 2070gcM	"[E]xperiencing a meaningful connection to our core selves, other humans, the world, and/or a greater power as expressed through our reflections, narratives and actions" (p. 57).[c]
Johnston & Mayers (2005) http://bit.ly/ 20FitAr	"Spirituality can be defined as the search for meaning and purpose in life, which may or may not be related to a belief in God or some form of higher power. For those with no conception of supernatural belief, spirituality may relate to the notion of a motivating force, which involves an integration of the dimensions of mind, body, and spirit. This personal belief or faith also shapes an individual's perspective on the world and is expressed in the way that he or she lives life. Therefore, spirituality is experienced through connectedness to God/a higher being and/or by one's relationship with self, others or nature" (p. 386).[a]
Boswell, Hamer, Knight, Glacoff, & McChesney (2007)	"[S]pirituality was defined broadly as a person's views of the world, particularly, how a person explains the world and the forces that impact her or his life" (p. 34).
Kroeker (2007)	"Spirituality is not finally a matter of technical expertise but of a shared humanity at its deepest level" (p. 66).
Townsend & Polatajko (2007)	"Spirituality is the essence of the person" (p. 30).
Wilding (2007) http://bit.ly/ 1VIN3FQ	"[Spirituality is] a life-sustaining phenomenon" (p. S67).[c]
Williams (2008) http://bit.ly/ 1SWxpJ5	"[S]pirituality is viewed as that which brings an individual a sense of peace and well-being while providing purpose and value. Spirituality as a source of personal power, vitality, and influence is a concept unique to each person, as it is perceived as an intrinsic source that provides personal meaning" (pp. 7–8).
McColl (2011)	"The desire for, or sensitivity to, the presence of spirit [and spirit as] the force that animates living things" (p. 18).

Note. [a]Summation of multiple definitions or descriptions from occupational therapy literature. [b]Summarized or used definitions from other sources. [c]Summation from research data or literature reviews.

(Egan & DeLaat, 1994; Townsend, 1993); however, in 1997, the *Canadian Journal of Occupational Therapy* and the *American Journal of Occupational Therapy* each published an issue dedicated to the subject, sharing multiple voices and perspectives about spirituality. This decision intentionally put the conversation about spirituality and occupational therapy in public view. Subsequent to these 1997 publications, authors continued to provide their interpretation of spirituality through proposed models and frames of references, through comparative literature reviews, or as a reflection of research results.

General Conceptualizations of Spirituality in Occupational Therapy

Beyond the initial point of defining or describing spirituality, authors have provided preliminary frameworks to better understand the multiplicity of ideas around the topic, referred to as *conceptualizations* in this chapter. In an extensive review of the occupational therapy literature, Unruh, Versnel, and Kerr (2002) critically reviewed the definitions of *spirituality* from diverse professional perspectives and classified them into the following seven major categories of understanding:

1. Relationship to God, a spiritual being, a higher power, or a reality greater than the self
2. Not of the self
3. Transcendence or connectedness unrelated to a belief in a higher being
4. Existential, not of the material world
5. Meaning and purpose in life
6. Life force of the person or integrating aspect of the person
7. Summative, or a combination of the aforementioned categories.

In addition to providing thematic categories, Unruh et al. (2002) suggested the following dimensions of spirituality that emphasize the origin from which spiritual definitions have been derived:

- *Secular:* Concerned with the affairs of the world that are not sacred, monastic, or ecclesiastical. This term is used to separate ideas about spirituality that are not related to sacred or religious ideas.
- *Sacred:* Traditionally defined as devoted to or especially acceptable to a deity or dedicated to or

reserved or appropriated for some person or purpose. This dimension of spirituality infers that there is something greater than the self without explicit reference to a belief in a higher being, gods, or God.
- *Theistic:* Refers to a belief in the existence of gods, especially God, who are supernaturally revealed to people.
- *Religious:* Refers to a particular system of faith and worship. Religions often have an explicit and exclusive theistic framework. However, it is possible for a religion to be multifaceted and inclusive of multiple secular, sacred, or theistic dimensions of spirituality.

Although these categories and dimensions help make distinctions about spirituality and place it in a larger, more inclusive world context, Unruh et al. (2002) concluded that the focus of spirituality in occupational therapy needed to be directed toward the way practitioners understand occupation and the application of occupational engagement. As an alternative to borrowing the concept of *spirituality* from other disciplines, they proposed using the concept of *occupational identity* as closely related to spirituality, arguing that a person "may center her or his occupational identity on occupations that are responsive to spiritual questioning" (p. 14).

The authors stressed that the primary focus for the occupational therapy practitioner is on occupations and personal identity. Select occupations may elicit aspects of spirituality, but spirituality, in and of itself, should not be the principal emphasis within the therapeutic process. Therefore, Unruh et al. (2002) promoted a shift in focus in occupational therapy from using general understandings and conceptualizations of spirituality to using spirituality as a way to identify occupations that provide meaning:

Understanding the client's spirituality may provide the occupational therapist with insight about the meaningfulness of occupations in the client's daily life and the way the client has constructed an occupational identity. Listening to the client will enable the therapist to understand what resources the client uses to manage daily occupational needs during health crises and challenges. Listening with sensitivity and respect to the client will support rather than hinder a person's spiritual struggle in such circumstances. Asking about spirituality, listening and understanding reflect a caring occupational therapy process rather than outcome goals of occupational therapy. (p. 14)

Unruh et al. (2002) added that "[t]argeting spirituality as an intervention goal may be beyond the occupational goals of evidence-based occupational therapy" (p. 14). Despite this caution, spirituality within the occupational therapy literature continued to be explored and further discussed, conveyed as personal and beyond the self (Howard & Howard, 1997) and deeply private (Kroeker, 2007) yet interrelated to others (Schulz, 2004), momentarily experiential (Toomey, 2011), and a process or life journey (McColl, 2011; Simo-Algado, Gregori, & Egan, 1997; Wilding, 2007). Spirituality encompasses feelings as well as beliefs and ideals (Phillips, 2003; Simo-Algado et al., 1997). It is experienced in mundane, everyday existence (Unruh, 1997) and in supernatural and extraordinary events (Collins, 2007).

Aspects of Spirituality in Occupational Therapy Literature

The definitions and descriptions in Table 3.1 can be further analyzed and categorized according to the different aspects of spirituality addressed. In this chapter, *aspects of spirituality* are select components connected in some way to the whole of spirituality. They include spirituality being part of the self, observable and tangible effects of spirituality, the paths to spirituality, and the contexts in which spirituality may be enhanced or promoted.

Internal and Internal–External Aspects of the Self

The first aspect of spirituality to be consistently discussed by authors is that spiritually is situated within and beyond the person. *Internal aspects* of a person's spirituality are inherent in or developed within the person (Figure 3.1). These aspects include beliefs (Low, 1997; Phillips, 2003; Williams, 2008) and values (Simo-Algado et al., 1997; Williams, 2008), personal culture (Baptiste, 2003), and worldviews (Boswell, Hamer, Knight, Glacoff, & McChesney, 2007; Smith, 2008).

Figure 3.1. Internal aspects of spirituality.

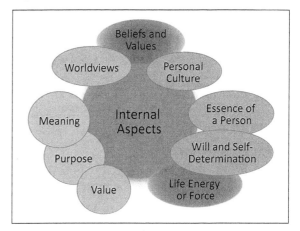

Figure 3.2. Internal–external aspects of spirituality.

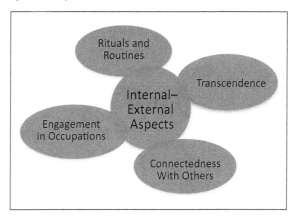

Internal aspects are also referred to as a life energy or life force (Egan & DeLaat, 1994; Wilding, 2007), the essence of a person (Egan & DeLaat, 1994; McColl, 2000), and will and self-determination (Law, Polatajko, Baptiste, & Townsend, 1997; Thibault, 1997; Williams, 2008). These aspects of spirituality provide meaning (McColl, 2000; Townsend, 1997b; Urbanowski, 1997; Urbanowski & Vargo, 1994; Vrkljan, 2000), purpose (Law et al., 1997; Williams, 2008), and value (Williams, 2008).

Internal–external aspects of spirituality are inherent qualities that become externalized, often observable, actions (Figure 3.2). Through these actions, internal aspects may expand, or new internal aspects may be cultivated. For example, a person may believe in the inherent goodness of all people. This internal aspect of the self may then be externally manifested by the person as he or she engages in daily encounters with others by openly approaching others and responding thoughtfully to the topics of conversation being discussed and any concerns. These encounters may further enhance a sense of connectedness with others, reinforcing and potentially strengthening additional beliefs about the goodness of all people. Internal–external aspects include rituals and routines (Phillips, 2003), connectedness with others (Egan & DeLaat, 1997; Kroeker, 2007; Law et al., 1997; Schulz, 2004; Thibault, 1997; Townsend, 1997a), transcendence (Howard & Howard, 1997; McColl, 2003, 2011), and engagement in occupations (Christiansen, 1997; Engquist, Short-DeGraff, Gliner, & Oltjenbruns, 1997; Hasselkus, 2002; Peloquin, 1997; Townsend, 1997b).

Although occupational therapy literature on spirituality does not include the terms *internal* and *internal–external aspects* of spirituality, it presents the notion that spirituality is part of the person and that all people have or embody spirituality (McColl, 2011; Townsend & Polatajko, 2007). Additionally, the phrase *mind–body–spirit* used in the literature equates with a perspective and recognition of the universality of spirituality, even though it is believed that the manifestation of spirituality is revealed differently in each person (Schulz, 2004; Williams, 2008).

Tangible Effects of Spirituality

Within the occupational therapy literature, spirituality is often associated with tangible benefits, such as future betterment, personal growth, meaning and purpose, and expanse of life (Figure 3.3). Some authors have portrayed these benefits to be inherent outcomes when a person engages in spiritual practices or meaningful occupations (McColl, 2011). In addition, some authors have shown that people seek spirituality when life challenges persist or are so difficult that relief through spirituality is not only desired but intensely sought (Beagan, Etowa, & Bernard, 2012; Smith & Suto, 2012).

Authors' discussions of the benefits of spirituality were primarily based on personal experience, either private or professional; observations made through the therapeutic process and relationships; or statements expressed by clients and research study participants. These discussions reflect the general belief that the experience of spirituality, however it might be realized, provides worth and value to a person. However, some authors acknowledged that the influence of spirituality may impede the therapeutic process or that some beliefs and ideals can negatively affect people (Kang, 2003; McColl, 2011).

Figure 3.3. Tangible benefits of spirituality.

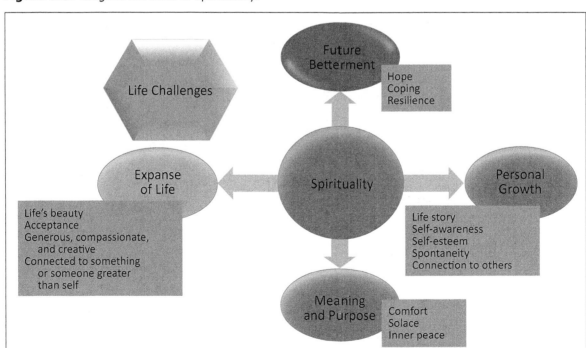

Future betterment

In some cases, spirituality provides an image of future betterment. *Hope,* a sense of possibility and the potential for a better or more fulfilling life or for ultimate healing, provides people with the ability to deal with the realities of life events and any harshness or pain experienced in life (Burgman, 2011; Schwartz & Fleming Cottrell, 2007; Tse, Lloyd, Petchkovsky, & Manaia, 2005; Wilding, 2007; Williams, 2008). *Coping* is the ability to handle a life event, and *resilience* is strength to deal with ongoing challenges of the life event. Hope, coping (Greenberg, 2004), and resilience (Schwartz & Fleming Cottrell, 2007) are often attributed to spirituality.

Personal growth

Spirituality is often associated with personal growth. Personal growth may include an understanding of ones' life story and trajectory and how one's life has contributed to others (Heuchemer & Josephsson, 2006), increased self-awareness (Boswell et al., 2007; Collins, 2007; Townsend, DeLaat, Egan, Thibault, & Wright, 1999), greater self-esteem (Collins, 1998; Tse et al., 2005), increased spontaneity (Greenberg, 2004), or a deeper connection to others (Boswell et al., 2007; Luboshitzky, 2008; Schulz, 2004; Wilding, 2007).

Meaning and purpose

Finding meaning and purpose is a process that can become focused and clear through spirituality (Donica, 2008). This process is often realized when a person achieves a sense of comfort, solace (Schwartz & Fleming Cottrell, 2007), and inner peace (Baker, 2008).

Expanse of life

The results of spirituality are recognized in the *expanse of life,* or the ability to put into perspective one's life experiences within the larger context of world events and others' lived realities. It may allow a person to recognize and acknowledge life's beauty beyond ordinary daily routines and during periods of suffering (Kronenberg, Pollard, & Sakellariou, 2011). In addition, a person may accept a life challenge and then let go of unnecessary burdens (Boswell et al., 2007; Luboshitzky, 2008); connect with something or someone greater than the self (Baker, 2008; Boswell et al., 2007); or become more generous, compassionate (Kang, 2003; Luboshitzky, 2008), or creative (Boswell et al., 2007).

Ways to Spirituality

Beyond the emphasis on the self within spirituality, the literature also discusses the processes or paths to spirituality, or ways to spirituality. The cover of the book *Spirituality and Occupational Therapy* (McColl, 2011) has an image that conveys this aspect of spirituality. The image is a small but gracefully arching red bridge in the middle of a beautiful lavish landscape. The picture was chosen to represent a path to and from spirituality. According to McColl (2011), the bridge symbolizes the activities that bring a person into a spiritual realm or place and contribute to the development and fulfillment of spirituality as well as the use of spirituality to enliven and understand life and occupations.

Several scholars have provided concrete examples of activities or meaningful occupations that may elicit or facilitate spiritual awareness and receptivity, such as engaging in silence and solitude (Thibault, 2011), reflection (Schulz, 2004), writing (Precin, 2006) and narrative or storytelling (Burgman, 2011; Howard & Howard, 1997; Schulz, 2004; Vrkljan, 2000), creative expression (Toomey, 1999, 2011), dreams (Collins, 2004), and prayer (Farah & McColl, 2008).

Such activities or occupations may also be more vigorous such as playing (Burgman, 2011), participating in active pursuits (Schulz, 2004; Unruh, 1997; Unruh & Elvin, 2004), and engaging in rituals and spiritual disciplines (Brémault-Phillips & Chirovsky, 2011a, 2011b; Luboshitzky, 2008). Alternatively, some authors have provided general descriptions of types of activities that a person may consider to be meaningful. For example, Kang (2003) used the terms *occupational abundance, occupational function, occupational balance,* and *occupational justice* to describe four distinct types of engagement that contribute to psychospiritual growth.

Some authors have gone beyond identifying select activities and occupations to characterizing life events and lived experiences of disability and illness (Schulz, 2004, 2005; Wilding, 2007) and suffering (Luboshitzky, 2008; Weskamp & Ramugondo, 2005) to understand the ways to spirituality. Whether

Figure 3.4. Ways to spirituality.

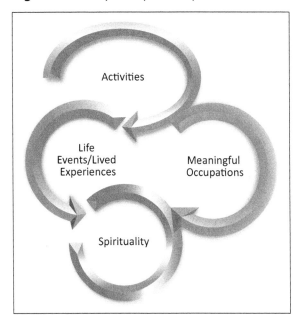

Figure 3.5. Spirituality within defined contexts.

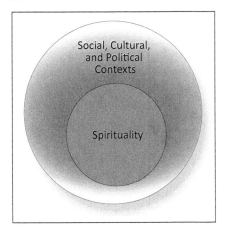

through select activities and occupations or life events and lived experiences, the authors discussed here have communicated an appreciation for doing or engaging in acts of doing that enliven or facilitate the possibility for spirituality (Figure 3.4).

Spirituality Within Defined Contexts

Some occupational therapy scholars have identified and described the specific contexts (e.g., social, cultural, political) within which people make meaning of and understand their spiritual beliefs, practices, and routines (Beagan et al., 2012; Kronenberg et al., 2011; Smith & Suto, 2012; Figure 3.5). However, according to the *Framework* (AOTA, 2014), spirituality is a client factor, which suggests that it is an internal aspect of a person, consistent with the first aspect of spirituality previously mentioned. Yet, the idea that occupational engagement, which is embedded in these specific contexts, is part of spirituality furthers the notion that spirituality is also embedded in these specific contexts (Beagan et al., 2012; Humbert, Bess, & Mowery, 2013; Smith & Suto, 2012).

Therefore, if spirituality is more than just a client factor and is also rooted within occupational engagement, it is important for occupational therapy practitioners to be sensitive to the contexts in which clients understand and practice spirituality and to client rituals and religious observances.

Although limited in quantity and scope, the articles listed in Table 3.1 add to the discussion of understanding spirituality within particular cultural groups and contexts. For example, Frank et al. (1997) addressed the rituals and routines of young Orthodox Jewish couples, and Smith-Gabai and Ludwig (2011) provided perspectives about observing the Jewish Sabbath. Tse et al. (2005) and Frank, Murphy, Kitching, Garfield, and McDarment (2008) provided insights into the beliefs and daily practices of indigenous people groups. Howard and Howard (1997), Schwartz and Fleming Cottrell (2007), and Williams (2008) discussed the Judeo-Christian perspective and influence on life meaning. Although these authors cautioned against generalizing their research to all groups of people, even within a specific and established cultural context, they illustrated how cultural contexts affect spirituality.

Therapy as Spiritual Practice

Occupational therapy scholars have started to share ways to understand spirituality within the context of therapy and to provide alternative ways to approach the topic within practice beyond considering spirituality solely as a client factor. This section highlights this expanding view.

Discussions about the dynamic among spirituality, life challenges, and engagement in occupations began to appear in the occupational therapy literature about 10 years ago. In particular, authors have proposed that spirituality not only provides a way to make sense of life and overcome difficult challenges but also offers the strength and capacity to fully engage in life (Schulz, 2005).

For example, Wilding, May, and Muir-Cochrane (2005) interviewed 6 people with mental illness about their perspectives on spirituality. The results indicated not only an expressed value of and appreciation for spirituality but also an acknowledgment of the need for spirituality in their lives. Without spirituality, the study participants believed that suicide was the only other option they had to deal with the immense challenges of living with severe mental illness. Therefore, spirituality within occupational therapy may provide concrete personal benefits to clients (Williams, 2008). In addition, it may reframe an understanding of disability (Boswell et al., 2007), sustain occupations (Wilding et al., 2005), and enhance the therapeutic relationship (Schwartz & Fleming Cottrell, 2007).

Psychospiritual Integration Frame of Reference

Kang (2003) offered a *psychospiritual integration* conceptual frame of reference in which spirituality was identified and explored through six dimensions:

1. Becoming
2. Meaning
3. Being
4. Centeredness
5. Connectedness
6. Transcendence.

Each of these dimensions helps form and shape personal and community fulfillment. According to Kang, *becoming* is the dynamic aspect of the person that is "associated with independence, personal growth, autonomy, and choice through active doing" (p. 97). *Meaning,* derived through narratives of occupational engagement, provides intrinsic knowing and "the creation of life themes" (p. 97). *Being* is the quality of being present and aware of self, others, and experiences. It is associated with not doing but opening up to "the wellspring of creativity, intuition, and love" (p. 98).

Centeredness, the core of being, provides people with a sense of who they are, their source of power and capacity, and a sense of where they have come from. Although centeredness may be focused on the self, *connectedness* allows a person to have a sense of belonging to the larger cosmos and recognizes the intricacies of and interrelationships with other living entities. *Transcendence* is twofold, encompassing both a drive and a goal for freedom, or the desire to be free from obstacles and limitations, allowing one to find ultimate meaning. Kang (2003) argued that in the psychospiritual integration perspective,

> spiritual order or fulfillment is said to exist when most or all the six dimensions of spirituality are observed in individuals or communities. Thus, when people are able to *become* what they want to be, to find authentic *meaning* and purpose in life, to *be* fully themselves in each moment, to abide in inner stability and knowledge of one's *centre,* to lovingly and compassionately *connect* with the larger matrix of life, and to *transcend* limitations of self and self's constructions, a condition of spiritual fulfillment is said to be present in them. (p. 98)

Kang (2003) highlighted engagement in occupation as a means by which a person may develop or enhance his or her spirituality, considering such occupations as spiritual occupations no matter what traditional category of occupation they fell into. Conversely, Kang also acknowledged that a person (or community) may not have the resources available or the opportunities to engage in spirituality to the capacity that strengthens and supports him or her through life events. Kang defined this condition as *spiritual disorder* or deprivation and suggested that occupational therapy intervention could be beneficial for overcoming this difficulty.

Transpersonal Perspective and Spiritual Emergency

Collins (2007) provided the occupational therapy community with insights into spirituality as it relates to a substantial shift in a person's consciousness, which may ultimately affect his or her views about self and life but initially be disruptive to his or her occupations. For example, a person may experience an out-of-body experience that gives him or her greater clarity about a universe beyond the physical and tangible world (e.g., near-death experience). That experience might bring such an intense emotional reaction that it immobilizes or constricts the person's ability to engage in familiar daily routines and activities.

Collins situated this perspective within a transpersonal lens with underlying assumptions that all people are spiritual beings, that they may experience reality beyond the tangible and "temporal and spatial boundaries" (p. 504) and that a significant spiritual experience may have profound meaning to a person.

The *transpersonal perspective* encourages openness to new experiences and new realities. As a person engages in and develops spiritual practices to enhance personal awareness and insights, he or she may encounter consciousness beyond the tangible, sometimes referred to as a *transcendent state*. Collins (2007) referenced this experience as **spiritual emergence,** or an enlightened state of consciousness with an expanded understanding of reality.

Transcendence may be intentionally pursued and viewed as a life-affirming experience. However, it may also result from a crisis and initially evoke panic and anxiety within the person experiencing the transcendent state. Collins (2007) described this state as an existential and spiritual crisis and labeled the experience as a **spiritual emergency.** The outward manifestation of a spiritual emergency may take on attributes more commonly associated with a break in reality or psychosis but should not be confused with a mental health diagnosis such as schizophrenia, mania, or substance-induced psychosis.

Although it may be difficult to imagine that feelings of anguish are a spiritual phenomenon or an experience that is not of this world, people who have written about it have provided insights into feelings of being overwhelmed and devastated but also about the spiritual clarity and enlightenment that followed. One contemporary example is Eckhart Tolle (2004), an author and spiritual teacher, who wrote about transitioning from despair and contemplation of suicide to profound personal and spiritual awakening. According to Collins (2007), occupational therapy can support a person's interpretation of his or her spiritual emergency and assist the person, when needed, to regain and engage in or reintegrate into his or her daily routines and activities to reestablish occupational identity.

Dealing With Suffering

Anthroposophy is a philosophy that explores fundamental questions of human existence, including issues related to suffering, pain, death, and evil and subsequent meaning making and self-awareness.

According to Luboshitzky (2008), seeking to explore and understand the meaning of suffering is a spiritual occupational practice. Luboshitzky stated that occupational therapy practitioners

> must realize that changing our own attitudes towards suffering can enable us to better help our clients in exploring meaning in their suffering and thus in their everyday life occupations as well. This process entails an attempt to accomplish the following objectives: to explore the purpose of one's suffering in relation to the unique meaning of one's life; to realize that the search for meaning is an individual task which each person must do alone; and to understand that even though one is not always able to change one's situation, one can always change one's attitude towards it. (p. 30)

Using the concepts of anthroposophy, Luboshitzky provided suggestions to the occupational therapy community about how practitioners may facilitate dialogue with and self-awareness in clients, including exploring the purpose or purposes for a person's life, supporting the engagement of valued rituals, promoting connectedness with others, acknowledging the value of letting go of images of who we should be and past dreams, accepting life circumstances and enjoying beauty despite suffering, and embracing a new life mission. Luboshitzky also suggested that before practitioners accompany clients through this journey they first examine their own understanding of pain and suffering, be open to their own and others' vulnerability, and be able to reaffirm life under difficult circumstances.

Kawa Model

The *Kawa Model* (Iwama, 2006) is an approach that elicits a person's perspectives about life's meaning by facilitating dialogue through the use of a river metaphor (i.e., *mizu,* or water, as a person's life energy or life flow). Iwama (2006) stated that "[f]luid, spirit, filling, cleansing and renewing, are only some of the meanings and functions commonly associated with this natural element" (p. 144). Iwama also stated that the role and purpose of occupational therapy is to "enhance life flow, regardless of whether it is interpreted at the level of the individual, institution, organization, community, or society" (p. 145).

In particular, the Kawa Model provides occupational therapy practitioners with an approach to discover how a client makes sense of his or her current life situation and life trajectory or journey. In addition, Iwama (2006) sought to provide a model that minimizes imposing concepts on clients. Although this model is not specifically linked to spirituality, Iwama stressed the importance of practitioners to respect a client's personal and larger worldviews and not impose predominate Western perspectives within the occupational therapy process. Being sensitive to diverse cultural perspectives, including how a client understands and uses spirituality, is paramount in client-centered care.

Discourse Analysis

Smith (2008) introduced the concept of *discourse analysis,* or the process and study of how language and concepts are used in practice, to shed further insight into spirituality and broaden the conversation beyond considering only the aspects of spirituality and the application of spirituality within practice. Discourse analysis has not been addressed formally in the broader occupational therapy literature. It stems from the idea that the underlying assumptions of occupational therapy's definitions and descriptions of spirituality need not only to be clearly articulated but also critiqued to formulate theoretical connections between spirituality and occupational therapy. Smith proposed the following questions to consider through discourse analysis:

- "What system of knowledge is being used to provide credibility for defining spirituality? Is a scientific system relevant/irrelevant? Is a religious system relevant/irrelevant?
- What are the situated meanings of the words and phrases that seem important when discussing spirituality? What professional model or institution is being reproduced or stabilized by the language?
- What is the main objective (activity) of the author/speaker regarding spirituality? Are there other objectives (sub-activities) at work (hidden or overt)? How do these constrain the language used?

- What value systems are being expressed by defining spirituality in a particular way? How are the benefits and values stabilized or transformed by the discourse?
- What aspects of gender, class, and/or race are relevant/irrelevant?
- What sorts of connections are made to previous ideas or texts on spirituality? How does the speaker/author bring about coherence between the past, future and present ideas?" (p. 50)

Smith challenges occupational therapy to move beyond universally accepted and simplistically promoted views of spirituality. By questioning the origins of the field's ideas and conceptualizations of spirituality and having a deeper appreciation for how it has defined and described the concept, occupational therapy can move toward a greater and deeper understanding of the topic, allowing the profession to broaden concepts and frameworks related to spirituality.

Summary

Authors often begin their work with a statement about the illusiveness of the term *spirituality* and some acknowledgment that it has no single definition. Some leave the construct open to interpretation, and others try to make peace with all of the conflict by combining thoughts and ideas into one mighty summation. Although there is no one definition of *spirituality* within occupational therapy (or in any other field investigated) or a consensus about how or whether the concept should be included in occupational therapy practice, the ideas presented in this chapter demonstrate a growing understanding of spirituality and occupation. In addition, these ideas validate that it is important to recognize spirituality in occupational therapy and continue the conversation. All of the authors discussed provided some recognition of the power and strength that spirituality can offer in the lives of people who suffer, know loss and pain, and seek something more than what most of life offers.

Some authors have asked occupational therapy practitioners to refocus their attention on occupation as the primary emphasis of therapy while still acknowledging the personal spirituality that people bring to therapy (Kronenberg et al., 2011; Smith, 2008; Unruh et al., 2002). Practitioners have also been asked to consider the intricacies of spirituality in the form of self-reflection, self-awareness, and psychological and transformational development (Collins, 2007; Kang, 2003), recognizing that therapy, through specific intentional and thoughtful spiritual approaches, can help provide guidance to clients through traumatic life events.

References

American Occupational Therapy Association. (2014). Occupational therapy practice framework: Domain and process (3rd ed.). *American Journal of Occupational Therapy, 68*(Suppl. 1), S1–S48. http://dx.doi.org/10.5014/ajot.2014.682006

Baker, L. M. (2008). A spring of hope: Fostering new life. *International Journal of Disability, Development and Education, 55,* 189–190. http://dx.doi.org/10.1080/10349120802033709

Baptiste, S. (2003). Culture as environment: Complexity, sensitivity, and challenge. In L. Letts, P. Rigby, & D. Stewart (Eds.), *Using environments to enable occupational performance* (pp. 81–95). Thorofare, NJ: Slack.

Beagan, B. L., Etowa, J., & Bernard, W. T. (2012). "With God in our lives he gives us the strength to carry on": African Nova Scotian women, spirituality, and racism-related stress. *Mental Health, Religion, and Culture, 15*(2), 103–120. http://dx.doi.org/10.1080/13674676.2011.560145

Boswell, B., Hamer, M., Knight, S., Glacoff, M., & McChesney, J. (2007). Dance of disability and spirituality. *Journal of Rehabilitation, 73*(4), 33–40. https://www.questia.com/library/journal/1G1-173463301/dance-of-disability-and-spirituality (no DOI available)

Brémault-Phillips, S., & Chirovsky, A. (2011a). Spiritual practices. In M. A. McColl (Ed.), *Spirituality and occupational therapy* (2nd ed., pp. 183–192). Ottawa, ON: CAOT Publications.

Brémault-Phillips, S., & Chirovsky, A. (2011b). The spiritual path. In M. A. McColl (Ed.), *Spirituality and occupational therapy* (2nd ed., pp. 151–158). Ottawa, ON: CAOT Publications.

Burgman, I. (2011). Spirituality in the lives of marginalized children. In F. Kronenberg, N. Pollard, & D. Sakellariou (Eds.), *Occupational therapies without borders: Towards an ecology of occupation-based practices* (Vol. 2, pp. 93–102). London: Elsevier Churchill Livingstone.

Chapparo, C., & Ranka, J. (Eds.). (1997). *Occupational Performance Model (Australia) monograph 1.* Sydney: Occupational Performance Network.

Christiansen, C. (1997). Acknowledging a spiritual dimension in occupational therapy practice. *American Journal of Occupational Therapy, 51,* 169–180. http://dx.doi.org/10.5014/ajot.51.3.169

Collins, M. (1998). Occupational therapy and spirituality: Reflecting on quality of experience in therapeutic interventions. *British Journal of Occupational Therapy, 61,* 280–285. http://dx.doi.org/10.1177/030802269806100614

Collins, M. (2004). Dreaming and occupation. *British Journal of Occupational Therapy, 67,* 96–98. http://dx.doi.org/10.1177/030802260406700207

Collins, M. (2007). Spiritual emergency and occupational identity: A transpersonal experience. *British Journal of Occupational Therapy, 70,* 504–519. http://dx.doi.org/10.1177/030802260707001202

Donica, D. K. (2008). Spirituality and occupational therapy: The application of the pyschospiritual integration frame of reference. *Physical and Occupational Therapy in Geriatrics, 27,* 107–121. http://dx.doi.org/10.1080/02703180802206082

Egan, M., & DeLaat, M. D. (1994). Considering spirituality in occupational practice. *Canadian Journal of Occupational Therapy, 61,* 95–101. http://dx.doi.org/10.1177/000841749406100205

Egan, M., & DeLaat, M. D. (1997). The implicit spirituality of occupational therapy practice. *Canadian Journal of Occupational Therapy, 64,* 115–121.

Engquist, D. E., Short-DeGraff, M., Gilner, J., & Oltjenbruns, K. (1997). Occupational therapist's beliefs and practices with regard to spirituality and therapy. *American Journal of Occupational Therapy, 51,* 173–180. http://dx.doi.org/10.5014/ajot.51.3.173

Farah, J., & McColl, M. A. (2008). Exploring prayer as a spiritual modality. *Canadian Journal of Occupational Therapy, 75,* 5–13. http://dx.doi.org/10.1177/000841740807500103

Frank, G., Bernardo, C. S., Tropper, S., Noguchi, F., Lipman, C., Maulhardt, B., & Weitze, L. (1997). Jewish spirituality through actions in time: Daily occupations of young Orthodox Jewish couples in Los Angeles. *American Journal of Occupational Therapy, 57,* 199–206. http://dx.doi.org/10.5014/ajot.51.3.199

Frank, G., Murphy, S., Kitching, H. J., Garfield, D., M., & McDarment, N. (2008). The Tule River Tribal history project: Evaluating a California tribal government's collaboration with anthropology and occupational therapy to preserve indigenous history and promote tribal goals. *Society for Applied Anthropology, 67,* 430–442. http://dx.doi.org/10.17730/humo.67.4.w605825710nu5v70

Greenberg, N. S. (2004). Spiritual spontaneity: Developing our own 9/11: One occupational therapist's spiritual journey across the 9/11 divide. *Occupational Therapy in Mental Health, 19,* 153–189. http://dx.doi.org/10.1300/J004v19n03_15

Hasselkus, B. R. (2002). *The meaning of everyday occupation.* Thorofare, NJ: Slack.

Heuchemer, B., & Josephsson, S. (2006). Leaving homelessness and addiction: Narratives of an occupational transition. *Scandinavian Journal of Occupational Therapy, 13,* 160–169. http://dx.doi.org/10.1080/11038120500360648

Howard, B. S., & Howard, J. R. (1997). Occupation as spiritual activity. *American Journal of Occupational Therapy, 51,* 181–185. http://dx.doi.org/10.5014/ajot.51.3.181

Humbert, T. K., Bess, J. L., & Mowery, A. M. (2013). Exploring women's perspectives of overcoming intimate partner violence: A phenomenological study. *Occupational Therapy in Mental Health, 29,* 246–265. http://dx.doi.org/10.1080/0164212x.2013.819465

Iwama, M. (2006). *The Kawa Model: Culturally relevant occupational therapy.* Philadelphia: Elsevier.

Johnston, D., & Mayers, C. (2005). Spirituality: A review of how occupational therapists acknowledge, assess, and meet spiritual needs. *British Journal of Occupational Therapy, 68,* 386–392. http://dx.doi.org/10.1177/030802260506800902

Kang, C. (2003). A psychospiritual integration frame of reference for occupational therapy, part 1: Conceptual foundations. *Australian Occupational Therapy Journal, 50,* 92–103. http://dx.doi.org/10.1046/j.1440-1630.2003.00358.x

Kroeker, P. T. (2007). In E. Townsend & H. Polatajko (Eds.), *Enabling occupation II: Advancing an occupational therapy vision for health, well-being, and justice through occupation* (p. 68). Ottawa, ON: CAOT Publications.

Kronenberg, F., Pollard, N., & Sakellariou, D. (Eds.). (2011). *Occupational therapies without borders: Towards an ecology of occupation-based practices, volume 2.* London: Elsevier Churchill Livingstone.

Law, M., Polatajko, H., Baptiste, S., & Townsend, E. (1997). Core concepts of occupational therapy. In E. Townsend (Ed.), *Enabling occupation: An occupational therapy perspective,* (pp. 29–56). Ottawa, ON: CAOT Publications.

Low, J. F. (1997). Religious orientation and pain management. *American Journal of Occupational Therapy, 51,* 215–219. http://dx.doi.org/10.5014/ajot.51.3.215

Luboshitzky, D. (2008). Exploring the spiritual meaning of suffering: A strategy of self-help, recovery, and hope. *Occupational Therapy in Health Care, 22,* 21–38. http://dx.doi.org/10.1080/J003v22n01_03

McColl, M. A. (2000). Spirit, occupation, and disability. *Canadian Journal of Occupational Therapy, 67,* 217–228. http://dx.doi.org/10.1177/000841740006700403

McColl, M. A. (2003). Section 4: Conclusions. In M. A. McColl (Ed.), *Spirituality and occupational therapy* (pp. 207–215). Ottawa, ON: CAOT Publications.

McColl, M. A. (2011). *Spirituality and occupational therapy* (2nd ed.). Ottawa, ON: CAOT Publications.

Peloquin, S. M. (1997). Nationally speaking—The spiritual depth of occupation: Making worlds and making lives. *American Journal of Occupational Therapy, 51,* 167–168. http://dx.doi.org/10.5014/ajot.51.3.167

Phillips, I. (2003). Infusing spirituality into geriatric health care: Practical applications from the literature. *Topics in Geriatric Rehabilitation, 19,* 249–256. http://journals.lww.com/topicsingeriatricrehabilitation/Abstract/2003/10000/Infusing_Spirituality_Into_Geriatric_Health_Care_.5.aspx

Precin, P. (Ed.). (2006). *Healing 9/11: Creative programming by occupational therapists.* Philadelphia: Haworth Press.

Puchalski, C., Ferrell, B., Virani, R., Otis-Green, S., Baird, P., Bull, J., . . . Sulmasy, D. (2009). Improving the quality of spiritual care as a dimension of palliative care: The report of the Consensus Conference. *Journal of Palliative Medicine, 12,* 885–904. http://dx.doi.org/10.1089/jpm.2009.0142

Schulz, E. K. (2004). Spirituality and disability: An analysis of select themes. *Occupational Therapy in Health Care, 18,* 57–83. http://dx.doi.org/10.1080/J003v18n04_05

Schulz, E. K. (2005). The meaning of spirituality for individuals with disabilities. *Disability and Rehabilitation, 27,* 1283–1295. http://dx.doi.org/10.1080/09638280500076319

Schwartz, L., & Fleming Cottrell, R. P. (2007). The value of spirituality as perceived by elders in long-term care. *Physical and Occupational Therapy in Geriatrics, 26,* 43–61. http://dx.doi.org/10.1300/J148v26n01_04

Simo-Algado, S., Gregori, J. M. R., & Egan, M. (1997). Spirituality in a refugee camp. *Canadian Journal of Occupational Therapy, 64,* 138–145. http://dx.doi.org/10.1177/000841749706400310

Smith, S. (2008). Toward a flexible framework for understanding spirituality. *Occupational Therapy in Health Care, 22,* 39–54. http://dx.doi.org/10.1080/J003v22n01_04

Smith, S., & Suto, M. J. (2012). Religious and/or spiritual practices: Extending spiritual freedom to people with schizophrenia. *Canadian Journal of Occupational Therapy, 79,* 77–85. http://dx.doi.org/10.2182/cjot.2012.79.2.3

Smith-Gabai, H., & Ludwig, F. (2011). Observing the Jewish Sabbath: A meaningful restorative ritual for modern times. *Journal of Occupational Science, 18,* 347–355. http://dx.doi.org/10.1080/14427591.2011.595891

Thibault, R. (1997). A funeral for my father's mind: A therapist's attempt at grieving. *Canadian Journal of Occupational Therapy, 64,* 107–114. http://dx.doi.org/10.1177/000841749706400306

Thibault, R. (2011). Occupational gifts. In M. A. McColl (Ed.), *Spirituality and occupational therapy* (2nd ed., pp. 111–120). Ottawa, ON: CAOT Publications.

Tolle, E. (2004). *The power of now.* Vancouver, BC: Namaste Publishing.

Toomey, M. A. (1999). The art of observation: Reflecting on a spiritual moment. *Canadian Journal of Occupational Therapy, 66,* 197–199. http://dx.doi.org/10.1177/000841749906600407

Toomey, M. (2011). Creativity: Spirituality through the visual arts. In M. A. McColl (Ed.), *Spirituality and occupational therapy* (2nd ed., pp. 233–240). Ottawa, ON: CAOT Publications.

Townsend, E. (1993). Occupational therapy's social vision. *Canadian Journal of Occupational Therapy, 60,* 174–184. http://dx.doi.org/10.1177/000841749306000403

Townsend, E. (1997a). Inclusiveness: A community dimension of spirituality. *Canadian Journal of Occupational Therapy, 64,* 146–155. http://dx.doi.org/10.1177/000841749706400311

Townsend, E. (1997b). Occupation: Potential for personal and social transformation. *Journal of Occupational Science, 4,* 18–26. http://dx.doi.org/10.1080/14427591.1997.9686417

Townsend, E., DeLaat, D., Egan, M., Thibault, R., & Wright, W. (1999). *Spirituality in enabling occupation: A learner-centered workbook.* Ottawa, ON: CAOT Publications.

Townsend, E. A., & Polatajko, H. J. (Eds.). (2007). *Enabling occupations II: Advancing an occupational therapy vision for health, well-being, and justice through occupation.* Ottawa, ON: CAOT Publications.

Tse, S., Lloyd, C., Petchkovsky, L., & Manaia, W. (2005). Exploration of Australian and New Zealand indigenous people's spirituality and mental health. *Australian Occupational Therapy Journal, 52,* 181–187. http://dx.doi.org/10.1111/j.1440-1630.2005.00507.x

Unruh, A. M. (1997). Spirituality and occupation: Garden musings and the Himalayan blue poppy. *Canadian Journal of Occupational Therapy, 64,* 156–160. http://dx.doi.org/10.1177/000841749706400112

Unruh, A. M., & Elvin, N. (2004). In the eye of the dragon: Women's experience of breast cancer and the occupation of dragon boat racing. *Canadian Journal of Occupational Therapy, 71,* 138–149. http://dx.doi.org/10.1177/000841740407100304

Unruh, A. M., Versnel, J., & Kerr, N. (2002). Spirituality unplugged: A review of commonalities and contentions, and a resolution. *Canadian Journal of Occupational Therapy, 69,* 5–20. http://dx.doi.org/10.1177/000841740206900101

Urbanowski, R. (1997). Spirituality in everyday practice. *OT Practice, 2,* 18–23.

Urbanowski, R., & Vargo, J. (1994). Spirituality, daily practice, and the occupational performance model. *Canadian Journal of Occupational Therapy, 61,* 88–94. http://dx.doi.org/10.1177/000841749406100204

Vrkljan, B. H. (2000). The role of spirituality in occupational therapy practice. *Occupational Therapy Now, 2*(2), 6–9.

Weskamp, K., & Ramugondo, E. L. (2005). Taking account of spirituality. In R. Watson & L. Swartz (Eds.), *Transformation through occupation* (pp. 155–167). London: Whurr Publishers.

Wilding, C. (2007). Spirituality as sustenance for mental health and meaningful doing: A case illustration. *Medical Journal of Australia, 186,* S67–S69. https://www.mja.com.au/system/files/issues/186_10_210507/wil11065_fm.pdf

Wilding, C., May, E., & Muir-Cochrane, E. (2005). Experience of spirituality, mental illness and occupation: A life-sustaining phenomenon. *Australian Occupational Therapy Journal, 52,* 2–9. http://dx.doi.org/10.1111/j.1440-1630.2005.00462.x

Williams, B. J. (2008). An exploratory study of older adults' perspectives of spirituality. *Occupational Therapy in Health Care, 22,* 3–19. http://dx.doi.org/10.1080/J003v22n01_02

CHAPTER 4.

SPIRITUALITY THROUGH THE LENS OF HEALTH CARE CHAPLAINCY

Priscilla Denham, MDiv, DMin, and Tamera Keiter Humbert, MA, DEd, OTR/L

Chapter Highlights

✧ Entering the health care setting
✧ The professional chaplain
✧ Reflecting on spirituality in health care
✧ Working premises of spirituality in health care

Key Terms and Concepts

✧ Chaplains
✧ Communication facilitators
✧ Ecclesiastical endorsement
✧ Grief
✧ Religion
✧ Specialized ministry
✧ Spiritual assessment

✧ Spiritual block
✧ Spiritual but not religious
✧ Spiritual injury
✧ Spiritual maturity
✧ Spirituality
✧ Verbatims

*C**haplains* are clergy or others endorsed by their faith group to provide interfaith spiritual care in various settings, such as hospitals, military facilities, retirement communities, and prisons. The foundational premise for a chaplain's work is that every person in a health care setting is a spiritual being, including patients, family members of patients, and staff. Although people may not identify with any religion, may be uncomfortable talking about spirituality, or may be antagonistic to religion and proclaim that they are not

spiritual in any way, all people are more than their bodily parts, mental processes, or conscious selves. Therefore, the entirety of who a person is includes the spirit.

This chapter briefly presents the education and training necessary to be a certified chaplain. It then gives a working definition of *spirituality* and discusses issues particularly pertinent in health care from the perspective of two chaplains from two faith traditions. The final section provides a behind-the-scenes look at what a chaplain does.

Entering the Health Care Setting

Illness, injury, aging, suffering, and the possibility of death confront most people with questions of the meaning of their life. What brings a person into a health care setting may raise profound questions about life's meaning, purpose, relationships, and priorities (Puchalski & Ferrell, 2010). It often elicits feelings of fear, grief, and helplessness. In addition, a traumatic accident or major health care concern may challenge a person's worldview and perspective of self. For example, the loss of a limb not only involves profound grieving but may also require the need to learn anew formerly "insignificant" daily tasks, such as brushing one's teeth.

I (first author) have been privileged to join many patients as they journeyed through these "shadows of death" seeking to discern their paths through complicated decisions regarding treatment. Many have struggled to find motivation to make such health care decisions that will result in a life very different from what they previously considered whole. For example, how does a person find meaning when recommendations for hip replacement surgery may end a running passion? How does a woman who wishes to breast feed her children accept a double mastectomy? How does a patient and significant others make the decision to end medical intervention?

I have observed that, regardless of the patient's physical outcome, the discussion and decisions regarding treatment are more helpful when the health care team recognizes the person as body and soul, that is, a whole person. Case Example 4.1, in which an injured mother enters the health care setting, illustrates the extreme circumstances in which chaplains and health care providers do their work.

The Professional Chaplain

The path to professional chaplaincy is multilayered and multidirectional. Chaplains come from many religious traditions. For hundreds of years, across religious traditions, prayers for healing and prayers for the dying were a routine part of ministry, whether at a patient's bedside or in a church. Even now, most Christian clergy make hospital visits when one of their parishioners is hospitalized.

However, in the past 100 years, with the increasing sophistication of medicine and treatment choices, complicated ethical decisions, and loosened ties to organized religion for many people, chaplaincy has become a specialized ministry with established standards and specialized prerequisites for those who choose to make ministry in a hospital their full-time professional work (Cobb, Puchalski, & Rumbold, 2012; Swift, 2014). Four primary requirements must be fulfilled to be a credentialed chaplain: (1) education, (2) documented relationship with an authorizing denomination or faith group, (3) training, and (4) experience.

Creating Standards

With the professionalization of chaplaincy as a specialized ministry, the importance of developing recognizable standards for quality care of patients and training chaplains across organizational boundaries has become a pressing need. Various organizations have developed to support the profession of chaplaincy, each working to articulate the standards necessary for excellence in the field. To bring best standards together, in 2004, the boards of six organizations involved in various aspects of pastoral care met to establish foundational documents. These documents, as follows, were intended to create a unified voice on professional pastoral care for these organizations, which represent more than 10,000 members who serve as chaplains, pastoral counselors, and pastoral care educators (Exhibit 4.1):

- *Common Code of Ethics for Chaplains, Pastoral Educators, and Students* (Association of Professional Chaplains [APC], 2004a)

Exhibit 4.1. *Chaplain Organizations*

- Association of Professional Chaplains
  www.professionalchaplains.org
- American Association of Pastoral Counselors
  www.aapc.org
- Association for Clinical Pastoral Education
  www.acpe.edu
- National Association of Catholic Chaplains
  www.nacc.org
- Neshama: Association of Jewish Chaplains
  www.najc.org
- Canadian Association for Spiritual Care
  www.spiritualcare.ca

Case Example 4.1. Interdisciplinary Collaboration of Care

The familiar number on the chaplain's pager told her something was urgent on the shock/trauma intensive care unit. "Chaplain, we could use your help up here. Bed 15 is waking up." As the chaplain moved through the hallways to the unit, she recalled what she had heard in the team meeting this week. "Bed 15" was a single mother, brought in over the weekend with multiple stab wounds from a robbery turned lethal. The team was still uncertain whether she could pull through.

What was troubling beyond her fragile physical status was that her only child had been killed in the break in, and no one knew whether the mother knew it. The social worker had been unsuccessful in tracing other family members for the previous 3 days while the patient was unconscious. And now she was waking up.

When the chaplain reached the nursing desk, she saw a knot of nurses discussing the issue. "We don't know what to say, chaplain. She is waking up for maybe 15 seconds and asks about her daughter. We are afraid that if we tell her that her daughter is dead, she will lose whatever will to live she has. But we don't want to lie to her either. So far, we have avoided saying anything because she is so heavily medicated for the pain, she falls back asleep quickly, but we will need to say something, probably by tomorrow. What is the best way to care for her? How can we help her want to live?"

The chaplain listened carefully for the next 30 minutes, observing and reflecting back the compassionate concern she heard around the circle. Some were deeply concerned about the ethical integrity of telling a patient the truth. Others were just as concerned that telling this patient that her daughter was dead would have a negative medical effect on the patient's own struggle toward healing.

The chaplain shared one of the earliest lessons she had been taught in her chaplaincy training: Patients do not ask a question until they are spiritually prepared to hear the answer—whether good or bad. Years of experience validated this teaching. The chaplain thought if the mother was strong enough to ask, she was ready to hear the truth told gently.

The nurses discussed when and how to support her in the telling. They decided on the next day. They thought the best team would be the chaplain, her assigned nurse for that shift, and any family member if the social worker could find one. They talked about how it would be hard for their patient to cry on the ventilator, but if the news was too painful, the heavy medication would let her go to sleep quickly after hearing. They also discussed how she would likely forget and ask again and again but that the nurse on duty could refer back to the original visit when the news was repeated. The chaplain walked away, proud of the hard work the team was doing to care for this woman, body and spirit.

The social worker was able to locate a sister living in a different city who traveled to share the painful news with the patient. The chaplain talked with the sister to prepare her for what she was about to see and how to give the news that the daughter had been killed. The chaplain and the assigned nurse for the day stood with the sister as she shared the news and were there to offer comfort and join in a prayer. In the days to follow, the patient did forget and asked again about her daughter, and whoever was attending to her that day would gently remind her of her sister's visit and the news.

- *Common Standards for Pastoral Educators/Supervisors* (APC, 2004b)
- *Common Standards for Professional Chaplaincy* (APC, 2004c)
- *Principles for Processing Ethical Complaints* (APC, 2004d).

Education

Chaplain candidates usually must complete an undergraduate degree from a college, university, or theological school accredited by the Council for Higher Education Accreditation and a graduate-level degree to provide a grounding in the profession. Graduate-level degrees, or the equivalent, for each faith group have different educational requirements. A typical seminary degree for a Christian is 3 years. Rabbis typically have a 6-year degree.

Formal training to become a Buddhist monk varies according to the location of the monastery and the type of Buddhism. However, the typical path of joining a *sangha* (i.e., religious community), finding a mentor, making the life changes to be accepted into a monastery, and then studying in the monastery often takes several years. Hindu and Muslim chaplain requirements vary in roles, length of study, and training requirements but generally entail the completion of a seminary or advanced degree (Isgandarova, 2010; Shirma, 2013).

Endorsement and Authorization

Chaplaincy is considered a form of **specialized ministry** (i.e., ministry done outside of a typical denominational congregational setting). Depending on the denomination or faith group, a chaplain may be ordained, licensed, or commissioned. This designation by an authorizing body of a denomination or faith group is often referred to as **ecclesiastical endorsement** by Protestant and Catholic groups.

Every denomination or faith group has its own standards and policies regarding authorization. Documentation of ecclesiastical endorsement ensures, for both the denomination and the setting in which the chaplain serves, that the chaplain is in good standing and has clear lines of accountability to the denomination as he or she provides ministry on behalf of that denomination.

Chaplains are usually required to renew endorsement every 1–5 years, depending on the authorizing body or credentialing organization. For example, the denominational requirement for chaplains in the American Baptist Churches/USA is that each year they make a report and receive a new letter of endorsement. The credentialing body of the Association of Professional Chaplains requires an updated letter of endorsement every 5 years.

Training

The minimum training required for certification by APC is four units of clinical pastoral education (CPE) accredited by the Association for Clinical Pastoral Education (ACPE), the United States Conference of Catholic Bishops Commission on Certification and Accreditation, or the Canadian Association for Pastoral Practice and Education. The standards for ACPE CPE are a minimum of 400 hours per unit. A unit has 100 hours of group and individual supervision by

a certified educator, which must include conceptual teaching and review of clinical case studies.

The remaining 300 hours must be spent in clinical ministry to patients, families, and staff. By ACPE standards, each unit requires learning goals, written clinical case studies (often called **verbatims**), documentation of reflective practice, and a final evaluation by both student and supervisor. A unit usually takes 3 months to complete (years ago, a unit was called a *quarter,* meaning a quarter of a year); therefore, four units is the equivalent of 1 year of training. The beginning unit includes basic skills, and the other three units include more advanced chaplaincy competencies.

Basic skills

In the beginning CPE unit, training emphasizes the basic skills of

- Developing self-awareness of gifts and limitations for spiritual care,
- Cultivating sensitivity to interfaith issues (i.e., learning how to do ministry with those of a different faith or no religious preference),
- Understanding the basic ethical and pastoral issues arising out of the clinical setting,
- Improving listening and reflection skills, and
- Learning to reflect pastorally on the human condition.

The ACPE standards broadly delineate these learning objectives as the areas of pastoral formation, pastoral competence, and pastoral reflection (ACPE, 2015). Because these areas of self-awareness and skills are helpful in any ministry context, many mainline denominations (e.g., some Lutherans, Episcopalians, many Associations of the United Church of Christ) require this beginning unit of CPE for their seminarians.

Chaplaincy competencies

Chaplaincy competencies are covered throughout the final three CPE units. These competencies include the ability to

- *Articulate a coherent conceptual understanding of pastoral care.* This competency includes having a rudimentary understanding of the social sciences, family systems, group dynamics, and organizational behavior to integrate pastoral identity and conduct, including communication skills, with other disciplines.

- *Understand the Common Code of Ethics* (APC, 2004a). This understanding ensures the appropriate use of pastoral authority and awareness and respect for the physical, emotional, and spiritual boundaries of others.
- *Develop pastoral skills.* These skills include establishing, deepening, and appropriately ending pastoral relationships; providing effective pastoral support to patients, families, and staff of an institution; providing spiritual care that respects diversity and differences of culture, gender, sexual orientation, and spiritual or religious practices; and eliciting the patient's, family's, and staff's personal understanding of their religious or spiritual resources (e.g., relationship to church or synagogue, artistic expression, meditation, significant relationships; Exhibit 4.2).
- *Establish professional identity as a chaplain in a specialized ministry setting.* This competency includes the chaplain's ability to promote the integration of spiritual care into the culture and service of the institution, establish and maintain professional interdisciplinary relationships, support and facilitate ethical decision making and care, document the patient's care in appropriate records, and foster collaborative relationships with community clergy and faith group leaders.

Experience as a Chaplain

The final step to becoming a board-certified chaplain is meeting with a committee that evaluates the applicant's readiness to be certified. In addition to the necessary documentation for education, authorization for ministry, and self- and supervisors' evaluations of a candidate's CPE units, the applicant must have completed a minimum of 1 year of experience as a chaplain beyond the year of supervision. Demonstration of the professional competencies are reviewed through papers the applicant writes to demonstrate how they were applied after training.

Exhibit 4.2. *Developing Pastoral Skills*

At the end of an advanced unit, I use the following list to assess ACPE students' ability to

- Initiate conversation
- Listen sufficiently to elicit and attend to presenting issues
- Draw a visit to a close with self-awareness
- Empathically respond
- Name underlying emotions heard and reflect them to the patient or family as appropriate
- Offer observations helpful to the situation
- Help conversation move beyond surface concerns or social chit-chat
- Ask open-ended questions to elicit sharing, reflections, or grief
- Clarify communication when necessary
- Elicit the patient's personal understanding of his or her religious or spiritual resources
- Offer appropriate prayer or readings
- Provide spiritual care to the patient's family
- Support staff as appropriate
- Work with diverse people (e.g., age, gender, religion, culture, sexual preference, socioeconomic status)
- Have knowledge and awareness of ethical considerations when raised by the patient or family
- Tolerate conflict and move toward resolution
- Implement crisis management
- Tell stories or elicit the patient's or families' stories
- Elicit a life review from the patient or family.

It is expected that these skills will become more fine-tuned as additional units and training are completed.

Source. Rabbi Leah Wald. Adapted with permission.

Reflecting on Spirituality in Health Care

In this section, two chaplains, one from a Protestant Christian tradition (first author) and one from a Jewish tradition (Leah Wald), consider spirituality. These chaplains have a combined experience of more than 50 years of working with people in various health care settings, including trauma hospitals, retirement communities, and psychiatric hospitals. Although this conversation was focused for purposes of this chapter, it is a part of an ongoing conversation between the minister and rabbi in several venues for close to 20 years.

Relationship Between Religion and Spirituality

Perhaps the most basic issue any chaplain must address is the relationship between religion and spirituality because many people connect the two. *Religion* is a set of shared rituals, traditions, and beliefs (and often history) that symbolize life-meaning values for the people who share them. *Spirituality* is a personal experience of connection to an ultimate meaning. Some people understand these concepts as equivalent to each other. They may see spirituality contained in the religious life of organized religion and might even understand their spirituality to be confined to that context. However, if a person considers nature, art, or working for justice to be sacred, religion may not be a part of that person's spiritual understanding at all. As a chaplain, I am particularly cautious to not assume that a person's identified religious connection (or lack thereof) is the same as that person's spiritual resource in his or her time of physical or psychological difficulty.

When a health care provider equates religion with spirituality, he or she may believe (or fear) that only designated religious professionals (e.g., clergy, chaplains, designated pastoral caregivers) should address a patient's spirituality. A referring health care provider may even assume that only clergy who match the patient's religious preference can (or should) provide spiritual care; however, that is not the case (Case Example 4.2).

In addition, health care providers who conflate religion and spirituality may assume that a patient who indicates no religious preference requires no spiritual care. This conclusion may be deeply wrong (Case Example 4.3) and cause a health care professional to miss a meaningful engagement with a patient who understands himself or herself as *spiritual but not religious.* In the United States, 30% of adults consider themselves "spiritual but not religious" (Bass, 2013, p. 66). As a growing number of people identify themselves this way, poll takers have even developed the shorthand of "SBNR" as a category of choice (Bass, 2013).

Case Example 4.2. Jewish Chaplain, Pentecostal Patient

A Jewish chaplain entered the room of a patient whose religious affiliation was with a Pentecostal church. The woman shared that she was seriously ill with a sexually transmitted disease and had been told she did not have long to live. She was able to discuss her situation with the chaplain but not with her family and church friends because she feared they would be critical of her on religious and moral grounds. Additionally, the patient was feeling pressured. Some church and family members had communicated the message that if her faith were strong enough, she could be healed.

The chaplain worked with the woman to help her sort through her own spiritual understanding of God's love and care, whatever the physical outcome. As the disease progressed, the chaplain also supported the woman in her evolving trust that she could tell her family the nature and predicted outcome of the disease. A few days before her death, the woman was able to talk openly with her family. They were heartbroken that she was dying and able to move from pressuring her to heal herself with faith to comforting and affirming her in her dying process.

Case Example 4.3. Spiritual Care Without God Talk

The chaplain walked into the room, introducing herself as she entered. "That's ok for you to keep going," the patient said with a smile, "I don't have anything to talk about with you. I don't believe in God."

Appreciating his frankness, yet aware that the staff believed he needed to talk about a recent diagnosis, the chaplain laughed. "Well, I've got time to talk, and if you don't mind, I'd like to hear about this God you don't believe in. I'm guessing I don't believe in him either." Then the patient laughed and they began to talk, moving first through a worn-out image of God from the patient's childhood and then on to the things that gave the man meaning and purpose in his adult life. From that base, the two then discussed his diagnosis and the treatment decisions he needed to make.

How Spirituality and Religion Connect

I (first author) see the connection of spirituality and religion as a Venn diagram with two circles overlapping, to a greater or lesser extent depending on a person's religious beliefs and their definition of spirituality (Figure 4.1). For some people, the circles may not overlap at all; Figure 4.2). It is my experience that in the spiritually mature person (discussed below), the circle of spirituality overlaps any and all differentiating circles of religion (Figure 4.3), conveying spiritual universalism (Case Example 4.4).

In other words, the spiritually mature person embraces and respects all religions and finds wisdom and truth in each one. For example, Mahatma Gandhi expressed his spiritual universalism when challenged by a critic. The man was concerned that Gandhi was too accepting of other religious perspectives and asked whether he was really a Hindu. Gandhi's response: "Yes, I am. I am also a Muslim, a Christian, a Buddhist, and a Jew" (Sen Gupta, 2008, p. 5).

Figure 4.1. The spirituality and religion connection: Spiritual and Religious.

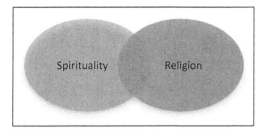

Figure 4.2. Spiritual but not religious.

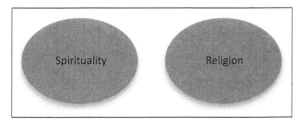

Figure 4.3. Spiritual maturity.

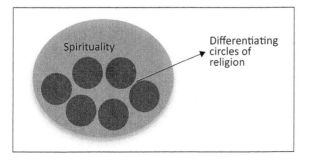

Case Example 4.4. Spiritual Support Across Religious Differences

A Christian chaplain had been told that a Jewish patient had only hours to live and had asked for prayer. The chaplain had called the rabbi who usually attended to patients in the hospital but was told he was out of town. The chaplain sat with the patient, listening to a bit of her life history, and then explained she would need to call another rabbi because the first person she called was unavailable. The elderly woman smiled and asked whether the chaplain would pray with her, saying "It's the same God." Although the patient was aware of the religious differences between herself and the chaplain and of the chaplain's inability as a Christian to offer traditional Jewish prayer, she asked for the spiritual comfort of prayer, which transcended their separate beliefs.

The following analogy is one I have used with health care professionals to help them understand the relationship between religion and spirituality: Spirituality is to religion as justice is to the law. The law and religion are the communally agreed upon articulated frameworks (or boundaries) within which people may legally or morally act. These frameworks are meant to reflect the underlying values of society or a religious community. Justice and spirituality, however, may transcend these frameworks and invite individual interpretation of social, legal, and moral actions.

A person's spiritual path may align with a particular religious community. Another person's spiritual path may be only loosely associated with a religious community and that person may be most comfortable remaining on the periphery of that religion. Yet another person may not be associated with any religious community. It is also possible (and not uncommon) for a person to attend a place of worship, be in prayer or meditation with others in that religious community, and not accept all the teachings while still finding genuine spirituality in such worship.

Another way to understand this analogy is through the example of the Quakers in the 1800s who helped slaves escape. According to the Dred Scott Decision in 1857 (*Dred Scott v. Sandford,* 60 U.S. 393), "harboring a 'fugitive from labor' was a violation of both the United States Constitution and of Federal Law. It wasn't just illegal; it was subversive, even treasonous" (Densmore, 2015). Yet, as early as the 1770s, Quakers were united on the idea that slaves had a natural right to freedom and that no Quaker should participate in slavery, which they considered a "national evil" (Densmore, 2015). Quakers rejected the legitimacy of slavery—it was not simply wrong, it was unjust, and no federal law could make it right.

Quakers challenged obedience to a law they did not consider just and accepted the legal consequences of breaking it. The person who makes a distinction between his or her personal beliefs in social principles (i.e., justice) and the legal manifestations of those principles (i.e., laws) mirrors the person who makes a distinction between his or her personal beliefs in the sacred (i.e., spirituality) and formally established belief systems and rituals around the divine (i.e., religion).

Application to the Health Care Setting

In the health care setting, where religious affiliation is charted and used as an identifier of need, it is particularly important not to confuse a lack of religious identity with a lack of spirituality or spiritual needs. Physical illness or injury often raises deep questions about the meaning of life and death. Therefore, spiritual questions may arise from the context of hospitalization that have been largely dormant in patients and their families. Moreover, people may want to feel God's presence in times of emotional trial, whether the religious "answers" of their past are sufficient to be a meaningful resource for the current event or not.

Working Premises of Spirituality in Health Care

As I (first author) have worked with clergy of multiple faiths and denominations, both in congregational work and health care settings, I have never experienced any two people having the exact same definition of spirituality. In the ongoing conversation with my colleague, Rabbi Leah Wald, we reflected on the definition of *spirituality* formed from our experiences working with patients, religious and nonreligious.

The rabbi defined it as "a sense of connection with something greater and beyond oneself that helps to give meaning to one's life, or a sense of connection with self, others, and something beyond." I defined *spirituality* as that place in oneself where the intimate (i.e., innermost sense of self or soul) and the transcendent (i.e., one's sense of the sacred) are joined, allowing one to feel or see an interrelationship with all others.

A person's spirituality may be experienced as feeling that he or she belongs in the moment and is at peace irrespective of the circumstances. Another way of seeing spirituality in health care is through a lens in which the ultimate meaning of a health-related event is understood within the holiness or wholeness of life.

Factors Affecting Spirituality

A foundational premise for the rabbi and me (first author) is that everyone is a spiritual being—each person has a specific spirit, an essence of that person that is unique to him or her. That spirit is the intangible summation of a person's mind, body, soul, and understanding of his or her relationship to the larger world (or universe). The result of this spirit results in the values, attitudes, and choices that a person makes.

A person's understanding of his or her spirituality and the ability to use it for meeting life's challenges vary. The depth and health of a person's spirituality is affected by his or her life experiences. Although a person's spirituality is not different on the basis of setting, context can affect how a person understands his or her spirituality as a meaningful resource for the needs of the moment. In ordinary circumstances, a person may be satisfied with the spiritual lessons he or she learned in childhood. When a crisis occurs or a traumatic event happens later in life, that same person may find the resources that worked when life was calm are now strained or tested when pain is severe.

A common example of this dilemma is a person whose early religious upbringing led him or her to believe that "being good" (however that was defined) would ensure God's protection from harm. The diagnosis of a disease or being in an accident may leave the patient shattered as he or she discovers the spiritual or religious lessons of childhood no longer seem true.

Body–Spirit Unity

Foundational to working with a patient's spirituality is the basic conviction that a human is a whole package.

The physical and spiritual aspects of a person cannot be separated out. The spirit of a person animates every part of him or her. Moreover, if therapists have a spiritual perspective on their work, for example, they could not work with an injured hand without also having some sense of what the injury (and healing) of that hand means to the patient. How the therapist relates to the patient as a whole affects the way treatment is approached and responded to.

Spirituality as Relational

For those who experience connectedness with another person, that relationship may be experienced as spiritual. A chaplain experienced spiritual care from her physical therapist when she was a patient during knee rehabilitation:

> It was painful doing the exercises necessary for recovery. What I realized very quickly, however, was that this therapist connected with me. It was clear she cared about me, not just teaching the physical tasks. The exercises were not just a painful burden to endure but actually became a joy. I looked forward to our sessions and wanted to please her. I felt we were working together for my healing—that my progress mattered to her. I soon discovered her other patients also felt this way. The difficult work—though not physically pleasant—lifted our spirits.

What the chaplain experienced during the therapy session was that she was recognized as a person and that the work being done together was meaningful beyond the physical recovery.

Consciousness and Mental Capacity

Chaplains assume that all people are spiritual beings, regardless of consciousness or mental capacity. However, being mindful that a person is a spiritual being may be difficult when he or she cannot communicate. For example, some patients may be unable to speak when on a ventilator or in a coma or because of limited cognitive ability or heavy medication. Even so, it is important for chaplains, and health care providers, to be attuned to these patients' spirituality through nuances of their nonverbal or physical communication to help them and their families during difficult situations (see Case Example 4.5).

Case Example 4.5. A Conversation With Many Levels

The chaplain in the shock/trauma intensive care unit (ICU) was called in to help a husband and wife who had been in a serious car accident. The husband, severely injured with multiple fractures and internal injuries requiring ventilation and high doses of pain medication, was in the ICU. The wife was also hurt and in another unit. For a few days, the chaplain made visits between the units. When the wife graduated to using a wheelchair, the chaplain spent time with both of them at the husband's bedside. Because the husband was on a ventilator and using heavy doses of pain medication, he could communicate only by writing a few words.

After several days, it became clear the husband's pain was increasing and his prognosis was decreasing. The young wife asked the chaplain and one of the trusted nurses to sit with her while she "discussed" with him what decisions he would have her make. From conversations with the wife, the chaplain observed that the couple seemed devoted to each other and were meaningfully connected to their faith community.

After the wife told her husband the medically relevant information, she asked whether he had thoughts about what he would want done or not done in terms of further treatments. Slowly, he began to trace out letters on the bedsheet: W-H-E-N i-n t-h-e c-o-u-r-s-e- o-f . . . . The wife and the chaplain began to laugh at the same time. The husband had started writing the prologue to the Declaration of Independence. Trying to express what he feared would be too painful for his wife to hear directly, the young man used his innate humor to indicate that he wanted to be set free from the tubes, alarm bells, and wires that trapped him in the bed, semiconsciousness, with no apparent positive value. His use of humor told his wife that he was not afraid to face death, and it was time to let him go.

Grief Work

Grief is the emotional and spiritual response to profound loss. I see grief as a kind of thread that weaves through a life. In my experience, whatever current loss is occurring, it pulls on the same emotional thread of other grief and losses in a person's life. For example, the loss of a spouse reverberates with the death of a parent, or losing the ability to walk may bring memories of an illness in childhood. Loss can be experienced on a spiritual level as a profound wound, often connecting with other losses in life.

Although grief may be largely resolved with successful treatment, greater grief work must be done when the end of treatment does not result in a return to anticipated functioning. The spiritual work that needs to happen to resolve problems with grief is a kind of reconstructive work, that is, for example, a reworking of the meaning and value of an injured hand if therapy does not result in a physical cure.

Spiritual Maturity

Spiritual maturity is when one can offer generativity and wisdom to others. It involves the recognition that a person's spiritual life, like his or her physical and emotional life, has a developmental trajectory. Spiritual maturity can vary. The earliest Christian writer, St. Paul, spoke to the issue of spiritual maturity in relation to a person's Christian journey when he said some need milk because they are not ready for meat. This metaphor suggests that a person's spirit is both whole and developing, just as a child is both a complete person and growing. It is also important to realize that a person's spiritual maturity is not necessarily correlated to his or her biological age, as anyone who has worked with pediatric patients is well aware.

When a chaplain works with patients, it is important to consider their level of spiritual maturity to better understand their needs (see Case Example 4.7). Note that many people are introduced to spirituality through religious images appropriate to their age as children, and some keep these images into adulthood with the result that this fixed spiritual understanding may stay at a simplistic level. Spiritual maturity,

---

Case Example 4.6. Loss as a Common Spiritual Wound

The chaplain and the employee assistance program director were running a grief support group for hospital employees. Although the group was initially designed to support people dealing with personal loss, during this time, the hospital was in turmoil because an institutional consolidation with a larger corporation was being revealed as destructive to patient care. Although all the staff participating in the group shared a variety of personal issues that were affecting their work performance (e.g., death of a parent, divorce, health issues of a loved one), a pall of depression caused by the consolidation was also apparent. Colleagues were being laid off without warning, supplies were monitored, and working relationships were ruptured when colleagues began looking for other jobs.

The chaplain knew there was a wide range of religious perspectives in the group, including an outspoken anti-religion person, but also noted the ability of everyone in the group to share a laugh. Deciding to use that spiritual path to help connect them, the chaplain and director worked together to be mindful of the things the group could laugh about. Although the group dealt with painful losses every week, there was also laughter in the room. Group members felt a kinship with others with different religious views and different losses because they had a spiritual bonding around the wry (but larger) perspective offered by humor.

Case Example 4.7. Understanding a Patient's Spiritual Maturity

Brought up in a religious framework that emphasized an image of God who kept a record of each person's sins, an 87-year-old woman with ovarian cancer confessed to the chaplain that she was sure she was being punished for having had an abortion more than 70 years earlier. Convinced that she would be judged, she had never shared this secret with any male clergy. Now, with a woman chaplain, and on the edge of death, she spoke. Although the patient was still sure that the cancer was a punishment, she was more at peace in believing she could meet God in a few days having done the ritual of confession, which she believed assured her of God's forgiveness.

Case Example 4.8. Understanding Other Professionals' Spiritual Maturity

In one hospital, the chaplains were the hospital's support team for rape survivors. One Monday morning, an 11-year-old girl was brought to the hospital, vomiting and with severe diarrhea. Her parents said she had been sent to the corner store for the Sunday paper the day before and had just wandered back this morning. Frightened and sick, the young girl explained how a man had physically forced her to perform oral and vaginal sex and then made her drink from a big bottle. Then, she said, she had gone to sleep.

The health care providers needed to know what was in the bottle. Ignoring the importance of the bottle's contents, the police officer assigned to the case insisted that because the girl had gone to sleep after the man raped her, "She must have wanted it." The officer's lack of spiritual maturity led him interpret the situation in a narrow, moralistic, judgmental way and kept him from asking the questions that would help him grasp the whole picture and therefore help the young survivor. The chaplain, however, while talking to the girl finally asked what was in the bottle. "I don't know. V-O-D-K-A were the letters on the bottle." Coming from a nondrinking family, the girl did not know what vodka was or that drinking half a bottle would make her "go to sleep."

Case Example 4.9. Anger as a Spiritual Block

The chaplain was asked to meet with a patient who had been in a car accident caused by a drunk driver. Although angry about the drunk driver who caused the accident (and possibly angry with God), the patient denied her anger. However, the patient indirectly expressed her anger by being persistently irritated, critical of staff, and uninvested in rehab, which slowed her recovery. While talking with the patient, the chaplain learned that she felt that anger was a sin and was also distressed that she "had been good," so it was unfair that she had been in an accident that wasn't her fault.

As the chaplain worked with the patient to understand that anger is a God-given emotion and to accept that bad things happen to good people, the patient's spirituality was challenged to grow into her present reality. Deeper spirituality resulted from directly addressing her anger, which reduced its indirect expressions. The patient was then able to stop projecting her anger and engage in treatment.

---

however, reflects a spiritual understanding that has developed through experiences of loss and wrestling with the complexities of life.

It is also important for chaplains to consider the spiritual maturity of other professionals involved with patients and how it may influence those patients. For example, Case Example 4.8 illustrates how a police officer's spiritual immaturity hindered helping a young rape survivor.

Spiritual Blocks and Injury

In addition to level of spiritual maturity, a spiritual block or injury may affect a person's spiritual journey. A *spiritual block* is when a person prejudges certain emotional responses, either their own or others', as wrong or unacceptable on the basis of his or her belief system. A *spiritual injury* is when a person feels blamed, disrespected, or hurt by another person's condemnation.

A spiritual block may present as a patient's refusal to recognize and acknowledge appropriate feelings in the context of injury or illness, such as anger, guilt, or despair. Note that the patient's feelings of anger, guilt, and despair may not be directly related to the physical condition or treatment outcomes of the patient, although hospitalization may be the precipitant for bringing these feelings to the surface. Some traditional religious teachings and some spiritual paths consider anger (a common reaction to a medical crisis) a negative or an incomplete action (see Case Example 4.9).

Spiritual injury may occur when a patient is not treated as a whole person. In an effort to be more fully recognized, the patient may express his or her sense of self in counterproductive ways. If the injury is severe (i.e., when it shames the patient and attacks his or her healthy sense of self), it may be assessed as spiritual distress and need to be addressed so the patient is able to heal. Although family, friends, and health care providers may help a patient spiritually, sometimes his or her spiritual injury may be best served by a chaplain, who is trained in spiritual

---

Case Example 4.10. Spiritual Injury

The patient was quietly fuming. The staff called the chaplain in to talk to the very silent man. As the chaplain pulled the story from him, the patient was able to say that he felt infantilized, talked down to, and told what to do as if he were a child. His response was to regress to extreme passivity. When the chaplain was able to demonstrate respect for his adult reasoning and abilities, the man was able to begin communicating with the staff. They then began talking to him on a more egalitarian basis, and he became cooperative and engaged in his treatment plan.

---

assessment and how to address it. For example, Case Example 4.10 describes a chaplain helping a patient who did not feel that his decision-making capacity as an adult was being honored.

What Chaplains Do

Although chaplains have a toolkit of competencies, skills, and experiences, each institution has its own unique needs and strengths, which affect what tasks take precedence. However, chaplains usually carry out certain basic tasks in any given week. In addition, chaplains work with both individuals and groups. Areas in which chaplains work include making spiritual assessments, exploring grief and hope, facilitating communication, serving as a resource for religious and interfaith issues, facilitating ethics and decision making, working as part of a team, serving as a bridge to the community, serving as a religious functionary, and providing a ministry of presence.

Making Spiritual Assessments

The aim of the chaplain's *spiritual assessment* is to be able to help the health care team understand the patient's and family's strengths and limitations and help the patient access his or her spiritual resources for healing. Whether done after being called for a consultation, as part of making rounds, or in response to a beeper sounding the arrival of a trauma or cardiac code, making a spiritual assessment is a foundational task for every chaplain. Such an assessment can be broadly defined as discovering what is profoundly meaningful to the patient. Chaplains use several formal assessment tools.

The FICA Spiritual History Tool (FICA; Puchalski & Romer, 2000), which explores the patient's faith and beliefs, importance of these beliefs to the patient, the patient's community connections to spiritual or religious groups, and how to address these issues during the patient's medical care, was one of the first spiritual assessment tools developed.

The HOPE Questions (HOPE; Anandarajah & Hight, 2001) examines the patient's sources of hope, strength, comfort, meaning, peace, love, and connection; the role of organized religion for the patient; the patient's personal spirituality and practices; and the effects of the patient's spirituality on medical care and end-of-life decisions. The HOPE more explicitly recognizes end-of-life issues as a spiritual concern than the FICA. Anandarajah and Hight described the HOPE as having the advantage of allowing an "open-ended exploration of an individual's general spiritual resources and concerns" (p. 85) without immediately focusing on either of the words *spirituality* or *religion*. The SPIRIT (Ambuel, 2000) explores the patient's spiritual belief system, personal spirituality, integration with a spiritual community, and ritualized practices and restrictions as well as these issues' implications for the patient's medical care and terminal events planning.

These assessment tools provide some common language in health care settings for spiritual issues. They ask questions that chaplains have been asking for decades to determine what is most meaningful to the patient, whether the patient's beliefs affect their health issues, whether the patient has a larger group or meaningful community that is supportive during his or her health crisis, and how the patient's beliefs and practices support or challenge the decisions to be made. Chaplains often use at least one of these assessment tools to gain insight into spiritual issues that may affect a patient's care. In addition, many chaplains have their own assessment criteria developed from their experience or unique to the institution they are serving.

Because a hospitalization rarely affects only the person hospitalized, chaplains also assess spiritual issues in relation to the family. This task is somewhat easier if the family is young and all members have similar beliefs. However, families in hospitals often include adults who may have different religions or spiritual practices and varying levels of connection to larger communities of support (religious or otherwise), which may require the chaplain to focus on multiple spiritual issues regarding medical treatment decisions.

This situation may be a challenge when what is profoundly meaningful to the patient is at odds with one or more of the family members.

Exploring Grief and Hope

When I conduct a spiritual assessment during a hospitalization, I always explore any grief issues involved. Dealing with grief may seem straightforward and logical, such as facing loss (or potential loss) of life when a patient has a dire diagnosis. However, it can also be complex, if it is tied to historical events (if a loved one died of the same disease) or involves anticipatory loss (if the result of the diagnosis affects future functioning). I have experienced people coping with grief on a spiritual continuum that ranges from hope to despair.

Particularly in health care, where hope is most often associated with medical success, it is important for chaplains to highlight spiritual hope, which is more encompassing than hope for a successful treatment (see Case Example 4.11). It is my

---

Case Example 4.11. Gardening as a Symbol of Hope

The chaplain entered the room of a man confined to the hospital until a heart could be found for a transplant. The chaplain was Jewish, and the patient was Roman Catholic. One clear task of the chaplain was ensuring that the patient was visited regularly by the priest to receive the sacrament, which was very important to the patient.

As weeks passed, the patient became despondent, losing hope that an appropriate heart would be found. Though he did not talk directly about his fear of no heart being found, he did express grief that he was not able to do his usual practice of gardening. The chaplain was an avid gardener herself, so—after gaining permission from the medical team—she brought in a tomato plant. Visitors and the medical staff became interested to see how the plant would do in the patient's window. When the patient pointed out the blossoms could not be fertilized inside, the chaplain took a paint brush and fertilized it with pollen from her own garden, and the plant set small fruit. For the patient, the growing plant became a symbol of God's presence and involvement in the patient's life even "in the captivity of a hospital room."

---

perspective that spiritual hope is associated with a connection to and a fuller unity with what is most meaningful to the patient, which may or may not involve physical longevity. For example, people can be clearly aware of impending death and maintain a sense of gratitude for their present condition and a joyful sense of looking forward (or contentment).

Facilitating Communication

Chaplains are often tasked with being *communication facilitators* by health care team staff, patients, and families because they are perceived as nonjudgmental and not invested in a specific outcome. Communication glitches may occur simply because a family lacks information or is not getting information in a language they understand. In addition, the patient's wishes may conflict with those of some family members, requiring the chaplain to help ease or resolve disagreements.

The patient (or family) may misunderstand hospital protocols and procedures because they are unfamiliar with related terms, concepts, or culture. For example, organ donation has historically created a cultural divide between the medical community and families because many families fear that if they agree to donate organs, the medical team will not work as hard to preserve life. This concern has been especially prevalent among African-American families (Brown, 2012).

Chaplains are skilled at identifying underlying issues and then finding common themes that are meaningful to all parties that can be discussed. Most people in the hospital setting (patients, family, and staff) are focused on the patient's physical issues. Although largely appropriate, conversations about medical issues may be inadequate for helping the patient discern what his or her wishes for treatment may or may not be (see Case Example 4.12).

Family members, thinking they are protecting the patient or "not taking away hope," may have only "cheerful" conversations with the patient and refuse to talk about the possibility that treatment may fail, despite the patient's desire and even need to do so. On the basis of separate conversations with the patient and the family, the chaplain may be aware that each is cognizant of the possibility of treatment failure yet is unwilling to "hurt" the other by discussing it directly. In this case, the chaplain can help the patient and family talk about their values and facilitate storytelling to help them

---

Case Example 4.12. The Grandmother With Only One Leg

The chaplain was called to the surgical interme-diate unit. "You have to make her understand, Chaplain. If she doesn't have her leg amputated, she will die." In the conversation with the elderly woman, the chaplain discovered that the dia-betic woman, who had already lost one leg, un-derstood clearly the implications of her refusal. However, the prospect of losing her remaining leg was too frightening.

As the conversation continued, the chaplain realized the woman associated the loss of her remaining leg with the loss of her relationship with her beloved grandson. She could cook for him only with difficulty, and he (moving into his teens) no longer wanted to just sit with her and talk. She was afraid if she lost her remaining leg, the small connection they had would be severed because she would be confined to a wheelchair.

Once the chaplain had assured her that she could refuse the operation if she wished, the con-versation continued, and the woman shared that she had other grandchildren, one still an infant. After expressing her grief, the woman came to the realization that she could provide value to her family, even without legs. She decided to have the operation.

Case Example 4.13. Medical Talk and Misunderstanding

The chaplain was sitting with the mother and aunt of the patient, a young man with severe head trauma as a result of a car accident. For several days, the two women had been hearing about various tests and procedures and discussing what they should do based on the latest report. A med-ical resident came to tell them that the patient was brain dead. Clearly uncomfortable, perhaps assuming they had known how such tests were interpreted, he told them, "The blood flow study was negative," and left the room quickly.

The two women turned to each other and began discussing how they would care for him at home. The chaplain realized that they had understood the report as good news of improvement. Excus-ing herself, she hurried down the hall to bring the resident back to explain in detail what *negative* meant in this case.

Case Example 4.14. Attending to Culture

Late one Friday afternoon, the chaplain was called to speak to a family who had just arrived from Israel. Coming to the hospital straight from the airport, the observant Jewish family was distressed that their loved one was on the 21st floor, and because the sun had just set, they could not push the electric call button for the elevator. The chaplain served as their Shabbas goy, handling the elevator and helping them find a hotel within walking range.

---

remember how they have handled painful situa-tions in the past, creating an atmosphere of sharing this emotional work together.

The chaplain is often present when bad news is delivered. Depending on the personality and personal comfort of the medical professional, he or she may retreat into "medical talk," and it becomes the task of the chaplain to help the family translate and un-derstand what is being said (see Case Example 4.13).

Serving as a Resource for Religious and Interfaith Issues

Chaplains serve as a resource for patients, family members, and staff for various religious or interfaith issues. For example, it is not uncommon for a pa-tient to ask his or her religion's position on organ donation or whether it is okay to refuse certain treatments. Therefore, chaplains help locate clergy

of the patient's faith or denomination. When that is not possible, the chaplain is then a researcher to help the patient make an informed decision. In addition, chaplains may support a religious practice for the patient or family members (see Case Example 4.14).

Facilitating Ethics and Decision Making

Hospitals have ethics committees staffed by multi-disciplinary members, usually including a chaplain or community clergymember. When an impasse oc-curs between the recommendations of the hospital

---

Case Example 4.15. Unresolved Family Secret

The chaplain was called to speak with a family (a husband and two young adult children) whose wife and mother was in the hospital on a ventilator. The doctors had just told the family that the patient was not likely to recover. The conversation was complex. The husband and children were wrestling with whether they should allow the ventilator be turned off or keep the patient on the ventilator for a few more days so her 19-year-old third child could make it to the hospital for a final farewell.

Complicating the issue was the fact that the third child had been adopted but never told. The patient and her husband had agreed they would tell their daughter when she was 21 years old. The husband felt he could not tell his daughter alone and that he could not tell her at the same time her mother was dying. The chaplain listened to their dilemma and helped them cope with their suffering. Observing the strength they shared as a family, the chaplain helped them come to their own understanding of what was most life-giving in this complex situation so they could make the best decision they could under the circumstances. Although there was no easy answer, they finally decided they would ask for continued medical care until the third child arrived, unless the patient began showing signs of being in pain.

Case Example 4.16. Helping the Team Assess a Family Member's Ability to Cope

"Chaplain, her son is going to die. The only thing keeping him going is the ventilator and drugs. But she keeps insisting God will cure him. The doctors are ready to turn off the ventilator, and it's going to be soon. We're afraid she will snap when it's turned off. Can you talk to her and tell us how we can help her take the news?"

The chaplain knew the woman. She came to the chapel daily, walking the perimeter, praying out loud for God's healing for her son. Trying to assess whether the mother was in complete denial, the chaplain gently asked what she thought her son's condition was. The mother explained that she belonged to a church that said, "You only have to ask, and it will be given to you." For the mother to agree with what the staff had been saying to her was to "tell the Devil she had given up." However, it became clear to the chaplain that the mother was realistic enough to recognize that her son had shown no improvement and that machinery was all that was keeping him breathing. The chaplain told the staff that they should be ready for grief but not a breakdown. The mother would believe he was dead when the breathing stopped with the ventilator.

---

staff or doctor and the wishes of the patient, a formal consultation is called. However, before an ethics committee becomes involved, many more intimate conversations occur among the chaplain, patient, and family members when competing values emerge or a clear choice is not evident (see Case Example 4.15).

Working as Part of a Team

Chaplains work as part of a hospital team that usually consists of the medical group or unit and other staff members. Because chaplains often serve on many medical teams within the hospital and the chaplain-to-bed ratio may be as high as 1:100 beds or more, they must be knowledgeable about numerous medical issues, flexible, able to juggle multiple cases, and able to handle both emergency and chronic patient situations. As a member of these teams, the chaplain plays an important role that includes giving educational support to staff to help them best care for patients and families (see Case Example 4.16).

Serving as a Bridge to the Community

Chaplains are a bridge to the community in several ways. The chaplain may contact the patient's clergyperson to let him or her know a visit would be welcome. If the patient is far away from his or her religious community, the chaplain may facilitate communication between the patient and the community. If the patient's clergyperson comes to the hospital, the chaplain may help him or her negotiate hospital rules and procedures, which can be confusing to those unfamiliar with such protocols. Even if the chaplain is unable to connect a patient with his or her religious community, many patients consider the chaplain to be like their home pastor, thus affording a sense of connection.

Serving as a Religious Functionary

Chaplains offer support with religious rituals or services. They often supply bibles or rosary beads when requested. Because community clergy are sometimes unable to come to the hospital at the time of urgent need, the chaplain may, for example, baptize a baby who will not live long enough for outside clergy to arrive. In addition, community clergy may be uncomfortable in hospital settings, especially in psychiatric hospitals where patients may "talk strange" and worship is sometimes chaotic, with congregants who claim to be God or the anti-Christ. In these cases, the chaplain offers interdenominational or interfaith services for worship or to memorialize a patient who has died. In addition, some people have been residents in facilities such as retirement communities or psychiatric hospitals for a long time and they no longer have connections with outside clergy. For these patients, the chaplain is their minister and their only access to valued sacraments and rituals (see Case Example 4.17).

Providing a Ministry of Presence

Chaplains may have tasks such as information gathering in the trauma bay. They sit with families in waiting rooms when families are frightened. They offer rituals to commemorate births and deaths. They pray at the bedside and at public meetings. They sit on ethics committees and institutional review boards.

However, what chaplains say they do the most is provide a ministry of presence. When they come to the patient's room their only agenda is to hear what is important to the patient. They listen to many different issues, hear stories of family quarrels and memories of great happiness, sit with those who are lonely, pray for courage and strength for those who ask, hear confessions, comfort children, and tell a good joke.

Chaplains work with teams to provide care for the whole person, acknowledging what life was like before and helping to envision a purposeful after. They honor grief and respect suffering. They help name what the patient may be unable to name for himself or herself. They try to help patients knit together the circumstances of the moment with the rest of their lives, creating a sense of meaning for living from the challenges they face.

Case Example 4.17. Communion for All

"You gonna have Communion today, Chaplain? We've gathered the guys into the dayroom." It was the first Wednesday of the month, the day the chaplain offered communion to the 25 men on this psychiatric unit. Most of them had Lutheran backgrounds and had never seen a female clergyperson, so the chaplain wore a clergy collar to help them understand she really was a minister.

She walked in with the bread and cup and saw Johnny sitting in a Posey vest. This patient was often in a straightjacket because he expressed his frustration by biting, often and hard. "Don't give him any, Chaplain," said the aide. "He's in a bad mood today, and he'll bite you." Because his hands were tied, the only way to offer the bread was to put it directly in his mouth. The chaplain was in a quandary. She respected the aide and her assessment, and she wasn't eager to be bitten, but she couldn't just walk past him either.

Beginning her walk around the room, murmuring "the body of Christ, broken for you," the Chaplain called each man by name as she gave him the small bit of bread. As she got closer to Johnny, she realized she had decided that if she were bitten, so be it. It was spiritually intolerable to think of just walking past him, excluding him from the blessing. Reaching him, she saw his eyes were closed as if in prayer. As she said "the body of Christ, broken for you, Johnny," the young man opened his mouth and carefully took the bread, saying Amen after he swallowed.

Summary

Experienced chaplains understand that their primary tools and skills are the values they embody and live. These tools and skills include

- A grounded sense of his or her own faith and source of spiritual nurture
- Genuine respect for other spiritual paths, including nonreligious ones
- The ability for listening to many levels of a story
- Warm compassion for loss and grief and the enduring power those wounds may have
- The willingness and desire to collaborate with others

- The humility that comes from an honest assessment of one's own gifts and limitations
- A nonjudgmental approach
- The wisdom that comes from integrating the painful lessons of one's own life experiences with the other aspects of one's life
- The ability to recognize, name, and reflect back those moments that are sacred in a person's story
- A love for providing companionship to people whose illness or injury changes life from what was expected to a journey into the unknown.

Disorienting distress, occasioned by a medical crisis or trauma, greatly affects a patient or family's recovery and healing. The role of the chaplain within the health care team is to provide insights into how patients and families can access their spiritual resources. Chaplains are trained to recognize and honor a wide range of spiritual expressions and interpret them for the health care team, providing guidance on how to best support patients through their treatment.

References

Ambuel, B. (2000). *Taking a spiritual history.* Retrieved from http://www.nhpco.org/resources/end-life-care--resources

Anandarajah, G., & Hight, E. (2001). Spirituality and medical practice: Using the HOPE questions as a practical tool for spiritual assessment. *American Family Physician, 63,* 81–89. http://www.aafp.org/afp/2001/0101/p81.html

Association for Clinical Pastoral Education. (2015). *Standards manual.* Retrieved from http://www.manula.com/manuals/acpe/acpe-manuals/2016/en/topic/standards

Association of Professional Chaplains. (2004a). *Common code of ethics for chaplains, pastoral educators, and students association of professional chaplains.* Retrieved from http://www.professionalchaplains.org/files/professional_standards/common_standards/common_code_ethics.pdf

Association of Professional Chaplains. (2004b). *Common standards for pastoral educators/supervisors.* Retrieved from http://www.professionalchaplains.org/files/professional_standards/common_standards/common_standards_pastoral_educators_supervisors.pdf

Association of Professional Chaplains. (2004c). *Common standards for professional chaplaincy.* Retrieved from http://www.professionalchaplains.org/files/professional_standards/common_standards/common_standards_professional_chaplaincy.pdf

Association of Professional Chaplains. (2004d). *Principles for processing ethical complaints.* Retrieved from http://www.professionalchaplains.org/files/professional_standards/common_standards/principles_processing_ethical_complaints.pdf

Bass, D. B. (2013). Christianity after religion: The end of church and the birth of a new spiritual awakening. New York: HarperOne.

Brown, E. (2012). African American present perceptions of organ donation: A pilot study. *Association of Black Nursing Faculty Journal, 23,* 29–33.

Cobb, M., Puchalski, C. M., & Rumbold, B. (2012). *Oxford textbook of spirituality in healthcare.* New York: Oxford University Press.

Densmore, C. (2015). *Quakers and the Underground Railroad: Myths and realities.* Retrieved from http://trilogy.brynmawr.edu/speccoll/quakersandslavery/commentary/organizations/underground_railroad.php#top

Dred Scott v. Sandford, 60 U.S. 393 (1857)

Isgandarova, N. (2010). The concept of compassionate engagement in Islam. *Yale Journal of Humanities in Medicine.* Retrieved from http://yjhm.yale.edu/essays/nisgandarova20100302.htm

Puchalski, C. M., & Romer, A. L. (2000). Taking a spiritual history allows clinicians to understand patients more fully. *Journal of Palliative Medicine, 3,* 129–137. http://dx.doi.org/10.1089/jpm.2000.3.129

Puchalski, C. M., & Ferrell, B. (2010). *Making health care whole: Integrating spirituality into patient care.* West Conshohocken, PA: Templeton Press.

Sen Gupta, S. (2008). *A man called Bapu.* Delhi: Pratham Books.

Shirma, R. D. (2013). *The necessity of a Hindu American chaplaincy.* Retrieved from http://theinterfaithobserver.org/journal-articles/2013/9/6/the-necessity-of-a-hindu-american-chaplaincy.html

Swift, C. (2014). *Hospital chaplaincy in the twenty-first century: The crisis of spiritual care on the NHS* (2nd ed.). London: Ashgate Publishing.

Part II.

UNDERSTANDING SPIRITUALITY THROUGH OCCUPATIONAL THERAPY LITERATURE

CHAPTER 5.

PHILOSOPHICAL CONCEPTIONS OF SPIRITUALITY IN THE OCCUPATIONAL THERAPY LITERATURE

Tamera Keiter Humbert, MA, DEd, OTR/L

Chapter Highlights

- ✧ Review and theoretical analysis
- ✧ Ontology
- ✧ Phenomenology
- ✧ Epistemology
- ✧ Cosmology
- ✧ Early foundational perspectives
- ✧ Contemporary perspectives.

Key Terms and Concepts

- ✧ Cosmology
- ✧ Epistemology
- ✧ Essence
- ✧ Intuition
- ✧ Meaning making

- ✧ Ontology
- ✧ Phenomenology
- ✧ Transcendence
- ✧ Wholeness

Within occupational therapy, *spirituality* has been defined, described, and conceptualized by many scholars over the past three decades. One approach to further understanding spirituality is to situate the topic in larger conversations related to philosophical and theological constructs (Bregman, 2006; Leibing, 2010).

It is a widely held belief in the occupational therapy community that to understand practice, practitioners must understand the theoretical perspectives that shape practice (Boyt Schell, Gillen, & Scaffe, 2014; Christiansen, Baum, & Bass-Haugen, 2005; Kielhofner, 2008). Considering theoretical perspectives relative to spirituality can strengthen understanding about the subject, allowing additional analysis, critique, and research opportunities. A review of the early foundational literature (from 1993 to 2004) and of contemporary literature (from 2005 to 2015) related to spirituality provides some understanding of the theoretical perspectives and assumptions initially promoted within the profession and those currently espoused.

This chapter reviews and analyzes how the occupational therapy literature conceptualizes spirituality. It briefly describes four philosophical or theological perspectives (i.e., ontology, phenomenology, epistemology, cosmology) and provides examples from the occupational therapy literature that represent these fundamental ideals or particular ways of knowing. Preliminary questions are posed for each perspective. Analysis then continues with the most contemporary definitions and descriptions of *spirituality* and additional considerations for the profession.

Review and Theoretical Analysis

The first step in the review and theoretical analysis entailed identifying and collecting occupational therapy literature that explicitly connected spirituality to practice and provided a conceptual framework about spirituality. Each article and text was read with the intention of deciphering what theoretical lens the author used. Primary clues came from the authors' descriptions or definitions of *spirituality* and through the context of their ideas. Four primary philosophical and theological perspectives were identified in the literature: ontology, phenomenology, epistemology, and cosmology. These perspectives are important to consider because they lay the groundwork for the application of and research on spirituality in practice.

Ontology

Ontology focuses on the nature of humankind, the universe, and a higher being. It consists of the beginning, the historical perspective, and the projected future conceptualizations depicting the core, and sometimes universal nature, of our being and existence. It attempts to answer the following questions:

- What is the essence of humankind?
- What is the essence of the universe?

- What is the essence of a higher being? (Davidson, 1997; Fisch, 1996; Nietzsche, 1998).

Contemporary language in spirituality also reflects the personal questions, What is our individual essence? Who are we? (O'Murchu, 1998). In this context, *essence* can be understood as our personal and unique qualities. The question of who we are surrounds ideas of our passions, keen interests and abilities, and unique talents and gifts that give us life and support communities with which we engage.

Several occupational therapy scholars have highlighted the ontological perspective in their definitions and understanding of *spirituality*, emphasizing the nature of humankind. For some, the primary focus is that spirituality is recognized as or associated with the core or essence of the person (see Exhibit 5.1).

Understanding ontology may entail recognizing the particular characteristics or qualities of another person. Perhaps a person has a keen awareness of

---

Exhibit 5.1. *Spirituality From the Ontological Perspective*

- "[T]he spirit is seen more simply as our truest selves which we attempt to express in all our actions" (Egan & DeLaat, 1994, p. 96).
- "[T]he spirit is not merely viewed as a component of the individual. Rather the spirit is seen as the essence of the person" (Egan & DeLaat, 1994, p. 101).
- "Spirituality and occupational therapy interconnect when we define spirit as the life force within us that tells us who we really are" (Gutterman, 1990, p. 236).
- "[W]hat I make, create, bring into being, is an expression of my own being—is 'so much of who I am.'... The spirit of [our] inner room emerges via ordinary but creative expressions" (Hasselkus, 2002, p. 108).
- "Human beings are viewed as non-linear, open, self-organising systems grounded in spirituality.... spirituality is viewed as a quality that ultimately makes us who we are and our universe what it becomes (Kang, 2003, p. 95).
- "May you realize in increasing measure the value of certain spiritual things, which are the real making of life.... [k]indness, humanity, decency, honor, good faith" (Kidner [1929, p. 385] as cited in Peloquin, 1997).

and ability to see beauty in the everyday activities of life. Without much thought, and even much time and energy, this person incorporates this disposition, this essence, into daily occupations and events throughout life.

For example, the memoir, *Riding the Bus With My Sister,* a story about an estranged sibling relationship, culminates with a sister recognizing the unique qualities of her younger sister (Simon, 2003). Through a commitment to spend more dedicated and focused time with her sister, Rachel Simon realizes that her sister Beth has cultivated important relationships with some of the city bus drivers and has the capacity to enlighten and touch others traveling with her on daily bus runs. Beth's essence is highlighted through these interactions and represented through the occupations Beth finds most meaningful and desirable, even when often misunderstood by others.

Gutterman (1990) identified an ontological perspective, stating, "Spirituality and occupational therapy interconnect when we define *spirit* as the life force within us that tells us who we really are" (p. 236, *italics added*). Do you seek adventure? Are you moved by compassion to assist others in need? Do you seek fairness and justice? What moves you to action? In the ontological perspective, answers to these questions point us to who we are and our unique essence.

Thomas Bessell Kidner (1929), a founder of the National Society for the Promotion of Occupational Therapy, portrayed spirituality as a process of enlightenment, self-awareness, and discovery of the essence of life by recognizing the value of "kindness, humanity, decency, honor, good faith" (as cited in Peloquin, 1997, p. 615). This view is aligned with the ontological perspective.

Beyond the general recognition of spirituality as encompassing the essence of a person and bringing attention to qualities that make up that essence, some authors attributed select occupations and activities to the formation of the essence of a person. Hasselkus (2002) discussed creative expression in relation to essence, describing how making, creating, and bringing into being is an expression of one's essence.

Some authors suggested the value of cultivating a person's existence within that essence, such as Kang (2003), who suggest spirituality is what makes people and the universe what it becomes. Coming to

an awareness and an appreciation of who we are, or our essence, is first facilitated through engagement in occupation and is then reflected back to us, reinforcing our particular qualities. As occupations are incorporated into life routines, and our essence is cultivated and developed, our existence, or life, is ultimately understood.

The question may arise of whether the essence, or truest part, of our being is made up of universal characteristics (e.g., kindness, humanity, decency) or whether our essence evokes personal attributes that ultimately influence our life. For example, can all people develop the same capacity for kindness and compassion? Is there, or should there be, a standard that all people should aspire to? If so, what would that standard be, and who would determine it? Conversely, do we recognize in ourselves how we uniquely experience and express compassion to others? Is that essence encouraged to develop and grow through our life events and occupational engagement? Recognizing the multiple ways our truest self, or our essence, may be displayed through all of humanity (i.e., past, present, and future and throughout various cultures) may generate diverse possibilities for and unlimited expressions of our essence.

In occupational therapy, what is the role of practitioners related to this ontological perspective? Is their role only to generally recognize the special or sacred, acknowledging the universal dignity of all people, or does it involve tapping into the essence of the individual client, facilitating his or her personal transformation within the therapy process?

Phenomenology

Phenomenology entails the meaning of life, the purpose of human existence, and what is important in and meaningful to people's lives as they construct an understanding about life (Exhibit 5.2). This perspective suggests that people have the ability to construct a personal and comprehensive sense of life and create a unique perspective in understanding the purpose of life and their purpose in life. Some overlap may exist between phenomenology and ontology, if ontology is understood to encompass unique characteristics of a person.

In an example of discovering one's personal sense of self and purpose of life, Martin Pistorius (2013) in *Ghost Boy* tells his story of being inflicted with

---

Exhibit 5.2. *Spirituality From the Phenomenological Perspective*

- "Spirituality relates to our thoughts, feelings and actions concerning the meaning that we make of our daily lives" (Egan & DeLaat, 1997, p. 116).
- "The client's spirituality, a source of inspiration, plays an influential role in directing what purposeful activities are identified as meaningful" (Engquist, Short-DeGraff, Gilner, & Oltjenbruns, 1997, p. 174).
- "Reflection upon one's life, the path it is taken, and the road ahead is an important process in meaning-making, and the basis for a narrative approach to addressing spirituality in occupational therapy" (Kirsh, 1996, p. 57).
- "Through engagement in occupations the children were able to look and find meaning in their experiences and give new meaning in their daily life" (Simó-Algado, Mehta, Kronenberg, Cockburn, & Kirsh, 2002, p. 69).
- "Spirituality is not merely a concept: it involves reflection and action in occupations that generate meaningful experiences" (Townsend, 1997b, p. 21).
- "Spirituality can be expressed through our engagement in occupations with personal meaning in our lives" (Unruh, 1997, p. 156).
- "The experience of meaning in everyday life activities" (Urbanowski & Vargo, 1994, p. 89).

---

a brain infection at age 12. He spends the next 9 years trapped in a body that cannot move or speak. Despite these limitations, he becomes more aware of events and begins to engage the world around him, trying to make sense of his physical, intellectual, and emotional challenges, the abuse he is subjected to, and ultimately his life desires and purpose. Through use of assistive technology, he shares his thoughts and beliefs about family, dedication, love, and what he has to offer to others, especially those who have no voice. Pistorius constructs his own perspective of who he is and what his purpose is in life, that is, to help others who do not have a voice.

A strength of phenomenology is that it allows for multiple perspectives about the meaning of life to develop through the engagement of occupations, interactions with others, and reflection (Porro,

2001; Silverman & Welton, 1988; Taylor, 1989). According to Pistorius,

> That moment was the one that drew all the other pieces together and made the jigsaw whole. I didn't know what each of those strangers had given me until one of them touched my broken, twisted, useless body and made me realize that I wasn't completely abhorrent.... Strangers can also rescue us—even if they don't know they're doing it. (p. 188)

Over the past two decades, phenomenology has been the most widely described and used theoretical perspective in occupational therapy literature concerning spirituality. Engquist, Short-DeGraff, Gilner, and Oltjenbruns (1997) stated that "the client's spirituality, a source of inspiration, plays an influential role in directing what purposeful activities are identified as meaningful" (p. 174). *Meaning making,* or the ability to make sense of life experiences and identify what is personally important, is a process that has been explicitly connected with the engagement in occupations (Townsend, 1997b; Unruh, 1997). Moreover, meaning making has been associated with daily life (Egan & DeLaat, 1997; Urbanowski & Vargo, 1994), the life journey (Kirsh, 1996), and life crises or challenging life events (Simó-Algado, Mehta, Kronenberg, Cockburn, & Kirsh, 2002). The following questions related to the phenomenology framework center on the idea of meaning making:

- Does all meaning making constitute spirituality?
- Is all meaning making grounded in spirituality?
- Are spirituality and meaning making different from meaning making of everyday occupations?

Epistemology

Epistemology involves seeking truth and knowledge as well as a way of knowing. Through this perspective, people come to an understanding about truth through their life experiences, insights, imagination, and wisdom (Exhibit 5.3). In the occupational therapy literature, epistemology is associated with rational thought and expressed actions through the development and refinement of values and beliefs (Luboshitzky & Gaber, 2001; Simó-Algado

Exhibit 5.3. *Spirituality From the Epistemological Perspective*

- "Whilst it is not the intention of this article to equate flow with spirituality, it is suggested that both share a common value, namely quality of experience" (Collins, 1998, p. 280).
- "By reaffirming the humanness of our patients and helping them to do the same as they progress in dealing with loss and finding a measure of wholeness, we acknowledge the spiritual aspects of occupational therapy" (Howard & Howard, 1997, p. 185).
- "Spirituality is a human phenomenon. . . . This complex dimension of human life includes values, attitudes, perspectives, beliefs, and emotions that constitute the inner core of a person" (Luboshitzky & Gaber, 2001, p. 71).
- "[W]e do not experience spirit through the usual human channels, but rather through transcendence, that is, an experience that goes beyond normal human experience" (McColl, 2000, p. 219).
- "[T]he opportunity to see universal truths in specific activities, to obtain a view of the whole cosmos in relation to a particular daily pattern of life, and to see one's life as a whole in relation to the grander scheme of things" (McColl, 2000, p. 222).
- "Spirituality can be viewed as a way of living which demonstrates essential values regarding the role of the individual in the world" (Simó-Algado, Gregori, & Egan, 1997, p. 139).
- "In the sessions, human values such as solidarity or love were recovered. Special attention was placed on working with feelings of hate and revenge, transforming them into human values" (Simó-Algado, Mehta, Kronenberg, Cockburn, & Kirsh, 2002, p. 69).

et al., 2002; Simó-Algado, Gregori, & Egan, 1997), through insights and awareness (Howard & Howard, 1997), and through transcendence or mystical knowing (Collins, 1998; McColl, 2000). The following questions pertain to spirituality viewed from an epistemological perspective:

- Does spirituality encompass all ways of knowing?
- Might spirituality be connected with and honored through **intuition,** an instinctive knowing beyond rational or conscious reasoning and a

way of knowing that is not yet represented in the occupational therapy literature?
- How does one come to understand truth; through those in authority, through traditions and heritage, or personal experiences?
- How do we respond to those with very different ways of knowing?
- What do we do with the conflict that might arise between different ways of knowing?

Epistemology encompasses both personal awareness and understanding (Armstrong, 1973; Holbrook, 1987; Miller & Cook-Greuter, 2000; Moser, 2002; Sloan, 1983) and collective understanding (Moser, 2002), potentially leading to hope, wholeness, or transcendence.

Hope

Desmond Tutu (2004), an African social activist, retired Anglican bishop, and Nobel Peace Prize winner and the Dalai Lama (1999), a Buddhist monk, spiritual leader, and Nobel Peace Prize winner, highlighted the importance of hope in times of extreme challenge, violence, and suffering. Through their life experiences, their study of religious and sacred texts, and their critical exploration of historical events, both have articulated what they believe to be truth in cultivating lives of love, forgiveness, generosity, and goodness. It is through this cultivation of truth that hope is generated, experienced, or known.

Wholeness

Wholeness is related to becoming mature, wise, complete, and well-rounded. Howard and Howard (1997) implied an epistemological perspective when stating, "By reaffirming the humanness of our patients and helping them to do the same as they progress in dealing with loss and finding a measure of wholeness, we acknowledge the spiritual aspects of occupational therapy" (p. 185). Here, *wholeness* is conceptualized as finding truth and understanding about loss.

Transcendence

Epistemology also concerns the experience of knowing that moves people to experience something beyond or greater than the self, often called *transcendence.*

McColl (2000) said, "We do not experience spirit through the usual human channels, but rather through transcendence, that is, an experience that goes beyond normal human experience" (p. 219).

For example, Sukey Forbes (2014) shared her story of great loss when her 6-year-old daughter died from a rare genetic disorder. Through her grief, Forbes tried to make sense of a world that had lost all meaning and purpose. She tried to make sense of her childhood and familial upbringing, how she had created and developed her role as a wife and mother, and how she attempted to understand the reason behind her daughter's death. Nothing made sense, and the grief was unbearable until she found a small porcelain angel in her daughter's linen closet and she "knew" that it was sign that her daughter was "okay." According to Forbes, this particular sign and others after it "made no sense according to any rules of the universe as I understood them. And yet it simply was" (p. 170).

In another example of transcendence, Jill Bolte Taylor (2009), a neuroanatomist and writer, described her physical and cognitive decline when she suffered a massive stroke. Elaborate descriptions of her near-death encounter and subsequent rehabilitation highlighted multiple experiences that brought clarity about the importance of her life and a connection to something beyond herself. She describes these transcendent experiences as Nirvana.

Cosmology

Cosmology is the idea that the universe is interconnected. This perspective acknowledges connectedness with others; nature; and, for some, a higher being (Exhibit 5.4). From this perspective, spirituality is developed through the awareness of and appreciation for the interconnectedness between humanity and the universe and through communal relationships (Cobb, 1988; O'Murchu, 1998).

For example, journalists Nicholas Kristof and Sheryl WuDunn (2009, 2014) have traveled the world interviewing people whose humanitarian efforts have made significant differences in others' lives. Despite, and often because of, personal experiences with violence, poverty, marginalization, and corruption, these people developed the desire to help others by building relationships and communities and developing programs that honor the avocational and vocational commitments of others to work for

Exhibit 5.4. *Spirituality From the Cosmological Perspective*

- "While this spiritual force underlies our uniqueness, it also allows us to connect with the rest of creation" (Egan & DeLaat, 1994, p. 96).
- "Meaning is constructed through our relationships with ourselves, other humans, inhabitants of the earth, the earth itself and, for many individuals, a higher power or Creator" (Egan & DeLaat, 1997, p. 116).
- "[T]hrough engagement in occupation, we experience meaningful connections to others in our social worlds. Occupations can nurture and release the spiritual aspects of our selves, enabling us to experience passion, reverence, and a sense of enlightenment in our lives" (Hasselkus, 2002, p. xii).
- "[S]pirit is not within the person, but instead is an energy that passes between people and the world. . . . I suggest spirit acts through us, rather than in us" (McColl, 2000, p. 218).
- "[T]he force that dissolves the boundaries between self and others, and helps us realize that other people and other parts of the world are real" (McColl, 2000, p. 222).
- "[A] definition for *spirituality* for occupational therapy could be experiencing a meaningful connection to our core self, other humans, the world, and a greater power as expressed through our reflections, narratives and actions" (Schulz, 2004, p. 72, *italics added*).
- "[A]n experience of connectedness to a universal order and even, at times, to a benevolent Will" (Thibeault, 2011, p. 104).
- ". . . inclusiveness as a community dimension of spirituality" (Townsend, 1997a, p. 146).
- ". . . connectedness with others and a wider community, to foster a sense of belonging" (Townsend, 1997a, p. 153).
- "[Spirituality] includes meaningful interaction with others. It is through the experience of meaningful interaction with the environment that our spirituality is expressed" (Urbanowski, 1997, p. 20).

the community's greater good. According to Kristof and WuDunn (2014),

> Kindness [is] a way of asserting our humanity, our connections to others, our basic decency and integrity. Participating in a cause larger

than yourself builds up our social networks, creates a sense of fulfillment, gets us out of bed in the morning with a bounce in our step, and helps makes a difference in the lives of others—even as it affirms a purpose for our own lives on earth. (p. 315)

Urbanowski's (1997) conceptualization of spirituality was expressed through a cosmological perspective and highlighted "meaningful interaction with others" (p. 20). Egan and DeLaat (1994) emphasized connecting with "the rest of creation" (p. 96).

McColl (2000) extended the concept of cosmology to include social justice and action, joining cosmological understanding with epistemology. She stated, "The spiritual connection between people is expressed in the quest to seek spiritual answers together . . . to extend social justice and liberation to all" (p. 220). *Occupational Therapy Without Borders* (Kronenberg, Algado, & Pollard, 2005) and its follow-up (Kronenberg, Pollard, & Sakellariou, 2011) highlighted occupational therapists' education, research, and work around the globe to address the needs of people who are underserved, marginalized, and neglected. The purpose of these texts was to bring awareness of these needs and, more important, to challenge the ethos (i.e., beliefs and attitudes) of individualistic and professional determination (i.e., competition and attitudes of superiority) and self-perseverance (i.e., survival at any cost) on the part of practitioners. Alternatively, Kronenberg et al. (2011) proposed that practitioners recognize "the inner place or source from which [they] operate individually and collectively" (p. 3) so that they may appreciate the diversity of beliefs, thoughts, and actions of all people and discover shared values.

One woman, living and working from a cosmological understanding, is Blondine Eya Nchama Uwimana. I met Blondine on a trip to Rwanda in 2005. I heard her story and met the many people affected by her desire to bring unity to a community suffering the aftermath of the Rwandan genocide. Blondine recognized the tremendous needs of orphaned children and women who were left destitute after the genocide and spent 6 months inviting both Hutu and Tutsi women to gather for tea and conversation. Her desire was to listen to the women and offer opportunities for voices and perspectives to be heard. Through these conversations, the need for viable food and water sources, education

for children, care and housing of orphans, and healing of a community became abundantly clear.

Blondine formed the Association Refuge for African Great Lakes Children, inspiring people to set aside their prejudices and unite to solve these problems. Blondine understood that, despite being on different political and cultural sides, the women were connected to each other as humans, women, and mothers. She fostered that powerful connection that can happen between people and within communities and was able to build that capacity for good.

The occupational therapy literature reviewed here recognizes some degree of interconnection among people, the environment, and a force beyond humans or all living creatures. However, the occupational therapy literature does not answer how people, the environment, and a greater force are interconnected or how their connection can be understood, appreciated, or used. Questions for occupational therapy practitioners include

- Is cosmology the grounding for social and occupational justice?
- If so, how can practitioners understand the interconnectedness among people, nature, and a greater force and promote it?
- Should the cosmological framework be introduced and used in practice outside of occupational justice and, if so, how might this occur?

Early Foundational Perspectives

In addition to addressing separate philosophical constructs, the early foundational literature (from 1993 to 2004) combined these perspectives to form a collective definition or description of *spirituality* (Exhibit 5.5). The interconnection among these combined philosophical constructs gives direction to answer the questions posed in the previous section of this chapter (i.e., the overlap of ontology and phenomenology) and provides a deeper understanding of life experiences. Personal experiences give meaning to life and may also provide some understanding of the truth about who we are, what our purpose is in this life, and how we are connected with others.

In my work with women who are overcoming domestic violence (Humbert, 2014; Humbert, Bess, & Mowry, 2013; Humbert, Engleman, & Miller, 2014), the women frequently emphasize these

Exhibit 5.5. *Spirituality From Combined Philosophical Perspectives in Early Foundational Literature*

Ontology/Epistemology
- "The fundamental orientation of a person's life; that which inspires and motivates that individual." (American Occupational Therapy Association [AOTA], 2002, p. 633).
- A context inherent to the individual "that influences personal beliefs, perceptions and expectations" (AOTA, 2002, p. 614).
- "Illness, injury, congenital disability, life crisis, or environmental disadvantage may engender a search for a new vision or revision of occupational identity along with renewed spiritual questioning" (Unruh, Versnel, & Kerr, 2002, p. 12).
- "Spirituality may be closely related to occupational identity for an individual. A person may center her or his occupational identity on occupations that are responsive to spiritual questioning" (Unruh et al., 2002, p. 13).

Ontology/Phenomenology/Cosmology
- "A pervasive life force, manifestation of a higher self, source of will and self-determination, and a sense of meaning, purpose and connectedness that people experience in the context of their environment" (Canadian Association of Occupational Therapists [CAOT], 1997, p. 182).
- "A pervasive life force, manifestation of a higher self, source of will and self-determination, and a sense of meaning, purpose and connectedness that people experience in the context of their environment" (Law, Polatajko, Baptiste, & Townsend, 1997, p. 43).

Phenomenology/Ontology
- "As spiritual beings, individuals are concerned with the nature, the meaning of life and their purpose and place in the universe" (CAOT, 2002, p. 18).

Epistemology/Phenomenology
- "[S]pirituality seemed to be viewed as a group of directing values that assisted individuals in deciding between different courses of actions, particularly courses of action with a potential impact on others. These values and their interpretation also seemed to provide individuals with meaning and purpose" (Egan & Swedersky, 2003, p. 531).

Ontology/Phenomenology
- "A case is made for acknowledging spirituality in clinical reasoning as a centralizing component of the patient's motivation and assignment of meaning in life" (Howard & Howard, 1997, p. 181).

Epistemology/Ontology
- "Spirituality is 'sensitivity to the presence of spirit': According to this definition, spirituality is a quality that human beings possess, to a greater or lesser degree, that allows them to be aware of the presence of spirit" (McColl, 2000, p. 218).

Phenomenology/Epistemology
- "Meaning derives from the opportunity to see universal truths in specific activities, to obtain a view of the whole cosmos in relation to a particular daily pattern of life, and to see one's life as a whole in relation to the grander schemes of things" (McColl, 2000, p. 220).
- [The garden is a] "spiritual enabler, making it possible to finding meaningfulness in life under extreme circumstances[, and] . . . spirituality may revolve around the possibility of hope, and transcendence beyond everyday visible existence" (Unruh, Smith, & Scammell, 2000, p. 76).

combined perspectives as they go through crisis intervention and begin their healing journey. For example, a woman coming to terms with domestic violence and identifying that she is in an abusive relationship may begin questioning her own understanding of truth (epistemology), particularly if what she has been taught about relationships and what she has experienced may be in conflict. Questioning who she is and how she is to respond within this relationship moves her to explore new possibilities of interaction and engagement (ontology). Connecting with other women who have experienced domestic violence often provides a sense of resilience and hope (cosmology). If she has children, her sense of meaning and identity as a mother informs her decisions about care and further intervention desired (phenomenology).

Working with women in the crisis shelter, I have recognized that all of the aforementioned concerns are intertwined and that as one aspect of spirituality is addressed through therapy, the other aspects are subsequently affected. It is frequently difficult to tease out one aspect of spirituality at a time; the role of the practitioner in this situation is to support where the women are in their personal healing journeys and honor the complexity of the healing process.

Connecting multiple philosophical perspectives leads to more robust and comprehensive definitions and descriptions of *spirituality*. However, the assumptions and beliefs about these interconnections should be scrutinized and possibly even challenged empirically. Questions that arise include

- How do these multiple perspectives intersect, and how do they influence each other?
- Does the essence of a person inform truth, or does truth inform the essence of the person?
- Is spirituality a developmental perspective that changes as maturation occurs through a lifetime?
- Is this conversation really within the realm and domain of occupational therapy (Hammell, 2001)?

Contemporary Perspectives

Like the early foundational literature, the literature reviewed from 2005 to 2015 was analyzed for philosophical and theological underpinnings (Exhibit 5.6). Elements of ontology, epistemology,

---

Exhibit 5.6. *Spirituality From Combined Philosophical Perspectives in Contemporary Literature*

Ontology
- Spirituality is the "essence of the person" (Townsend & Polatajko, 2007, p. 30).
- Spirit is "the force that animates living things" (McColl, 2011, p. 18).

Phenomenology/Epistemology
- "Values, beliefs, and spirituality influence a client's motivation to engage in occupations and give his or her life meaning. Values are principles, standards, or qualities considered worthwhile by the client who holds them. Beliefs are cognitive content held as true" (Moyers & Dale, 2007, p. 28; AOTA, 2008, p. 633).
- "Spirituality is understood as the timeless and universal search for meaning, and the desire for wholeness or an integrated self-thinking, feeling, and acting in the presence of the 'numinous'" (Kirsh, 2011, p. 202).
- Rituals (populations) are "[s]hared social actions with traditional, emotional, purposive, and technological meaning contributing to values and beliefs within the group or population" (AOTA, 2014, p. S27).
- Rituals (personal) are "[s]ymbolic actions with spiritual, cultural, or social meaning contributing to the client's identity and reinforcing values and beliefs. Rituals have a strong affective component and consist of a collection of events (Fiese, 2007; Fiese et al., 2002; Segal, 2004)" (AOTA, 2014, p. S27).

Phenomenology/Epistemology/Ontology
- "Spirituality relates to the acknowledgment of an individual's sense of meaning and purpose in life, which may, or may not be expressed through religious doctrine, beliefs and practices. Spirituality involves a unity of body, mind, and spirit and relationship with someone or something beyond ourselves that sustains and comforts us" (Tse, Lloyd, Petchkovsky, & Manaia, 2005, p. 181).

Epistemology
- Rituals (personal) are "symbolic actions with spiritual, cultural, or social meaning. Rituals contribute to a client's identity and reinforce the client's values and beliefs (Fiese et al., 2002; Segal, 2004)" (AOTA, 2014, p. S8).
- "Habits, routines, roles, and rituals can support or hinder occupational performance" (AOTA, 2014, p. S8).
- Rituals (populations) are "shared social actions with traditional, emotional, purposive, and technological meaning, contributing to values and beliefs within the population" (AOTA, 2008, p. 644).

(Continued)

Exhibit 5.6. *Spirituality From Combined Philosophical Perspectives in Contemporary Literature (Cont.)*

- Spirituality is "having coherent beliefs about the higher purposes, the meaning of life, and the meaning of the universe" (Pentland & McColl, 2011, p. 142).
- Values, beliefs, and spirituality are "clients' perceptions, motivations, and related meaning that influence or are influenced by engagement in occupations." Values are "acquired beliefs and commitments, derived from culture, about what is good, right, and important to do" (Kielhofner, 2008), and beliefs are "cognitive content held as true by or about the client" (AOTA, 2014, p. S22).

Ontology/Epistemology
- "Spirituality is a person's views of the world, particularly, how a person explains the world and the forces that affect her or his life" (Boswell, Hamer, Knight, Glacoff, & McChesney, 2007, p. 34).
- "Spirituality is often conceptualized as being about creating and expressing one's inner self, and the values and beliefs that matter at our core" (Unruh, 2011, p. 250).

Ontology/Phenomenology
- "Spirituality is sensitivity to the presence of spirit, and . . . spirituality resides in persons, is shaped by the environment, and gives meaning to occupations" (CAOT, 2007, p. 374).
- "Spirituality is viewed as that which brings an individual a sense of peace and well-being while providing purpose and value. Spirituality as a source of personal power, vitality, and influence is a concept unique to each person, as it is perceived as an intrinsic source that provides personal meaning" (Williams, 2008, p. 8).

Epistemology/Cosmology
- Religious observance (i.e., participating in religion) involves "an organized system of beliefs, practices, rituals, and symbols designed to facilitate closeness to the sacred or transcendent" (Moreira-Almeida & Koenig, 2006, p. 844; AOTA, 2014, p. S20).

Ontology/Cosmology
- Spirituality is "an experience of connectedness to a universal order and even, at times, to a Benevolent Will. As elusive as it may sound, this experience rests at the very core of my existence" (Thibault, 2011, p. 104).

Epistemology/Cosmology/Phenomenology
- "Engaging in activities that allow a sense of connectedness to something larger than oneself or that are especially meaningful, such as taking time out to play with a child, engaging in activities in nature, and helping others in need" (Spencer, Davidson, & White, 1997; AOTA, 2014, p. S20).

Cosmology/Phenomenology
- "Hope . . . requires a vision of how things could be and the anticipation of achievement. The author believes that hope involves having some understanding of how as individuals we are connected to the universe, a core element of spiritual well-being" (Ramugondo, 2005, p. 320).
- "Personal spirituality . . . is the developmental 'engine' that propels the search for connectedness, meaning, purpose and contribution" (Baptiste, 2011, p. 241).
- Spirituality is "[t]he aspect of humanity that refers to the way individuals seek and express meaning and purpose and the way they experience their connectedness to the moment, to self, to others, to nature, and to the significant or sacred" (Puchalski et al., 2009, p. 887; AOTA, 2014, p. S22).

Epistemology/Phenomenology/Ontology/Cosmology
- Spirituality is "the personal quest for understanding answers to ultimate questions about life, about meaning and about relationship with the sacred or transcendent, which may (or may not) lead to or arise from the development of religious rituals and the formation of community" (Moreira-Almeida & Koenig, 2006, p. 844; AOTA, 2008, p.633).

Note. AOTA = American Occupational Therapy Association; CAOT = Canadian Association of Occupational Therapists.

phenomenology, and cosmology are still articulated in the occupational therapy literature; however, the language around such descriptions has evolved. Spirituality is now discussed with some explanation about how these philosophical perspectives might be connected or experienced. For example, linkages are made among the mind, body, and spirit (Tse, Lloyd, Petchkovsky, & Manaia, 2005). Articles also discuss how spirituality is experienced through the environments and occupations people engage in (AOTA, 2008, 2014; CAOT, 2007), and some descriptions of spirituality recognize the potential connection with other life forces such as universal order, benevolent will, and the sacred (AOTA, 2008, 2014; Boswell, Hamer, Knight, Glacoff, & McChesney, 2007; Ramugondo, 2005; Thibault, 2011).

In the occupational therapy literature, the experience of spirituality is beginning to be labeled with words such as *vision, hope,* and *well-being* (Ramugondo, 2005), *peace* (Williams, 2008), *anticipation* (Ramugondo, 2005), *comfort* (Tse et al., 2005), *understanding* (AOTA, 2008), *vitality* and *strength* (Williams, 2008), *wholeness* (Kirsh, 2011), *creating* (Unruh, 2011), and *desire* and *quest* (AOTA, 2008; McColl, 2011). These terms suggest more than a general recognition of spirituality within a person or a simple definition of spirituality; they imply a benefit to or outcomes from spirituality and people's active involvement with or reciprocal response to spirituality. Moreover, spirituality in this literature is described as timeless (Kirsh, 2011), universal (Kirsh, 2011), and personal and individual (Baptiste, 2011; Williams, 2008), emphasizing both the uniformity (i.e., consistency between all people) and uniqueness of spirituality.

In analyzing the various ways spirituality has been depicted in contemporary occupational therapy literature, when spirituality is directly connected to religious beliefs and practices, the associated philosophical framework tends to be related to epistemology and the establishment and integration of beliefs and values (AOTA, 2002, 2008, 2014). Spirituality understood from a more global perspective tends to reflect an ontological framework (McColl, 2011; Townsend & Polatajko, 2007; Thibault, 2011), an ontological perspective integrated with phenomenology (CAOT, 2007; Williams, 2008), or a phenomenological framework that may then expand to include a cosmological viewpoint (AOTA, 2014; Baptiste, 2011; Thibault, 2011).

Critique

Although the occupational therapy literature includes diverse philosophical and theological perspectives of spirituality, it is unclear how aware the authors have been of any philosophical or theoretical underpinnings. In addition, it is unclear whether or not the authors had any intention of focusing on a particular philosophical or theoretical perspective, because no philosophical or theological statements were made in the literature reviewed.

The review of the early foundational and contemporary literature demonstrates the multiplicity of understandings of and the complexity in formulating concepts about spirituality. However, the review of the contemporary literature shows a general construct of spirituality that strongly encompasses elements of ontology (i.e., essence of the self), phenomenology (i.e., meaning making), and cosmology (i.e., connectedness).

Much of the occupational therapy literature on spirituality focuses on a phenomenological viewpoint, whether the literature is empirical or descriptive in nature. Because definitions of terms, such as *meaning, meaning making,* and *meaningful occupations,* are ambiguous in the literature related to phenomenology, further analysis is required.

Summary

The theoretical constructs surrounding spirituality as represented in the occupational therapy literature have pointed to elements of ontology, epistemology, phenomenology, and cosmology, each with distinct applications for research and practice. Despite this diversity in understanding, authors have often subsumed multiple perspectives into one definition or description of spirituality, portraying the complexity of the topic.

References

American Occupational Therapy Association. (2002). Occupational therapy practice framework: Domain and process. *American Journal of Occupational Therapy, 56,* 609–639. http://dx.doi.org/10.5014/ajot.56.6.609

American Occupational Therapy Association. (2008). Occupational therapy practice framework: Domain and process

(2nd ed.). *American Journal of Occupational Therapy, 62,* 625–683. http://dx.doi.org/10.5014/ajot.62.6.625

American Occupational Therapy Association. (2014). Occupational therapy practice framework: Domain and process (3rd ed.). *American Journal of Occupational Therapy 68*(Suppl. 1), S1–S48. http://dx.doi.org/10.5014/ajot.2014.682006

Armstrong, D. M. (1973). *Belief, truth, and knowledge.* Cambridge, UK: Cambridge University Press.

Baptiste, S. (2011). Work: Understanding spirituality and work. In M. A. McColl (Ed.), *Spirituality and occupational therapy* (2nd ed., pp. 241–248). Ottawa, ON: CAOT Publications.

Boswell, B., Hamer, M., Knight, S., Glacoff, M., & McChesney, J. (2007). Dance of disability and spirituality. *Journal of Rehabilitation, 73,* 33–40. http://bit.ly/1Q9tIiR

Boyt Schell, B. A., Gillen, G., & Scaffe, M. (Eds.). (2014). *Willard and Spackman's occupational therapy* (12th ed.). Philadelphia: Lippincott Williams & Wilkins.

Bregman, L. (2006). Spirituality: A glowing and useful term in search of a meaning. *Omega, 53*(1–2), 5–26. http://dx.doi.org/10.2190/40NU-Q4BX-9E9K-R52A

Canadian Association of Occupational Therapists. (1997). *Enabling occupation: An occupational therapy perspective.* Ottawa, ON: CAOT Publications.

Canadian Association of Occupational Therapists. (2002). *Enabling occupation: An occupational therapy perspective* (2nd ed). Ottawa, ON: CAOT Publications.

Canadian Association of Occupational Therapy. (2007). *Enabling occupation II: Advancing an occupational therapy vision for health, well-being, and justice through occupation.* Ottawa, ON: Author.

Christiansen, C. H., Baum, M. C., & Bass-Haugen, J. (Eds). (2005). *Occupational therapy: Performance, participation, and well-being.* Thorofare, NJ: Slack.

Cobb, J. B., Jr. (1988). Wholeness centered in spirit. In H. Newton Malony, M. Papen-Daniels, & H. Clinebell (Eds.), *Spirit-centered wholeness beyond the psychology of self* (pp. 225–245). Lewiston, NY: Edwin Mellon Press.

Collins, M. (1998). Occupational therapy and spirituality: Reflecting on quality of experience in therapeutic interventions. *British Journal of Occupational Therapy, 61,* 280–285. http://dx.doi.org/10.1177/030802269806100614

Dalai Lama. (1999). *Ethics for the new millennium.* New York. Berkley Publishing.

Davidson, A. I. (Ed). (1997). *Foucault and his interlocutors.* Chicago: University of Chicago Press.

Egan, M., & DeLaat, M. D. (1994). Considering spirituality in occupational practice. *Canadian Journal of Occupational Therapy, 61,* 95–101. http://dx.doi.org/10.1177/000841749406100205

Egan, M., & DeLaat, M. D. (1997). The implicit spirituality of occupational therapy practice. *Canadian Journal of Occupational Therapy, 64,* 115–121. http://dx.doi.org/10.1177/000841749706400307

Egan, M., & Swedersky, J. (2003). Spirituality as experienced by occupational therapists in practice. *American Journal of Occupational Therapy, 57,* 525–533. http://dx.doi.org/10.5014/ajot.57.5.525

Engquist, D. E., Short-DeGraff, M., Gilner, J., & Oltjenbruns, K. (1997). Occupational therapist's beliefs and practices with regard to spirituality and therapy. *American Journal of Occupational Therapy, 51,* 173–180. http://dx.doi.org/10.5014/ajot.51.3.173

Fiese, B. H. (2007). Routines and rituals: Opportunities for participation in family health. *OTJR: Occupation, Participation and Health, 27,* 41S–49S. http://dx.doi.org/10.1177/15394492070270S106

Fiese, B. H., Tomcho, T. J., Douglas, M., Josephs, K., Poltrock, S., & Baker, T. (2002). A review of 50 years of research on naturally occurring family routines and rituals: Cause for celebration? *Journal of Family Psychology, 16,* 381–390. http://bit.ly/23XKyoW

Fisch, M. H. (1996). *Classic American philosophers.* New York: Fordham University Press.

Forbes, S. (2014). *The angle in my pocket: A story of love, loss, and life after death.* New York: Viking.

Gutterman, L. (1990). A day treatment program for persons with AIDS. *American Journal of Occupational Therapy, 44,* 2324–237. http://dx.doi.org/10.5014/ajot.44.3.234

Hammell, K. W. (2001). Intrinsicality: Reconsidering spirituality, meaning(s), and mandates. *Canadian Journal of Occupational Therapy, 68,* 186–194. http://dx.doi.org/10.1177/000841740106800307

Hasselkus, B. R. (2002). *The meaning of everyday occupation.* Thorofare, NJ: Slack.

Holbrook, D. (1987). *Education and philosophical anthropology.* Cranbury, NJ: Associated University Press.

Howard, B. S., & Howard, J. R. (1997). Occupation as spiritual activity. *American Journal of Occupational Therapy, 51,* 181–185. http://dx.doi.org/10.5014/ajot.51.3.181

Humbert, T. K. (2014). Use of the Kawa Model: Understanding women's recovery from intimate partner violence. In E. Bellamy (Ed.), *Partner violence: Risk factors, therapeutic interventions and psychological impact.* New York: Nova Science.

Humbert, T. K., Bess, J., & Mowry, A. (2013). Exploring women's perspectives of overcoming intimate partner violence: A phenomenological study. *Occupational Therapy in Mental Health, 29,* 246–265. http://dx.doi.org/10.1080/0164212X.2013.819465

Humbert, T. K., Engleman, K., & Miller, C. E. (2014). Exploring women's expectations of recovery from intimate partner violence: A phenomenological study. *Occupational*

Therapy in Mental Health, 30, 358–380. http://dx.doi.org/ 10.1080/0164212X.2014.970062

Kang, C. (2003). A psychospiritual integration frame of reference for occupational therapy. Part 1: Conceptual foundations. *Australian Occupational Therapy Journal, 50,* 92–103. http://dx.doi.org/10.1046/j.1440-1630.2003.00358.x

Kidner, T. B. (1929). Address to graduates. *Occupational Therapy and Rehabilitation, 8,* 379–385.

Kielhofner, G. (2008). *Model of Human Occupation: Theory and application* (4th ed.). Philadelphia: Wolters Kluwer.

Kirsh, B. (1996). A narrative approach to addressing spirituality in occupational therapy: Exploring personal meaning and purpose. *Canadian Journal of Occupational Therapy, 63,* 55–61. http://dx.doi.org/10.1177/000841749606300107

Kirsh, B. (2011). Narrative: What makes narratives spiritual and how can we use them in OT? In M. A. McColl (Ed.), *Spirituality and occupational therapy* (2nd ed., pp. 201–208). Ottawa, ON: CAOT Publications.

Kristof, N., & WuDunn, S. (2009). *Half the sky: Turning oppression into opportunity for women worldwide.* New York: Vintage Books.

Kristof, N., & WuDunn, S. (2014). *A path appears: Transforming lives, creating opportunity.* New York: Alfred A. Knopf.

Kronenberg, F., Algado, S. A., & Pollard, N. (2005). *Occupational therapy without borders: Learning from the spirit of survivors.* London: Elsevier/Churchill Livingstone.

Kronenberg, F., Pollard, N., & Sakellariou, D. (2011). *Occupational therapies without borders: Towards an ecology of occupation-based practices, Volume 2.* London: Elsevier/Churchill Livingstone

Law, M., Polatajko, H., Baptiste, S., & Townsend, E. (1997). Core concepts of occupational therapy. In Canadian Association Occupational Therapists (Ed.), *Enabling occupation: An occupational therapy perspective* (pp. 29–56). Ottawa, ON: CAOT Publications.

Leibing, A. (2010). Looking over the neighbor's fence: Occupational therapy as an inspiration for (medical) anthropology. *Ethos, 38,* 1–8. http://dx.doi.org/10.1111/j.1548-1352.2010.01139.x

Luboshitzky, D., & Gaber, L. B. (2001). Holidays and celebrations as a spiritual occupation. *Australian Occupational Therapy Journal, 48,* 66–74. http://dx.doi.org/10.1046/j.1440-1630.2001.00251.x

McColl, M. A. (2000). Spirit, occupation and disability. *Canadian Journal of Occupational Therapy, 67,* 217–228. http://dx.doi.org/10.1177/000841740006700403

McColl, M. A. (Ed.). (2011). *Spirituality and occupational therapy* (2nd ed.). Ottawa, ON: CAOT Publications.

Miller, M., & Cook-Greuter, S. R. (Eds.) (2000). *Creativity, spirituality, and transcendence: Paths to integrity and wisdom in the mature self.* New York: Ablex.

Moreira-Almeida, A., & Koenig, H. G. (2006). Retaining the meaning of the words religiousness and spirituality: A commentary on the WHOQOL SRPB group's "A cross-cultural study of spirituality, religion, and personal beliefs as components of quality of life." *Social Science and Medicine, 63,* 843–845. http://dx.doi.org/10.1016/j.socscimed.2006.03.001

Moser, P. K. (Ed.). (2002). *The Oxford handbook of epistemology.* New York: Oxford University Press.

Moyers, P. A., & Dale, L. M. (2007). *The guide to occupational therapy practice* (2nd ed.). Bethesda, MD: AOTA Press.

Nietzsche, F. (1998). *Beyond good and evil: Prelude to a philosophy of the future.* New York: Oxford University Press.

O'Murchu, D. (1998). *Reclaiming spirituality: A new spiritual framework for today's world.* New York: Crossroads Publishing.

Peloquin, S. M. (1997). The spiritual depth of occupation: Making worlds and making lives. *American Journal of Occupational Therapy, 51,* 167–168. http://dx.doi.org/10.5014/ajot.51.3.167

Pentland, W., & McColl, M. A. (2011). Occupational choice. In M. A. McColl (Ed.), *Spirituality and occupational therapy* (2nd ed., pp. 141–149). Ottawa, ON: CAOT Publications.

Pistorius, M. (2013). *Ghost boy.* Nashville, TN: Nelson.

Porro, P. (2001). *The Medieval Concept of Time: The scholastic debate and its reception in early modern philosophy.* Boston: Brill.

Puchalski, C., Ferrell, B., Virani, R., Otis-Green, S., Baird, P., Bull, J., . . . Sulmasy, D. (2009). Improving the quality of spiritual care as a dimension of palliative care: The report of the Consensus Conference. *Journal of Palliative Medicine, 12,* 885–904. http://dx.doi.org/10.1089/jpm.2009.0142

Ramugondo, E. L. (2005). Unlocking spirituality: Play as a health-promoting occupation in the context of HIV/AIDS. In F. Kronenberg, S. A. Algado, & N. Pollard (Eds.), *Occupational therapy without borders: Learning from the spirit of survivors* (pp. 313–325). New York: Elsevier Churchill Livingstone.

Schulz, E. K. (2004). Spirituality and disability: An analysis of select themes. *Occupational Therapy in Health Care, 18,* 57–83. http://dx.doi.org/10.1080/J003v18n04_05

Segal, R. (2004). Family routines and rituals: A context for occupational therapy interventions. *American Journal of Occupational Therapy, 58,* 499–508. http://dx.doi.org/10.5014/ajot.58.5.499

Silverman, H. J., & Welton, D. (Eds.). (1988). *Postmodernism and continental philosophy.* Albany, NY: State University of New York Press.

Simó-Algado, S., Gregori, J. M. R., & Egan, M. (1997). Spirituality in a refugee camp. *Canadian Journal of Occupational Therapy 64,* 138–145. http://dx.doi.org/10.1177/000841749706400110

Simó-Algado, S., Mehta, N., Kronenberg, F., Cockburn, L., & Kirsh, B. (2002). Occupational therapy intervention with children survivors of war. *Canadian Journal of Occupational Therapy, 69,* 205–218. http://dx.doi.org/10.1177/000841740206900405

Simon, R. (2003). *Riding the bus with my sister.* New York: Plume.

Sloan, D. (1983). *Insight-imagination: The emancipation of thought and the modern world.* Westport, CT: Greenwood Press.

Spencer, J., Davidson, H., & White, V. (1997). Help clients develop hopes for the future. *American Journal of Occupational Therapy, 51,* 191–198. http://dx.doi.org/10.5014/ajot.51.3.191

Taylor, C. (1989). *Sources of the self: The making of the modern identity.* Cambridge, MA: Harvard University Press.

Taylor, J. B. (2009). *My stroke of insight: A brain scientist's personal journey.* New York: Viking.

Thibeault, R. (2011). Occupational therapy values. In M. A. McColl (Ed.), *Spirituality and occupational therapy* (2nd ed., pp. 103–110). Ottawa, ON: CAOT Publications.

Townsend, E. (1997a). Inclusiveness: A community dimension of spirituality. *Canadian Journal of Occupational Therapy, 64,* 146–155. http://dx.doi.org/10.1177/000841749706400311

Townsend, E. (1997b). Occupation: Potential for personal and social transformation. *Journal of Occupational Science, 4,* 18–26. http://dx.doi.org/10.1080/14427591.1997.9686417

Townsend, E. A., & Polatajko, H. J. (2007). *Enabling occupation II: Advancing an occupational therapy vision for health, well-being and justice through occupation.* Ottawa, ON: CAOT Publications.

Tse, S., Lloyd, C., Petchkovsky, L., & Manaia, W. (2005). Exploration of Australian and New Zealand indigenous people's spirituality and mental health. *Australian Occupational Therapy Journal, 52,* 181–187. http://dx.doi.org/10.1111/j. 1440-1630.2005.00507.x

Tutu, D. (2004). *God has a dream: A vision of hope for our time.* New York: Doubleday.

Unruh, A. M. (1997). Reflections on . . . spirituality and occupation: Garden musings and the Himalayan blue poppy. *Canadian Journal of Occupational Therapy, 64,* 156–160. http://dx.doi.org/10.1177/000841749706400312

Unruh, A. (2011). Appreciation of nature: Restorative occupations. In M. A. McColl (Ed.), *Spirituality and occupational therapy* (2nd ed., pp. 249–256). Ottawa, ON: CAOT Publications.

Unruh, A. M., Smith, N., & Scammel, C. (2000). The occupation of gardening in life-threatening illness: A Qualitative Pilot Project. *Canadian Journal of Occupational Therapy, 67,* 70–77. http://dx.doi.org/10.1177/000841740006700110

Unruh, A. M., Versnel, J., & Kerr, N. (2002). Spirituality unplugged: A review of commonalties and contentions, and a resolution. *Canadian Journal of Occupational Therapy, 69,* 5–20. http://dx.doi.org/10.1177/000841740206900101

Urbanowski, R. (1997). Spirituality in everyday practice. *OT Practice, 2,* 18–23.

Urbanowski, R., & Vargo, J. (1994). Spirituality, daily practice, and the occupational performance model. *Canadian Journal of Occupational Therapy, 61,* 88–94. http://dx.doi.org/10.1177/000841749406100204

Williams, B. J. (2008). An exploratory study of older adults' perspectives of spirituality. *Occupational Therapy in Health Care, 22,* 2008, 3–19. http://dx.doi.org/10.1080/J003v22n01_02

CHAPTER 6.

THE MEANING OF MEANING: THINKING ABOUT PHENOMENOLOGY AND MEANING

Tamera Keiter Humbert, MA, DEd, OTR/L

Chapter Highlights

◇ Meaning and occupational therapy
◇ General constructs of meaning
◇ Critique of general constructs of meaning
◇ Aspects of meaning making and occupations
◇ Critique of aspects of meaning making and occupations
◇ Dynamic relationships of meaning making in specific contexts and occupations
◇ Next steps.

Key Terms and Concepts

◇ Collective meaning making
◇ Culture
◇ Engagement
◇ Entity
◇ Epistemology
◇ Global themes of meaning
◇ Identity
◇ Meaning and occupations
◇ Meaning making
◇ Moral meaning making
◇ Narrative identity

◇ Occupational form
◇ Occupational self
◇ Occupational value
◇ Ontology
◇ Phenomenology
◇ Psychospiritual integration
◇ Spiritual meaning making
◇ Transpersonal event
◇ ValMO Model
◇ Valued occupations

Literature specifically related to occupational therapy and spirituality identifies four philosophical perspectives—ontology, phenomenology, epistemology, and cosmology— and a combination of these concepts. Of these, phenomenology is the predominant conceptualization of spirituality in occupational therapy literature.

Phenomenology is the study of or focus on personal experience and understanding. It is consistent with the emphasis on and promotion of meaning as core to occupational therapy.

A comprehensive analysis of the literature (published from 1993 to 2015) specifically related to phenomenology, or meaning making, as it relates directly or indirectly to the construct of spirituality was conducted to determine how authors defined, understood, and promoted the development of the phenomenological perspective, or meaning, within a person's life through occupational therapy practice. This chapter highlights three distinct, and increasingly complex, conceptualizations derived from that analysis, including (1) general constructs of meaning, (2) aspects of meaningful occupations, and (3) the dynamic relationships of meaning making with and within specific contexts and occupations.

Meaning and Occupational Therapy

The occupational therapy profession often references the meaning of activities and the meaning of a person's life no matter what influences and catastrophes interrupt that life (Boyt Schell, Gillen, & Scaffe, 2014; Christiansen, Baum, & Bass-Haugen, 2005). Practitioners use the phrase *meaningful and purposeful activities* (American Occupational Therapy Association [AOTA], 2014; Hinojosa & Blount, 2014; World Federation of Occupational Therapists, 2012) to articulate occupational therapy's belief that the value and meaning people place on their occupations, roles, and activities provide a basis for occupational therapy intervention in client-centered practice (Boyt Schell et al., 2014; Christiansen et al., 2005; Hinojosa & Blount, 2014; Townsend & Polatajko, 2007).

General Constructs of Meaning

The occupational therapy literature includes three general constructs of meaning: (1) an important or significant entity, (2) meaning and occupations, and (3) meaning making. Table 6.1 provides the terms used for each construct in the occupational therapy literature. This section discusses each of the constructs in detail.

Important or Significant Entity

In the first general construct of meaning, the literature refers to meaning and meaningfulness as attributed to something of importance or significance to a person. Authors used the word *meaningful* to represent an important or significant experience (Collins, 1998), event (Romanoff & Thompson, 2006; Schoessow, 2010; Zecevic, Magalhaes, Madady, Halliagan, & Reeves, 2010), activity (Mack, 2002; Pizzi & Briggs, 2004), or relationship (Baker, 2008) as it was perceived by the person. The experience, event, activity, and relationship are collectively defined as an *entity.* In addition, specific times, places, people, actions, and affective components (e.g., emotions) are often associated with the experience, event, activity, or relationship.

Although an occupation may be associated with the valued entity, it is not the primary focus of meaningfulness and an explicit connection may not exist between engagement in the associated occupation and the entity. For example, someone might identify a wedding or union as a significant or meaningful event in his or her life. The event holds the meaning and the occupations engaged in may be part of or subsumed in the event. The focus or expressed meaning is in the wedding and not the activities or occupations involved in the wedding.

Valued occupations, as described broadly in the literature, are single or collective activities that represent a general recognition of enjoyment, importance, pleasure, or appreciation (Allen, Kellegrew, & Jaffe, 2000; Griffith, Caron, Desrosiers, & Thibeault, 2007). For example, someone might say that he enjoys going to the beach, listening to music, attending seminars, or being with friends. The engagement in any of these activities holds some significance for the person, and the person recognizes that importance. References to *meaning* and *meaningful* occupations in this part of the literature are general in nature and imply some worth or value to the person (AOTA, 2014).

Meaning and Occupations

The second general construct of meaning, *meaning and occupations,* focuses on the engagement of occupations and the value or meaning placed on an occupation or an aspect of an occupation. The central focus shifts in the literature from having a general perspective of value connected with an entity or activity to highlighting the engagement in

Table 6.1. General Constructs of Meaning Depicted in the Occupational Therapy Literature

General Construct	Term Used	Author/Link
Important or significant entity	Meaningful experience	Collins (1998) http://bit.ly/1TaHIZS
	Meaningful event/ life	Romanoff & Thompson (2006) http://bit.ly/1W8aDfb
		Schoessow (2010) http://bit.ly/20GfmLQ
		Zecevic, Magalhaes, Madady, Halliagan, & Reeves (2010) http://bit.ly/1Q44Gve
	Meaningful activity	Mack (2002) http://bit.ly/1PzNAWR
		Pizzi & Briggs (2004) http://bit.ly/1mDP22h
	Meaningful relationship	Baker (2008) http://bit.ly/1K9Yaaa
	Valued occupation	Allen, Kellegrew, & Jaffe (2000) AOTA (2014) http://bit.ly/1NOHU9o
		Griffith, Caron, Desrosiers, & Thibeault (2007) http://bit.ly/1UZ2Ksp
Meaning and occupations	Meaningful occupations (life/ daily/mundane)	Hannam (1997) http://bit.ly/1KByPWD Hasselkus (2002) Hocking (1997) http://bit.ly/1QnHAAk Pereira & Stagnitti (2008) http://bit.ly/1W8aDfb Reid (2010) http://bit.ly/1oidsiP Romanoff & Thompson (2006) http://bit.ly/1W8aDfb Thompson & MacNeil (2006) http://bit.ly/1U4pZ5S
	Meaningful routines/rituals	Luboshitzky & Gaber (2001) http://bit.ly/1St9xwJ
		Romanoff & Thompson (2006) http://bit.ly/1W8aDfb
	Meaningful therapeutic occupation	Fieldhouse (2003) http://bit.ly/1POChXw
		Schulz (2005b) http://bit.ly/23UV8Nv
	Meaningful, purposeful occupations	AOTA (2011) http://bit.ly/1T10TnD
		Tse, Lloyd, Petchkovsky, & Manaia (2005) http://bitly.1KWDDpF
	Meaningful life occupations	AOTA (2011) http://bit.ly/1T10TnD

(Continued)

Table 6.1. General Constructs of Meaning Depicted in the Occupational Therapy Literature (*Cont.*)

General Construct	Term Used	Author/Link
Meaning making	Meaning of occupations	AOTA (2011) http://bit.ly/1T10TnD
		AOTA (2014) http://bit.ly/1NOHU9o
		Hannam (1997) http://bit.ly/1KByPWD
		Hasselkus (2002)
		Nelson (1988) http://bit.ly/1QTfxeN
		Stadnyk (2011) http://bit.ly/1o0jncY
	Meaning and purpose in life	AOTA (2011) http://bit.ly/1T10TnD
		Boswell, Hamer, Knight, Glacoff, & McChesney (2007) http://bit.ly/1Pj2X8c
		Collins (1998) http://bit.ly/1TaHIZS
		Ivarsson & Müllersdorf (2009) http://bit.ly/1VhGxpx
		Kirsh (1996) http://bit.ly/1T3QAiM
		Lloyd & O'Connor (2007) http://bit.ly/1TaJGti
		Luboshitzky (2008) http://bit.ly/20mj6wJ
		McColl (2011)
		Moyers (1997) http://bit.ly/23UXcVO
		Schulz (2005a) http://bit.ly/20mj6wJ
		Schwarz & Fleming Cottrell (2007) http://bit.ly/20vpTWA
		Tse, Lloyd, Petchkovsky, & Manaia (2005) http://bit.ly/1R5g9y9
		Wilding (2007) http://1.usa.gov/1Rmg3nA
		Wilding, May, & Muir-Cochrane (2005) http://bit.ly/1ooGD4c
	Meaning and purpose of/to life	do Rozario (1994) http://bit.ly/1o0lRYF
		McColl (2000) http://bit.ly/1V12KIk
		McColl (2011)

(*Continued*)

Table 6.1. General Constructs of Meaning Depicted in the Occupational Therapy Literature (*Cont.*)

General Construct	Term Used	Author/Link
	Meaning and purpose of/to life	Simó-Algado, Mehta, Kronenberg, Cockburn, & Kirsh (2002) http://bit.ly/20vMySX
		Urbanowski & Vargo (1994) http://bit.ly/23TpK23

Note. AOTA = American Occupational Therapy Association.

occupation and the *meaning* associated with that occupation. Although the link between *meaning* and *occupation* is stronger than in the first general construct in this subcategory of the literature, references and descriptions still tend to be vague or elusive. For example, according to the *Occupational Therapy Practice Framework* (3rd ed.; AOTA, 2014) **engagement** in occupation is described as

> performance of occupations as a result of choice, motivation, and meaning within a supportive context and environment. Engagement includes objective and subjective aspects of clients' experiences and involves the transactional interaction of the mind, body, and spirit. (p. S4)

Several authors have identified a central component of occupation and meaning within occupational therapy practice (Boyt Schell et al., 2014; Christiansen et al., 2005; Hinojosa & Blount, 2014; Nelson, 1988). The concept presented in the literature is that each person experiences occupations in his or her own way and attributes value and meaning about those occupations based on their experiences. Other occupational therapy scholars have clarified the significance of meaning and occupations, such as the recognition that a person may find unique meanings held within daily, mundane activities and objects (Hannam, 1997; Hasselkus, 2002; Hocking, 1997; Peloquin, 1997; Pereira & Stagnitti, 2008; Reid, 2010; Thompson & MacNeil, 2006).

Meaning and objects

Meaning and occupations includes objects. Particular objects used in the completion of occupations may have significant meaning for the person using the objects. For example, the use of a particular tea cup may provoke intense feelings, past memories, or contribute to how and when the cup is actually used (Hannam, 1997). Hocking (1997) presented the following perspective to better understand the interconnectedness between a person and objects and to link meaning to both personal and social contexts of that interconnectedness:

> Meaning may be ascribed at a personal level, such as valuing an object because your daughter gave it to you. Societal meaning is ascribed in interaction with other people, and includes notions such as who has priority use of the object, who has responsibility for its care, what kinship or friendship tie is it evidence of, or what social sign or signal it embodies such as masculinity, wealth, or social status. (p. 29)

Meaning and activities

Romanoff and Thompson (2006) suggested that everyday activities can transcend ordinary meaning to include powerful, rich experiences. For example, brushing hair may become more than a grooming task completed as part of a morning routine; it may symbolize self-expression and a creative outlet. In addition, in meaning and activities, meaning and value are highlighted as being associated with ongoing and established routines and rituals (Romanoff & Thompson, 2006).

Meaningful and purposeful occupations are attributed to ongoing life occupations as the occupations, rituals, and routines are integrated over time (AOTA, 2011; Luboshitzky & Gaber, 2001; Tse, Lloyd, Petchkovsky, & Manaia, 2005). The use of meaningful occupations within the therapeutic context may provide an avenue for clients to gain insights, expand perspectives when dealing with a disability (Schulz, 2005b), and promote further discovery and integration of health and well-being (Fieldhouse, 2003).

Meaning Making

The third general construct of meaning, ***meaning making,*** is the intentional process a person undertakes to become aware of, make connections to, and articulate how he or she makes sense of personal experiences (Aubin, Hachey, & Mercier, 1999; Hasselkus, 2002; Lloyd & O'Connor, 2007). When considering meaning making and occupations, occupational therapy practitioners must first understand that select occupations hold different connotations for different people (Hannam, 1997).

For example, for some, meal preparation may signify the value and importance of a caregiver role. For others, it may be a creative outlet that is not considered a responsibility but an opportunity to expand the self, experiment, and craft new recipes. For yet others, it may be associated with getting nutrition for health. Stadnyk (2011) stated, "Occupations are complex and may hold contradictory (social–political–cultural) meanings" (p. 194). The occupational therapy literature on meaning making recognizes unique personal perspectives and how a person understands and articulates the way he or she makes sense of occupations (AOTA, 2011, 2014).

More broadly, meaning making encompasses an internal process of understanding and making sense of occupations over time and within a shared culture. Romanoff and Thompson (2006) stated,

> Human beings are makers of meaning. We are able to anticipate the events of our day and move orderly and predictably through our lives because of our ability to attribute causality and imbue events with meaning. Meaning construction, the process by which we make sense of our world, is an inherently social act. The perceptions and constructs through which we experience ourselves and our world are shaped from expectancies and core beliefs developed through unique experiences and shared culture. (p. 309)

The literature related to meaning making and occupational therapy indicates a connection among occupational engagement, the process of meaning making, and understanding purpose in life. Because occupational therapy scholars consider occupations to be not only tasks but also experiences that contribute to a person's collective journey, ongoing meaning making for occupations contributes to the

Figure 6.1. Exchange between occupational engagement and meaning and life meaning.

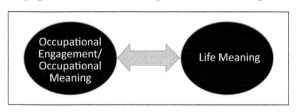

overall purpose of a person's life (Hasselkus, 2002; Wilson, 2011).

For example, Moyers (1997) stated that "the person attempts to discover his or her purpose or reasons for being in the world and clarifies within the schemes the importance of interpersonal relationships, daily events, and goals" (p. 211). Moreover, while occupations provide meaning to a person throughout life (influenced by socio–cultural–political contexts and personal development or life experiences), *life meaning*—the process of making sense of one's life—is influenced by those occupations (Schwarz & Fleming Cottrell, 2007), creating an exchange between occupational engagement and meaning and life meaning (Figure 6.1).

Wilding, May, and Muir-Cochrane (2005) further expressed a reciprocal relationship between meaning making and purpose but with a slightly different slant, considering spirituality the impetus for meaning making. They stated, "Spirituality provided meaning to occupations which results in participants experiencing purposeful and satisfying doing" (p. 5).

Other literature on phenomenology or meaning making has focused not only on a person's personal lived experiences and engagement in occupations but also on his or her reflective processes (Froehlich & Nelson, 1986; Kirsh, 1996; Schulz, 2005b). Moreover, Romanoff and Thompson (2006) stated, "Attention is given to the discovery of meaning in life experience through a process of reflection, nonjudgmental examination, interpretation, and narration" (p. 310).

The majority of the occupational therapy literature that focuses on meaning making highlights the role of occupations in life purpose (Kirsh, 1996; Schwarz & Fleming Cottrell, 2007). This focus includes how people make sense of their occupations and experiences and understand their inherent value and then make meaning of their collective experiences and ultimately life (Hasselkus, 2002). However, McColl (2000) identified the importance of taking an even broader perspective of meaning making, stating,

> If we speak specifically of the opportunity for transcendence in everyday activities, then we recognize that meaning is not characteristic of specific activities. Rather, meaning derives from the opportunity to see universal truths in specific activities, to obtain a view of the whole cosmos in relation to a particular daily pattern of life, and to see one's life a as whole in relation to the grander schemes of things. (p. 220)

Within this subcategory of meaning-making literature, authors have recognized the importance of engagement in life events, experiences, and occupations within the context of spirituality, reflection, or a universal perspective and how they relate to life purpose. In particular, this perspective may be helpful when people are trying to make meaning of difficult life events and circumstances such as death, disability, crisis, and chaos (Tse et al., 2005).

Critique of General Constructs of Meaning

A basic premise of occupational therapy is that meaning and occupations have a shared relationship. This concept leads to the question of whether practitioners should attend to desired occupations or the meaning of those occupations. Each suggests a different theoretical stance, particularly related to spirituality. These theoretical perspectives are based on whether engagement in occupation facilitates meaning making or whether meaning (life or purpose) dictates the occupations chosen. If engagement in occupation promotes meaning, then a phenomenological perspective could be rightfully proposed. Conversely, if occupations are chosen because they are meaningful, then the perspectives of *epistemology* (i.e., knowing) and *ontology* (i.e., perceiving existence) might be more applicable.

Collins (1998) did not explicitly define the term *meaning* when it was initially associated with experience; however, Collins (2007) later described *meaning* in the context of a *transpersonal event* in which a person experiences a life-changing and often dis-

orienting experience. An example of a transpersonal event might include attending a conference or retreat and discovering great insight into one's life and awareness of how to proceed with major life decisions.

In another example, people dealing with addictions sometimes describe a "rock-bottom" experience in which they cry out in desperation for help and receive great comfort, a sense of peace, and renewed strength. These feelings or states of peace and strength are described as coming from someplace beyond themselves. This experience, labeled by Collins as a *spiritual event,* is considered to have an epistemological or even ontological basis. According to Collins (2007), occupations and routines can be disrupted by the intensity of the transpersonal event or the disorientation that follows this transpersonal and highly unusual event. Reestablishing occupations may be needed and provided through therapeutic intervention and therefore become the primary focus in occupational therapy. However, the meaning of the event holds significance for the person, not the engagement in occupations. In other words, meaning is not necessarily discovered through engagement in occupations but through the transpersonal event.

The question then arises whether multiple theoretical aspects are present when the terms *meaning* and *meaningful* as well as *meaningful occupations* are broadly used. Moreover, does the philosophical emphasis change depending on the context in which these terms are used? If the term *meaningful occupations* is used without this philosophical understanding, practitioners do not know what is being promoted or what philosophical theories underpin the term.

Aspects of Meaning Making and Occupations

Beyond a general connection of occupations and meaning making, the occupational therapy literature articulates specific aspects of meaningful occupations. The assumption shared by this literature is that occupations are meaningful (i.e., full of meaning) and their meaning or how they are meaningful can be described. For this subcategory of literature, reviewed articles were divided between meaningful aspects of occupations related to the self and to the collective (Table 6.2).

Table 6.2. Aspects of Meaningful Occupations in the Literature

Aspect	Term Used	Author/Link
Self	Meaning and self or identity	Christiansen (1999) http://bit.ly/1QnGiFx Fieldhouse (2003) http://bit.ly/1POChXw Griffith, Caron, Desrosiers, & Thibeault (2007) http://bit.ly/1UZ2Ksp Kirsh (1996) http://bit.ly/1T3QAiM Romanoff & Thompson (2006) http://bit.ly/1W8aDfb Sakellariou & Simó-Algado (2006) http://bit.ly/1KlTRJ0 Schulz (2005a) http://bit.ly/2070gcM Shearsmith-Farthing (2001) http://bit.ly/1ooK0bs Vrkljan & Miller-Polgar (2001) http://bit.ly/1SdZM5r Wilson (2011)
	Occupational value or beliefs	Eklund, Erlandsson, & Persson (2003) http://bit.ly/20zDWZs Helbig & McKay (2003) http://bit.ly/1SGbshK Hvalsøe & Josephsson (2003) http://bit.ly/1KD8Z4s Persson, Erlandsson, Eklund, & Iwarsson (2001) http://bit.ly/1SGbNAV Williams (2008) http://bit.ly/1SWxpJ5
	Culturally meaningful occupations	Hannam (1997) http://bit.ly/1KByPWD Hocking (2009) http://bit.ly/1Qpwo6a Romanoff & Thompson (2006) http://bit.ly/1W8aDfb Simó-Algado, Mehta, Kronenberg, Cockburn, & Kirsh (2002) http://bit.ly/20vMySX Wilson (2011)
	Spiritual meaning	Boswell, Knight, & Hamer (2001) http://bit.ly/20IGDNG Frank et al. (1997) http://bit.ly/1TaLO4p Kroeker (1997) http://bit.ly/1SG9U7s Pentland & McColl (2011) Smith-Gabai & Ludwig (2011) http://bit.ly/1O1vHOD Wilding, May, & Muir-Cochrane (2005) http://bit.ly/1ooGD4c

(Continued)

Table 6.2. Aspects of Meaningful Occupations in the Literature (*Cont.*)

Aspect	Term Used	Author/Link
	Global themes, meaning, or universal truths	Jackson, Carlson, Mandel, Zemke, & Clark (1998) http://bit.ly/20zIizO Persson, Erlandsson, Eklund, & Iwarsson (2001) http://bit.ly/1SGbNAV
Collective	Meaning with others	Cipriani et al. (2010) http://bit.ly/1QTmVqt Fieldhouse (2003) http://bit.ly/1P0ChXw Frank et al. (1997) http://bit.ly/1TaLO4p Greenberg (2003) http://bit.ly/23V1FI6 Hannam (1997) http://bit.ly/1KByPWD Heuchemer & Josephsson (2006) http://bit.ly/20TvExE Hvalsøe & Josephsson (2003) http://bit.ly/1KD8Z4s Moylan, Carey, Blackburn, Hayes, & Robinson (2015) http://bit.ly/20IC1XV Smith-Gabai & Ludwig (2011) http://bit.ly/1O1vHOD
	Shared meaning and conflicting meaning	Romanoff & Thompson (2006) http://bit.ly/1Wo5aBi Heuchemer & Josephsson (2006) http://bit.ly/20TvExE
	Meaning and traditions	Frank et al. (1997) http://bit.ly/1TaLO4p Tzanidaki & Reynolds (2011) http://bit.ly/1PVsGRB

Aspects of Meaning Related to the Self

Literature related to meaning making that is particularly focused on describing occupational engagement portrays an interconnection between the doing of occupations and a context of awareness of or influence on the individual person. The underlying assumptions are that self-identity, values, beliefs, and culture have reciprocal relationships with occupational choice and engagement. For some scholars, personal identity or self-identity is closely related to occupational engagement. Thus, the process of giving meaning to occupation involves a connection between a person's *identity*, or self-image, and the engagement of select occupations (Christensen, 1999; Fieldhouse, 2003; Shearsmith-Farthing, 2001; Wilson, 2011).

Occupational self

Griffith et al. (2007) described *meaningful occupations* as "activities that are particularly enjoyed, appreciated and/or considered important.... [They] allow expression of an identity that each person holds dear and wants to convey to others" (p. 83). Additionally, Vrkljan and Miller-Polgar (2001) articulated that occupations are "a source of meaning; choice; and control, balance and satisfaction" (p. 242) that is used in reestablishing some control or readjusting expectations and personal self-images when confronted with a major life challenge.

Vrkljan and Miller-Polgar used the term *occupational self* to convey this interplay or interdependence between the person and engagement in occupations. Therefore, as a person engages in select occupations, identity is established, enhanced, developed, or reestablished. In addition, as self-identity is formulated or reconstructed during or after an illness, select occupations are chosen to enhance that identity. Thus, the construction of meaning involves both process and outcome.

Narrative identity

Kirsh (1996) promoted the idea that identity develops and is reconfigured over the course of a lifetime. Kirsh used the term *narrative identity* to describe how people use life experiences and personal stories to formulate a sense of meaningfulness and life purpose. Likewise, narrative identity is an essential element for ongoing personal well-being and life satisfaction (Christensen, 1999). In addition, the importance of life narratives is reinforced when coming to terms with illness or end of life because creation and re-creation of these narratives can promote healing during these circumstances (Romanoff & Thompson, 2006).

Occupational value

Persson, Erlandsson, Eklund, and Iwarsson (2001) provided a comprehensive framework highlighting layers of meaning making (i.e., *micro,* or select activities; *mesa,* or developing occupations; *macro,* or integrated occupations) and promoted the concept of *occupational value,* attributing significance to a particular occupation as a prerequisite to meaning making and occupational engagement. According to Persson et al., people view occupations as valuable to themselves within varying intrinsic degrees (concrete value, symbolic value, self-reward value) and make meaning of occupations within the context of these values.

Although not using the language of occupational value, Williams (2008) also referenced the interplay among occupations, self-identity, and the connection of values when she stated, "occupations are selected that agree with personal views on life" (p. 14). Although limited literature relates to the constructs of values and occupational engagement, several authors have recognized that values play some part in meaning making (Eklund, Erlandsson, & Persson, 2003; Helbig & McKay, 2003; Hvalsøe & Josephsson, 2003) and that the formation and ongoing shaping of identity is linked with the selection of and engagement in occupations (Persson et al., 2001).

Figure 6.2. Occupational engagement and the person within the cultural context.

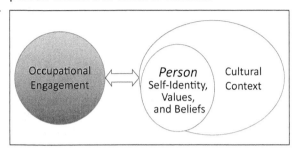

Culture

Culture entails beliefs, perspectives, rituals, and routines (AOTA, 2014) and is an important context that influences both what a person does and how a person makes meaning of life experiences (Hannam, 1997; Hasselkus, 2002; Romanoff & Thompson, 2006; Simó-Algado, Mehta, Kronenberg, Cockburn, & Kirsh, 2002; Wilson, 2011). Although the preliminary literature that was reviewed for spirituality and meaning making is limited in describing how culture influences occupations and occupational choices, it gives some attention to the importance of recognizing both cultural contexts and occupational engagement for the individual person when providing intervention (Figure 6.2). In addition, Romanoff and Thompson (2006) articulated the symbolic importance of creating, using, and re-creating rituals and routines because they provide people with a sense of belonging and identity.

Spiritual meaning making

How do occupational engagement and meaning making influence identity and the ongoing formulation of personal spiritual meaning making? Often described as *spiritual meaning* or *global meaning,* **spiritual meaning making** involves the individual person, the cultural context, and occupational engagement as well as the person's life events and continuing development of spiritual meaning (Figure 6.3). Spiritual meaning making assumes that as a person engages in occupations, life events, and rituals, spiritual meaning is further developed, deepened, or enhanced (Frank et al., 1997; Hasselkus, 2002; McColl 2011; Smith-Gabai & Ludwig, 2011).

Spiritual meaning making also assumes that meaning is individualized and unique. Pentland and McColl (2011) stated, "For some, spiritual meaning is associated with the concept of a higher

Figure 6.3. Occupational engagement, the person, cultural context, and spiritual meaning making.

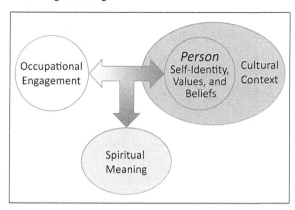

being and may conform to religions or faith traditions. For others, spiritual meaning derives from a sense of connection—with others, with nature, with the past, present, and future" (p. 147).

Spiritual meaning making depends on occupational engagement. Hasselkus (2002) stated, "Engagement in occupation is one primary way for us to 'be' in the world. We can think of occupation as a vehicle by which our internal world is expressed in our external world . . . [, and] our spiritual consciousness is given expression in our daily worldly lives" (p. 112). For example, Frank et al. (1997) highlighted the spiritual meaning that Orthodox Jews placed on regularly engaged occupations (e.g., prayer) and rituals (e.g., observing the Sabbath) and stated, "The two dimensions of existence [spirituality and occupation] cannot be separated but rather define each other" (p. 205). Engagement in select occupations provided self- and community identity and reinforced and enlivened spiritual meaning.

Engaging in valued occupations and constructing a new personal self-identity can play a part in making sense of the world in light of a disability, which may promote acceptance, personal growth, and comfort and facilitate spiritual meaning (Boswell, Knight, & Hamer, 2001). In a related study, Wilding et al. (2005) articulated the mutual relationships between spirituality and occupational engagement with people dealing with mental health concerns. The authors stated, "Spirituality is a form of Being that provides the meaning, which underpins purposeful and satisfying doing, and spirituality provide[s] meaning to occupations, which

results in participants experiencing purposeful and satisfying doing" (p. 5).

Kang (2003) offered a *psychospiritual integration (PSI)* frame of reference for spiritual meaning making that identified the following six dimensions of occupational engagement and spirituality:

1. Becoming
2. Meaning
3. Being
4. Centeredness
5. Connectedness
6. Transcendence.

The literature presents several diverse ways in which these six constructs flow together (Kang, 2003; Wilcock & Townsend, 2014), but further investigation is needed about how they precisely relate to the topic of spirituality and their application to real-world experiences. The PSI frame of reference also provides a model for assessing and providing intervention for people and communities, but Kang's conclusions are inadequately supported by empirical evidence.

Global themes

Meaning making continues and enlarges throughout a person's life. Jackson, Carlson, Mandel, Zemke, and Clark (1998) presented the idea of global themes of meaning, which gives credence to a lifetime of developing personal meaning making. Jackson et al. described *global themes of meaning* as "emerging from a compilation of ideologies . . . and the person's particular interpretive slant applied to life situations" (p. 328). They suggested that the self is constantly constructed and revealed through occupations. Persson et al. (2001) extended the concept of global themes of meaning to also include people allowing perspectives to develop, being open to transformation through the discovery of meaning, and connecting to others and society.

Aspects of Meaning Related to the Collective

Beyond recognizing personal awareness and the impact of occupational engagement and meaning making, occupational therapy literature describes *collective meaning making,* which is meaning making that is influenced by or within a group or community context (Cipriani, 2010; Fieldhouse, 2003; Frank et al., 1997; Greenberg, 2003; Hannam, 1997; Smith-Gabai & Ludwig, 2011). Hvalsøe and Josephsson (2003) reported on the conditions necessary to find meaning in occupations beyond the personal level. Engagement in occupations needs to support restoration and creation of life toward a new normality (after injury or disability), bring intrinsic satisfaction and acknowledgment from others, and facilitate an experience of positive feelings and a sense of well-being.

Heuchemer and Josephsson (2006) and Romanoff and Thompson (2006) highlighted the importance of collective meaning making for a person to deal with a major life event or transition and elaborated on the challenges that occur when conflict exists among the people who are involved in a shared experience. For example, a person may be working on goals to remain sober, employed, and living in permanent housing. The ability to achieve and sustain such goals may be highly dependent on the strength of a community network; however, disagreements between different support systems about how to accomplish these goals may undermine the person's success.

Critique of Aspects of Meaning Making and Occupations

This chapter is only a start to the conversation about meaning and occupations and should not be considered an exhaustive examination. Most of the literature reviewed tends to be informative and conceptual in nature, and there is little empirical evidence in this literature to suggest that these ideas are experienced universally, from either a personal or collective perspective.

Self-Identity and Occupational Identity

Concepts related to self-identity and occupational identity have been described in the occupational therapy literature (other than the literature specifically related to spirituality and meaning making), but the constructs offered have been associated more with ontological concepts (Christiansen, 1999; McCuaig

& Frank, 1991; Rudman & Dennhardt, 2008) and transpersonal perspectives (Christiansen, 1999; Collins, 2004, 2007) than with phenomenology. From an ontological perspective, occupations are secondary to the understanding of personal experiences. Meaning is first attributed to people's personal perspectives of who they are and how they experience life; occupations are subsequently chosen and have meaning because the occupations are associated with people's perspectives.

It is not explicitly clear or universally articulated how phenomenology intersects with ontology and transpersonal experiences. For example, can engagement in occupations transform personal perspectives about life and purpose? In addition, no empirical evidence explains how identity changes over time through occupational engagement (Christiansen, 1999), and all of the meaning making associated with identity changes and the social contexts that influence identity are not fully understood.

For example, Kroeker (1997) provided the concept of *moral meaning making,* that is, the ability to make sense of ethical quandaries and embody virtues, as part of self-identity, collective identity, and spirituality. Although Kroeker comes from a philosophical perspective and not an occupational therapy perspective, the concept of moral meaning making presented suggests another aspect of self-identity and spirituality that has not been represented or fully understood in occupational therapy literature.

Culture and Occupation

Ideas in the occupational therapy literature related to culture and occupation have predominantly come from a Western mindset. Although the literature acknowledges that culture affects how people make meaning of occupations (Hannam, 1997; Hocking, 2000), the concept of culture being embedded within occupations and meaning has only recently been considered (Iwama, 2006, 2007; Iwama, Thomson, & Macdonald, 2009). Understanding the complexity of culture, occupational engagement, and meaning making is particularly limited as it relates specifically to spirituality (Iwama, 2006), worldviews (Smith, 2008), and occupational identity (Phelan & Kinsella, 2009; Rudman & Dennhardt, 2008). This area needs further investigation.

Occupational Doing and Engagement

Spiritual meaning making may entail more than just doing occupations. The literature contains multiple references to occupations and the implicit and explicit understanding of doing occupations. However, in the articles reviewed that were specifically related to spirituality and meaning making in this subcategory of the literature, occupations went beyond the act of doing and included the concept of *being* while engaging in occupations and making sense of life and experiences (Thibeault, 1997; Wilding et al., 2005). The occupational therapy literature has numerous references to occupation as it relates to doing and being (Hasselkus, 2002; Watson, 2006), belonging (Rebeiro, Day, O'Brien, Semeniuk, & Wilson, 2001), doing–being–becoming (Lyons, Orozovic, Davis, & Newman, 2002), being-in-becoming (Rudman & Dennhardt, 2008), and becoming through doing (Hocking, 2005).

Although multiple scholars promote the idea of meaning making and engagement in occupations (Nelson, 1988) and meaning making and life purpose (Hasselkus, 2002), only a few proposals exist about how these processes happen. For example, the *ValMO Model* (i.e., Value Dimensions, Meaning, and Complexity in Human Occupation Model) provides a way to analyze the complexity of meaning making, occupational engagement, and occupational value by categorizing the three levels of perspectives of occupations (i.e., macro, meso, micro) and emphasizing an ongoing process of integrating these levels (Persson et al., 2001). However, the model has limited application and research related to it (Eklund et al., 2003).

Dynamic Relationships of Meaning Making in Specific Contexts and Occupations

Examining the literature that attempts to explicitly link meaning making, occupations, and spirituality might lead to a better understanding of what is meant by *phenomenology* and how it applies to occupational therapy. This section describes empirical literature that highlights meaning making of select occupations, changes in the self through and within occupations, meaning making and spirituality within select contexts, and the meaning of

spirituality and occupational engagement. These studies have begun to shape a preliminary understanding of phenomenology as it applies to the engagement of occupations.

Meaning Making of Select Occupations and Populations

Literature within the field has focused on the meaning of specific occupations with select populations (Table 6.3). The articles reviewed here acknowledge that study participants could make meaning of chosen and valued occupations and that some of the participants also had an appreciation of and explicit connection to a spiritual element within that meaning. When the connection was made between meaning and spirituality, its articulation tended to be vague or general (Lloyd, Wong, & Petchkovsky, 2007; Pereira & Stagnitti, 2008; Unruh, Smith, & Scammell, 2000) or associated with God (Frank et al., 1997; Tzanidaki & Reynolds, 2011). This literature also recognizes that although study participants could provide diverse and comprehensive meanings of valued and engaged occupations, the authors provided limited viewpoints about the dynamic interplay among self-identity, engagement in occupations or life, and meaning making.

Reinventing, Co-Creating, and Clarifying Self and Occupations

Beyond the ability to make meaning of a select occupation, people can make meaning of their lived experiences, the occupations they engage in, and how these occupations influence their self-identity (Table 6.4). Engagement in occupations assists people living and dealing with issues and life challenges, such as mental health concerns, physical illness, injury, disability, injustice, aging, and death and dying, altering their self-perception or identity.

Living with mental illness

In a study by Hvalsøe and Josephsson (2003), people living with a mental illness shared their perspectives on meaningful occupations. Their descriptions included occupations that supported restoration and normalcy, feelings of autonomy, future positive images of engaging in occupations, personal values, roles and identity, intrinsic satisfaction and positive acknowledgment from others, productivity

Table 6.3. Meaning Making of Select Occupations and Populations

Occupation/ Author/Link	Population	Theme	Spirituality Reference
Owning pets (Allen, Kellegrew, & Jaffe, 2000) http://bit.ly/ 1SPQmxD	Men with HIV/ AIDS (*n* = 7)	Emotional component of pet ownership Daily routines and responsibilities	—
Engaging in religious practices and rituals (Frank et al., 1997) http://bit.ly/ 1TaLO4p	Orthodox Jewish couples (*n* = 4)	Observing the Sabbath Studying and praying Keeping a kosher home	Spirituality is experienced through the orchestration of concrete acts in time and opportunities to bind with God (p. 205).
Making and having a cup of tea (Hannam, 1997) http://bit.ly/ 1KByPWD	Women from a community group (*n* = 5)	Meaning through the reasons for drinking tea Meaning through the senses Meaning through objects used Meaning through temporality Meaning through social context Meaning through changes in lifestyle	—
Working in a training garden (Jonasson, Marklund, & Hildingh, 2007) http://bit.ly/ 1oEL2ju	People with a neurological condition completing outpatient rehabilitation (*n* = 14)	Beneficial Productive Voluntary Complicated	—
Engaging in art (Lloyd, Wong, & Petchkovsky, 2007) http://bit.ly/ 23w0QFt	People with a mental health condition involved in a community arts program (*n* = 8)	Expression Self-discovery Empowerment Self-validation Spirituality: Meaning and purpose; acceptance and hope	Having a belief in a higher being, a sense of meaning and purpose, connectedness to nature and humanity, and altruism (p. 210).
Engaging in leisure occupations (Pereira & Stagnitti, 2008) http://bit.ly/ 1W8aDfb	Well-elderly Australian Italians (*n* = 10)	Link between leisure activities, subjective experiences, and health	Spiritual health and engagement in bocce.
Using creativity in occupational therapy practice (Schmid, 2004) http://bit.ly/ 1Se5AMc	Occupational therapists with 10–26 years of experience working in rehabilitation, mental health, and hospice (*n* = 3)	Creativity being part of everyday practice Use of creativity as a conscious approach Creativity involves risk taking Creativity through the use of expressive arts in therapy	—

(Continued)

Table 6.3. Meaning Making of Select Occupations and Populations (*Cont.*)

Occupation/ Author/Link	Population	Theme	Spirituality Reference
Making traditional arts and crafts (Tzanidaki & Reynolds, 2011) http://bit.ly/ 1PVsGRB	Older women living in rural Crete (*n* = 12)	Deep respect for Cretan traditions of art and craft making Personal satisfaction of art making Experiencing and expressing continuity of self in later life Making social connections through art making Appreciating the financial aspects of art making Art making as a means of coping with the challenges of later life Experiencing spirituality within art and craft making	Connection with God.
Gardening (Unruh, Smith, & Scammell, 2000) http://bit.ly/ 23V3GEc	Women with breast cancer (*n* = 3)	Physical elements of the garden Interaction with living things Meeting personal needs Reflections about life Coping through gardening	Spirituality and reflecting on life processes. Garden as a "spiritual enabler, making it possible to find meaningfulness in life under extreme circumstances" (p. 76). "Spirituality may revolve around the possibility of hope, and transcendence beyond everyday visible existence" (p. 76).

Note. — = not applicable.

and accomplishment, social engagement, and contributions to society. Additionally, participants acknowledged the desire to be recognized as a valuable person, have a sense of well-being, be safe and in control, and create balance in everyday activities. The focus on identity and occupations in this study highlighted the interconnection between the two and the value of autonomy, as self-identity, by the participants. Hvalsøe and Josephsson stated,

> The element of being supported as an autonomous person, which is closely related to identity, is identified as a major theme in this study. Several of the informants stressed that they were not in a position to take full autonomy for granted but had, instead, constantly

to fight either to hold onto partial autonomy or to move towards full autonomy. (p. 68)

The authors furthered their analysis by advocating the potential role of intervention in supporting occupations of personal choice related to productivity, social engagement, and other nonstigmatizing occupations with the goal of increased well-being, personal satisfaction, and strengthened identity.

Living with physical disability

Living with physical disabilities over the course of a lifetime affect self-identity, and engagement in occupations can also influence and change identity. Although occupational therapy literature recognizes

Table 6.4. Reinventing, Co-Creating, and Clarifying Self and Occupations

Context/Author/Link	Population	Theme/Concept
Physical disability (Boswell, Knight, & Hamer, 2001) http://bit.ly/20IGDNG	Women ages 35–55 years living with severe physical disabilities (*n* = 6)	Essential nature of the spirituality–disability interaction. Disability as a frame of reference for spirituality. Spirituality as a frame of reference for disability.
Homelessness and addiction (Heuchemer & Josephsson, 2006) http://bit.ly/20TvExE	Women in recovery (*n* = 2)	Homelessness as a specific lived plot (i.e., story, narrative). Social relationships influence lived plots. Change through employment Acting out a new plot.
Mental illness (Hvalsøe & Josephsson, 2003) http://bit.ly/1KD8Z4s	People receiving mental health services (*n* = 4 women ages 41–63 years; *n* = 4 men ages 24–45 years)	Engagement supporting restoration and creation of the life world (i.e., existence, purpose) toward normality. Engagement bringing intrinsic satisfaction and acknowledgment of others. Engagement facilitating positive feelings and a sense of well-being.
Aging and autonomy loss (Griffith, Caron, Desrosiers, & Tibeault, 2007) http://bit.ly/1UZ2Ksp	Community-dwelling older adults with autonomy loss (*n* = 6 women ages 67–89 years; *n* = 2 men ages 70 and 72 years)	Identity and meaningful occupations. Adjusting identity in the context of loss and autonomy. Social, psychological, and spiritual aspects of adjusting identity. Engagement in life.
Life-threatening illness (Unruh & Elvin, 2004) http://bit.ly/1Qpzqre	Women with breast cancer in early 50s 2–4 years after diagnosis (*n* = 3)	Attraction of dragon boat racing. Physical and emotional well-being. Competition as positive energy. Dragon boat racing as social support. Transcendence, connectedness, or oneness. Re-occurrence of breast cancer and death of team members: fear, identification (of the possibility of re-occurrence or death) and coping, increasing public awareness of breast cancer.
Life-threatening illness (Vrkljan & Miller-Polgar, 2001) http://bit.ly/1SdZM5r	Women with breast cancer ages 51, 52, and 56 years (*n* = 3)	Doing = living. Deconstruction of occupational self. Transition. Reconstruction of occupational self.

the connection between engagement in meaningful occupations and self-identity, and the desire to engage in such meaningful occupations, it also supports realigning, or shifting, self-identity through meaningful occupations. For example, Boswell et al. (2001) interviewed 6 women living with physical disabilities and asked them to share their perceptions of disability, spirituality, and identity. The authors made clear the reciprocal relationship between spirituality and self-identity and emphasized the changing and evolutionary concepts of self as described by the participants, stating,

> As with other major life experiences, their experience of disability offered a frame of reference within which they interpreted the world and within which their spiritual beliefs emerged.... Each of the women came to view disability as an integral part of herself that often precipitated or demanded a search for personal growth and spiritual meaning.... From the onset of their disability and continuing to the present time, these women experienced events or encounters that led to periods of questioning themselves, their worldviews, or both.... During adulthood, many of the participants continued to experience events or encounters specifically related to religious issues. These experiences evoked questions concerning their perceptions of self as a person with disability. (p. 22)

Community-dwelling older adults

Identity continues to change throughout life and through the aging process. Griffith et al. (2007) furthered the notion of an evolutionary and dynamic self-identity in the later stages of adult life that is influenced by others and engagement in occupations. They stated,

> People have numerous names for themselves according to the social environment in which they find themselves. One's identity is not expressed with others, it is also a function of these interactions. Social interactions are essential for the creation of one's identity. (p. 87)

Griffith et al. presented self-identity as emerging from engagement in meaningfully chosen occupations

that change over time and according to ability, such as in the case of older adults who "have identities that are no longer tied to performing the occupations of self-care, productivity and leisure, but rather to a sense of being active in life despite physical limitations" (p. 88).

Life-threatening illness

Like the community-dwelling older adults in Griffith et al.'s (2007) study, women in the Vrkljan and Miller-Polgar (2001) study identified the necessity to abandon occupations as a result of the psychological and physical ramifications of breast cancer. However, the women also went through a transition in understanding who they were by taking control of their lives and rearranging meaningful occupations. By engaging in new or adapted occupations, the women "found that their diagnosis no longer defined their sense of self, rather it became a part of it" (p. 242). The authors further articulated,

> Thus, the findings of this present study support the notion that in a period of personal crisis, such as a life-threatening diagnosis, occupational engagement may provide the means through which "reconstructive" messages are relayed to the occupational self. It is through this engagement in meaningful occupations that individuals may perceive messages that emphasize health and well-being, rather than the confines that may be imposed by illness. (p. 242)

Like these women dealing with breast cancer and creating a new self-identity through engagement in occupations (Vrkljan & Miller-Polgar, 2001), Unruh and Elvin (2004) described the use of competitive boat racing as a way women with breast cancer redefined their self-identity and projected it to the community as they portrayed new images of women dealing with breast cancer and advocated for awareness. They stated,

> The most prevalent theme . . . was the way in which dragon boat racing enabled [the women] to make a positive interpretation of their negative experience of breast cancer; it was also a key element of the public message that they wanted to convey to other women.

Their comments suggested that as they became involved with dragon boat racing, they also began to reappraise the cancer experience as a challenge, something that could be overcome. (p. 147)

Homelessness and addiction

In a study conducted with women recovering from homelessness and addiction (Heuchemer & Josephsson, 2006), the women frequently came into conflict with other's perspectives and meanings, creating an opportunity for the women to reflect and consider alternative meanings for their occupations and routines. According to Heuchemer and Josephsson, actively engaging in change, reshaping meaning, and living out that new meaning were part of addiction recovery. In addition, the engagement in spirituality by the participants provided some indication about the influence of spirituality on occupation and self-identity. Heuchemer and Josephsson stated, "Spirituality

gave one participant the possibility of creating a new plot that related to the continuity and coherence of her life" (p. 166).

Meaning and the Construct of Spirituality in Challenging Contexts

Multiple studies have demonstrated an explicit connection between meaning and spirituality within the context of challenging life situations (Table 6.5; *Note.* "Time Frame in Meaning Making" column is discussed later in this chapter. There is some recognition that people's perspectives can and do change over time and with the course of intervention). Although 3 of the studies highlighted the use of spirit and spirituality in making meaning of lived experiences, that was not their main focus (Beauregard & Solomon, 2005; Humbert, Bess, & Mowery, 2013; Lorenzo, 2003). However, the primary intent of the remaining studies reviewed in this literature subcategory focused on understanding spirituality from a select perspective and context

Table 6.5. Meaning and the Construct of Spirituality Within Select Contexts

Context/ Author/Link	Population	Theme	Time Frame in Meaning Making	Definition of Spirituality by Author
HIV (Beauregard & Solomon, 2005) http://bit.ly/ 1RPrGUU	Women with HIV ages 40–44 years (*n* = 5),	Fearing disclosure Experiencing challenges Having supportive networks Coping positively with HIV	Unknown but length of time after diagnosis 1–15 years	Spirituality and a belief in a higher power provided a sense of encouragement and support (p. 118).
Physical disability (Boswell, Hamer, Knight, Glacoff, & McChesney, 2007) http://bit.ly/ 1Pj2X8c	Adults with physical disabilities (*n* = 13; 7 men and 6 women)	Purpose Awareness Connections Creativity Acceptance	10+ years with physical disability	A person's views of the world, particularly how a person explains the world and the forces that affect his or her life (p. 34).
Physical disability (Boswell, Knight, & Hamer, 2001) http://bit.ly/ 20IGDNG	Women with severe physical disabilities ages 35–55 years (*n* = 6)	Essential nature of the spirituality–disability interaction Disability as a frame of reference for spirituality Spirituality as a frame of reference for disability	Unknown but reference to an evolution of religious affiliations throughout lifetime	An inner belief system concerning how the world works.

(Continued)

Table 6.5. Meaning and the Construct of Spirituality Within Select Contexts (*Cont.*)

Context/ Author/Link	Population	Theme	Time Frame in Meaning Making	Definition of Spirituality by Author
Domestic violence (Humbert, Bess, & Mowery, 2013) http://bit.ly/ 1mqh9lw	Women in recovery from intimate partner violence ages 24–59 (*n* = 6)	Relationships Starting over Spirituality Expansion of self Forward movement	Unknown but in active intervention or shelter for 1.5–3 months	Expressed as movement past the abuse through faith, hope, and refuge (p. 257).
Disability (Lorenzo, 2003) http://bit.ly/ 1PlMYra	South African women with disabilities	Struggles: "I'm left with nothing" Sadness: "My soul doesn't rest" Strength: "I became one of them" Spirit: "We can do things to develop ourselves"	Unknown but narrative storytelling developed over a period of time and through multiple workshops	A spirit of doing, ability, being, change, and compassion.
Mental illness (MacGillivray, Sumsion, & Wicks-Nicholls, 2006) http://bit.ly/ 1WQ2Y6s	Adolescents with mental illness (*n* = 11)	An intangible part of the self Knowing yourself and the process of getting to know yourself better Personal beliefs and values Personal dreams and their pursuit Search for meaning and purpose	Unknown	Experience, expression, and evolution of meaning about self, others, and the world (p. 295).
Childhood- and adult-onset disability (Schulz, 2005a) http://bit.ly/ 20mj6wJ	People with Judeo-Christian perspective with childhood-onset disabilities (mean years with disability, 41.6; *n* = 6) People with Judeo-Christian perspective with adult-onset disabilities (mean years with disability, 13; *n* = 6)	*Childhood-onset disability* Connecting and expressing for purpose and meaning Disability as a vehicle to discover God's plan *Adult-onset disability* Connecting and expressing through feelings and actions Disability as a learning experience	Unknown	Experience of a meaningful connection to the core self, other humans, the world, or a greater power as expressed through reflections, narratives, and actions (p. 1284).

(Continued)

Table 6.5. Meaning and the Construct of Spirituality Within Select Contexts (*Cont.*)

Context/ Author/Link	Population	Theme	Time Frame in Meaning Making	Definition of Spirituality by Author
Aging in long-term care facility (Schwarz & Fleming Cottrell, 2007) http://bit.ly/ 20vpTWA	Elders residing in a long-term care facility ages 66–88 years receiving occupational therapy services 1.5–6 months (*n* = 5)	Meaning and purpose Coping and positive outlook Reliance and dependence Comfort and consolation Hope for recovery Therapeutic rapport	Unknown but participants reflected on the use of spirituality throughout their life challenges	A context inherent to the person that influences personal beliefs, perceptions, and expectations; however, no definition of spirituality was provided to the participants.
Mental illness (Wilding, May, & Muir-Cochrane, 2005) http://bit.ly/ 1ooGD4c	People with mental illness ages 35–55 years (*n* = 6)	Spirituality is life-sustaining Spirituality saves one from death Spirituality sustains occupations Spirituality sustains mental health and well-being	Unknown	Spirituality might or might not include religion; a connection to other people or a community; a sacred space; an important relationship with oneself or one's higher self; or belief in the healing power of crystals, witchcraft, or love or mysticism (p. 3); however, participants were asked to define *spirituality* as it was relevant and meaningful to them.
Aging (Williams, 2008) http://bit.ly/ 1SWxpJ5	Well-elderly with a Christian background (*n* = 3)	Perceptions of spirituality: Principle-based and intrinsic Integration of spirituality in daily life: Motivation and meaning Spirituality and personal needs: Strengths and inspiration Spirituality and chosen occupations: Perspectives on life	Unknown but all participants actively involved in religiously affiliated activities; 2 reported lifetime involvement	That which brings a sense of peace and well-being while providing purpose and value to a person (p. 7).

(Boswell, Hamer, Knight, Glacoff, & McChesney, 2007; Boswell et al., 2001; MacGillivray, Sumsion, & Wicks-Nicholls, 2006; Schulz, 2005a; Schwarz & Fleming Cottrell, 2007; Wilding et al., 2005; Williams, 2008).

Living with HIV

In a preliminary article that shed light on the experiences of women who were living with HIV, Beauregard and Solomon (2005) identified spirituality as one component of coping that brought strength and resources to the women. The focus of spirituality in this article was clearly a higher power. They stated, "Spirituality and a belief in a higher power provided a sense of encouragement and support. The higher power combated the feelings of isolation and gave them strength to cope with the everyday challenges" (p. 188). Although this study did not set out to understand the experience of spirituality as understood by the women, it provided some information about the role of spirituality in their lives.

Recovering from intimate partner violence

Humbert et al. (2013) identified the value and importance of spirituality as a way to cope with intimate partner violence. They stated, "Spirituality was expressed as movement past the abuse through faith, hope and refuge" (p. 257). Although some of the women expressed spirituality as a belief in a higher power, it was also communicated through their optimism for a brighter future and through the support of other women and staff at the shelter.

Living with a physical disability

In a study by Lorenzo (2003), South African women shared narratives about living life with a disability. They expressed struggles and sadness as well as strengths and spirit that enabled them to move beyond their challenges and grief. Spirituality was found in a higher power and through the ability to do, the ability to develop skills, and the support of other women. Spirituality was couched in terms of a spirit of doing, spirit of ability, spirit of being, spirit of change, and spirit of compassion.

Reflecting further on the understanding of spirituality as a central and powerful dynamic in relation to understanding the disability experience, Boswell et al. (2001) stated,

> The women in this study portrayed spirituality as a vehicle for changing their lives in a significant way. One participant described her spiritual views as providing direction to her life, a direction that moved her closer to God.... The women who participated in this study clearly viewed spirituality as a springboard for meaning and acceptance of disability and reflected on their perceptions of themselves as persons with disabilities. (p. 23)

Boswell et al. (2007) expressed the intricate and essential role that spirituality can play in the lives of people with disabilities. They stated, "The interaction of spirituality and disability unfolded in the lives of these participants is a dance in which both partners influence the direction and rhythm of the steps" (p. 39). In addition, the authors discussed a multidimensional relationship between the themes associated with spirituality (purpose, awareness, connections, creativity, and acceptance) and the lived experience of disability.

Aging

Williams (2008) conducted a study on the meaning of spirituality through the perspectives of three well elderly participants. The intrinsic and central component of spirituality, as understood by the participants, was the powerful connection among spirituality, life events, values, and identity. Williams stated,

> Spirituality, as perceived by the participants, creates purposefulness and is used as an adaptive measure to adjust to life's challenges. It often provides a means of negotiation to deal with life's disruptions, particularly those that threaten well-being, while serving as a filter through which value is assigned. Spirituality, though complex and often ambiguous, has a definite impact on who we are, what we become, and how this is accomplished. (p. 16)

To further ideas of spirituality and meaning making, Schwarz and Fleming Cottrell (2007) explored the perspectives of 5 elders on the integration of spirituality by occupational therapists and their rehabilitation services within a faith-based, long-term-care facility. The participants discussed not only the meaning of spirituality to their life context, including its contribution to hope, comfort, coping, and purpose, but also its effect on the therapeutic relationship. According to one participant, the occupational therapist was "a role model because she implemented spirituality, believing that the experience helped strengthen [the resident's] religious beliefs and convictions" (p. 52). In addition, the authors stated,

> All of the participants reflected that the therapist's use of a holistic approach to intervention, which considered their physical, mental and spiritual well-being, allowed them to better appreciate the value of their [occupational therapy] services. Consideration of the spiritual context in a setting which typically emphasizes only physical rehabilitation needs was viewed as effective for strengthening the therapeutic relationship between each participant and the occupational therapist. (p. 53)

Living with mental illness

Wilding et al. (2005) described the powerful influence and meaning that spirituality had for people diagnosed with a mental illness. Spirituality offered a sense of hope and a way to cope with the resulting challenges of mental illness. They discussed how participants strongly asserted that "spirituality was *vital* to life, and that without spirituality, death was the only option" (p. 6). The study emphasized the connection between being and doing, stating that participants

> believed that spiritual forces in the Universe assisted them. Spirituality provided guidance and help, which meant that participants were not alone, but that they could tap into an "energy source" that was bigger than each individual and that also helped each participant to act in the world. (p. 7)

Wilding et al. concluded that participants' perspectives of spirituality went beyond using spirituality as a coping mechanism to deal with the challenges of living with mental illness to defining themselves foremost as spiritual beings living a rich and full life.

In a study of adolescents receiving mental health services, the elements of spirituality deemed most important or critical to the adolescents were related

to the individual and lifelong pursuits of self-discovery and understanding (MacGillivray et al., 2006). Elements related to religion and external pursuits, activities, and relationships were considered less relevant.

Childhood- vs. adult-onset disability

Schulz (2005a) identified a distinct difference in how some of the participants in her study made meaning of spirituality, particularly between participants who had a childhood-onset disability and those with an adult-onset disability. Participants with a childhood-onset disability framed their meaning of spirituality around a connection to a higher being and that relationship as a central force in shaping their understanding about disability and life.

Participants with an adult-onset disability made meaning of spirituality through more personal avenues of expression. The meaning of a higher power shifted from an intrinsic and central focus to an entity that a person may connect with as he or she would connect with others and the world. The emphasis of spirituality in this instance is first on connecting the self to spirituality through personal feelings and then expressing that spirituality through actions and making further connections to a higher being, others, and the world.

Meaning of Spiritual and Occupational Engagement

The interconnection and intersection among context, occupations, and meaning making culminate in a discussion of how people dealing with life challenges have engaged in select occupations related to spirituality and have used that spirituality to make meaning of their lives and attend to life challenges. Three articles that addressed this interconnection were found in the literature (Table 6.6). This limited but important collection of articles suggests some interplay among engagement in occupations, empowerment and ability to make meaning of lived experiences, and meaning making of spiritual experiences within the context of life challenges.

Spiritually related occupations

Beagan and Etowa (2011) interviewed 41 African Nova Scotian women who experienced racism and

Table 6.6. Meaning of Spiritual and Occupational Engagement

Context/ Author/Link	Population	Theme	Spirituality Defined by Participants	Spirituality Defined by Author
Racism and oppression (Beagan & Etowa, 2011) http://bit.ly/ 1RmxJ2G	African Nova Scotian women (mean age, 51 years; *n* = 41)	Experiencing racism Occupations related to spirituality Meanings and functions of spiritually related occupations	Spiritual occupations include bible reading, formal relationship with a church community, volunteering, and private and solitary activities (e.g., prayer, meditation, singing, listening to music).	Spiritual occupations were those that were identified as such by the participants (primarily religious pursuits; p. 278).
Aging and autonomy loss (Griffith, Caron, Desrosiers, & Thibeault, 2007) http://bit.ly/ 1UZ2Ksp	Community-dwelling older adults with autonomy loss (*n* = 6 women ages 67–89 years; *n* = 2 men ages 70 and 72 years)	Identity and meaningful occupations Adjusting identity in the context of loss and autonomy Social aspects of adjusting identity Psychological aspects of adjusting identity Spiritual aspects of adjusting identity Engagement in life	Spirituality is related to religion, although the two are not exactly the same. Religion focuses on how to live morally correct lives; spirituality refers to a belief in a greater power that has a positive influence on people. Prayer and meditation are means to connect with this greater power.	The authors did not define *spirituality* and instead offered the following explanation to the participants: "The word *spirituality* seems to mean different things to different people. Tell me how you would define the word *spirituality*" (p. 82).
Schizophrenia (Smith & Suto, 2012) http://bit.ly/ 1JIBoWW	People with schizophrenia ages 39–59 years with length of illness 7–40 years (*n* = 9)	Religious or spiritual practices: Doing to nurture spirituality Religious or spiritual agency: Freedom to think in spiritual terms	Not defined	Core dimensions of spirituality were identified: Religious/spiritual (R/S) practices are activities that nurture spirituality. R/S principles are beliefs/ value statements adopted from surrounding societal discourse. R/S agency is the sense of freedom to choose among the spiritual options in the public discourse. Psychotic R/S experiences are not deliberately sought out and when articulated to others require an explanation. R/S role taking is a means to represent spirituality to others.

oppression and asked the women to share their meaning of their valued occupations. In the study, the authors first identified the occupations that participants found meaningful. Select activities were then identified as spiritually related occupations and were predominantly religious-based activities. These activities included Bible reading, having a formal relationship with a church community and engaging in church social events, volunteering, and engaging in private and solitary activities (e.g., prayer, meditation, singing, listening to music). Beagan and Etowa stated that although church-related activities and spirituality-related occupations brought support to the women, the value of the occupations was in the connection to others and in their own personal meaning making.

The authors noted that the spiritual occupations were key to surviving racism for the women, stating "For these particular women, spiritual resources and occupations were key not only to living a moral life, but to surviving racism" (p. 285). They found that spirituality and engagement in spirituality provide not only the ability to cope with ongoing challenges but the strength to overcome them. Study results highlighted the intersection of engaging in spirituality and spiritually related occupations and reconstructing personal meaning and beliefs.

Spiritual occupations valued but not central

One article in this subcategory of literature highlighted that spiritual occupations are valued but not central to the engagement of occupations and meaning construction. Griffith et al. (2007) identified the spiritual aspect of occupation, identity, and adaption as perceived by community-dwelling elderly who have lost autonomy through their inability to carry out previously valued occupations. The participants identified prayer and meditation as their primary spiritual activities and related the importance of these activities in their daily lives; however, spiritual occupations were not central to their meaning of occupations (i.e., how they made sense of all of their other occupations in light of the spiritual occupations) or central to their identity.

Nevertheless, study participants described a "transpersonal dimension" of spirituality, which was the "connection to a reality beyond the human condition" (p. 88). In addition, "the ability [of spirituality]

to positively transform lives was central to the experience of the study participants" (p. 88). Like the study by Beagan and Etowa (2011), the study by Griffith et al. underscores aspects of transpersonal and transcendent being as connected with spirituality, meaning making of challenging life situations, and engagement in occupations.

Smith and Suto (2012) echoed the doing of spiritual or religious practices with people with schizophrenia. Engaging in centering prayer, communal prayers, and meditation nurtured spirituality and brought emotional equilibrium and a sense of respect and hope to these people. Additionally, the authors noted that the participants experienced *spiritual agency,* or the freedom to think in spiritual terms as a result of engaging in religious and spiritual practices.

Next Steps

What people actually do within the occupations associated with spirituality is not completely described in much of the occupational therapy literature beyond descriptions of occupations such as praying, meditating, reading sacred texts, and attending church services. Therefore, Hocking (2009) encouraged occupational therapy practitioners to conduct further research to expand their knowledge about the meaning of occupations to better understand what is really involved in an occupation and the depth of the occupation. She stated,

> Enhanced knowledge of occupations will inform occupational therapists by explicating the meaning, demands, and context of their clients' occupations, better equipping therapists to use occupation therapeutically. Informed by well-founded knowledge that exceeds personal experience, therapists will be altered to the situated meanings of occupations that vary across gender, generations, and cultures. Thus informed, therapists will be better placed to make decisions about supporting continued engagement or supporting withdrawal from an occupation. (p. 148)

Practitioners need to be cautious about how they understand and use occupations within intervention and as they conduct occupational profiles with clients. In particular, practitioners must be sensitive to the various ways people understand spirituality, what occupations or aspects of occupations people consider to be spiritual, and the meaning derived from those spiritual occupations.

Occupational therapy practitioners need to consider meaning making within the client's personal temporal and developmental contexts. In other words, beyond understanding the actual occupations people engage in (Hocking 2009), practitioners also need to understand the life stage and perspective of the client engaged in an occupation as he or she makes meaning of that occupation. Nelson (1988) defined ***occupational form*** as consisting of "an objective set of circumstances, independent of and external to a person" (p. 633) that can be used to describe select occupations. He further espoused the idea that meaning making is connected to occupational form. Meaning making, however, is understood in retrospect, is time specific, and interrelated to a person's developmental structure. Nelson stated that "meaning is constituted by the interaction between occupational form and the individual's developmental history (a 'looking back")" and that "meaning involves reflection" (p. 636).

Points of time or levels of occupations (Nelson, 1988) provide varying personal interpretations of meaning and need to be considered to understand the empirical literature on meaning and engagement in occupations. More precisely, as practitioners read about study participants making meaning of a select occupation or occupations, or making meaning of spirituality or their personal life challenges, they should ask themselves at what point did that meaning occur and did it change over time or will it change in the future? For example, Table 6.5 provides information, although limited, about the time frame of participants' meaning making about their lived experiences. The implications for understanding, interpreting, and applying the results of empirical literature are a better appreciation for the dynamic personal and temporal contexts in the process of meaning making.

Occupational therapy practitioners need to better understand how transformation occurs and how it affects meaning making within the scope of practice. The reviewed literature suggests that the engagement in occupations has a bearing on how a person makes meaning of life and modifies or changes his

or her meaning of experiences or life (Beagan & Etowa, 2011; Boswell et al., 2001; Griffith et al., 2007; Vrkljan & Miller-Polgar, 2001). Additionally, as part of the occupational therapy process, meaning perspectives and schemes can be reframed and reordered to facilitate images of hope and purpose (Hasselkus, 2002; Heuchemer & Josephsson, 2006; Mattingly & Fleming, 1994; Ramugondo, 2005; Simó-Algado & Burgman, 2005; Townsend & Polatajko, 2007). The empirical occupational therapy literature lacks an explicit explanation of how meaning making occurs in real-world situations and practice scenarios and how to facilitate meaning making through occupational therapy intervention.

Lastly, the limited, but important studies focusing on the meaning of spirituality as perceived by people with disabilities need to be considered in light of the definitions of spirituality that researchers established for their studies (see Table 6.5). The definitions of spirituality provided, or not provided, by the researchers to the participants may have potentially influenced the responses received and the final data analyzed. Although some authors indicated that the description of spirituality came from the participants and was part of the data analysis (Beauregard, & Solomon, 2005; Humbert et al., 2013), one study provided no definition of spirituality to participants (Schwarz & Fleming Cottrell, 2007) and one asked participants for their definitions while still providing a description of spirituality (Wilding et al., 2005). These various methodological decisions may have potentially biased the participants' responses or the final data analysis.

Summary

The construct of spirituality within the occupational therapy literature is diverse, and even when focused attention is given to one aspect, such as phenomenology, the intricacies are considerable. The literature reviewed, particularly the empirical literature, puts a premium on the intersection of occupational engagement and self-identity formation or the evolution of self-identity. Meaning is associated with this intersection; however, spirituality may or may not be associated with that meaning.

When spirituality is connected to the intersection of occupational engagement and self- or community identity, it is either understood in the context of how a person engages in occupations that are considered spiritual or religious practices or makes sense of life challenges through the engagement of occupations. The focus in these instances is on personal context and the use of select occupations.

What is not clear from this literature review is how spirituality is understood beyond phenomenology. For example, if spirituality is understood to encompass a cosmological viewpoint, how and when does this occur and how might it be affected (or not) by the occupations engaged in? If spirituality is associated with multiple ways of knowing (epistemology), how do occupations and the engagement in occupations highlight such experiences? What might the implications be for occupational science and occupational therapy practice? To answer these questions, occupational therapy must carry out ongoing analysis of topics such as the theoretical underpinnings of spirituality, continue dialogue about the multiple aspects of spirituality presented in the literature, and conduct research to further extrapolate the multiple constructs of spirituality and the engagement of occupations.

References

Allen, J. M., Kellegrew, D. H., & Jaffe, D. (2000). The experience of pet ownership as a meaningful occupation. *Canadian Journal of Occupational Therapy. 67,* 271–278. http://dx.doi.org/10.1177/000841740006700409

American Occupational Therapy Association. (2011). The role of occupational therapy in end-of-life care. *American Journal of Occupational Therapy, 65*(Suppl.), S66–S75. http://dx.doi.org/10.5014/ajot.2011.65S66

American Occupational Therapy Association. (2014). The occupational therapy practice framework: Domain and process (3rd ed.). *American Journal of Occupational Therapy, 68*(Suppl. 1), S1–S48. http://dx.doi.org/10.5014/ajot.2014.682006

Aubin, G., Hachey, R., & Mercier C. (1999). Meaning of daily activities and subjective quality of life in people with severe mental health illness. *Scandinavian Journal of Occupational Therapy, 6,* 53–62. http://dx.doi.org/10.1080/110381299443744

Baker, L. M. (2008). A spring of hope: Fostering new life. *International Journal of Disability, Development and Education, 55,* 189–190. http://dx.doi.org/10.1080/10349120802033709

Beagan, B. L., & Etowa, J. B. (2011). The meaning and functions of occupations related to spirituality for African Nova Scotian women. *Journal of Occupational Science, 18,* 277–290. http://dx.doi.org/10.1080/14427591.2011.594548

Beauregard, C., & Solomon, P. (2005). Understanding the experience of HIV/AIDS for women: Implications for occupational therapists. *Canadian Journal of Occupational Therapy, 72,* 113–120. http://dx.doi.org/10.1177/000841740507200206

Boswell, B., Hamer, M., Knight, S., Glacoff, M., & McChesney, J. (2007). Dance of disability and spirituality. *Journal of Rehabilitation, 73,* 33–40.

Boswell, B. B., Knight, S., & Hamer, M. (2001). Disability and spirituality: Reciprocal relationships with the implications for the rehabilitation process. *Journal of Rehabilitation, 67*(4), 20–25. http://connection.ebscohost.com/c/articles/5711101/disability-spirituality-reciprocal-relationship-implications-rehabilitation-process

Boyt Schell, B. A., Gillen, G., & Scaffe, M. (Eds.). (2014). *Willard and Spackman's occupational therapy* (12th ed.). Philadelphia: Lippincott Williams & Wilkins.

Christiansen, C. (1999). Defining lives: Occupation as identity: An essay on competence, coherence, and the creation of meaning [Eleanor Clark Slagle Lecture]. *American Journal of Occupational Therapy, 6,* 544–558. http://dx.doi.org/10.5014/ajot.53.6.547

Christiansen, C. H., Baum, M. C., & Bass-Haugen, J. (Eds.). (2005). *Occupational therapy: Performance, participation, and well-being.* Thorofare, NJ: Slack.

Cipriani, J. (2010). Experience and meaning of group altruistic activities among long-term care residents. *British Journal of Occupational Therapy, 73,* 269–276. http://dx.doi.org/10.4276/030802210X12759925468989

Collins, M. (1998). Occupational therapy and spirituality: Reflecting on quality of experience in therapeutic interventions. *British Journal of Occupational Therapy, 61,* 280–285. http://dx.doi.org/10.1177/030802269806100614

Collins, M. (2004). Dreaming and occupation. *British Journal of Occupational Therapy, 67,* 96–98. http://dx.doi.org/10.1177/030802260406700207

Collins, M. (2007). Spiritual emergency and occupational identity: A transpersonal experience. *British Journal of Occupational Therapy, 70,* 504–519. http://dx.doi.org/10.1177/030802260707001202

do Rozario, L. (1994). Ritual, meaning, and transcendence: The role of occupation in modern life. *Journal of Occupational Science, 1,* 46–53. http://dx.doi.org/10.1080/14427591.1994.9686385

Eklund, M., Erlandsson, L., & Persson, D. (2003). Occupational value among individuals with long-term mental illness. *Canadian Journal of Occupational Therapy, 70,* 276–284. http://dx.doi.org/10.1177/000841740307000504

Fieldhouse, J. (2003). The impact of an allotment group on mental health clients' health, wellbeing, and social networking. *British Journal of Occupational Therapy, 66,* 286–296. http://dx.doi.org/10.1177/030802260306600702

Frank, G., Bernardo, C. S., Tropper, S., Noguchi, F., Lipman, C., Maulhardt, B., & Weitze, L. (1997). Jewish spirituality through actions in time: Daily occupations of a young Orthodox Jewish couple in Los Angeles. *American Journal of Occupational Therapy, 57,* 199–206. http://dx.doi.org/10.5014/ajot.51.3.199

Froehlich, J., & Nelson, D. L. (1986). Affective meaning of life review through activities and discussion. *American Journal of Occupational Therapy, 40,* 27–33. http://dx.doi.org/10.5014/ajot.40.1.27

Greenberg, N. S. (2003). Spiritual spontaneity. *Occupational Therapy in Mental Health, 19,* 153–189. http://dx.doi.org/10.1300/J004v19n03_15

Griffith, J., Caron, C. D., Desrosiers, J., & Thibeault, R. (2007). Defining spirituality and giving meaning to occupation: The perspective of community-dwelling older adults and autonomy loss. *Canadian Journal of Occupational Therapy, 74,* 78–90. http://dx.doi.org/10.2182/cjot.06.0016

Hannam, D. (1997). More than a cup of tea: Meaning construction in an everyday occupation. *Journal of Occupational Science, 4,* 69–74. http://dx.doi.org/10.1080/14427591.1997.9686423

Hasselkus, B. R. (2002). *The meaning of everyday occupation.* Thorofare, NJ: Slack.

Helbig, K., & McKay, E. (2003). An exploration of addictive behaviours from an occupational perspective. *Journal of Occupational Science, 10,* 140–145. http://dx.doi.org/10.1080/14427591.2003.9686521

Heuchemer, B., & Josephsson, S. (2006). Leaving homelessness and addiction: Narratives of an occupational transition. *Scandinavian Journal of Occupational Therapy, 13,* 160–169. http://dx.doi.org/10.1080/11038120500360648

Hinojosa, J., & Blount, M.-L. (2014). Occupation, activities, and occupational therapy. In J. Hinojosa & M.-L. Blount (Eds.), *The texture of life: Occupations and related activities* (4th ed., pp. 1–16). Bethesda, MD: AOTA Press.

Hocking, C. (1997). Person–object interaction model: Understanding the use of everyday objects. *Journal of Occupational Science, 4,* 27–45. http://dx.doi.org/10.1080/14427591.1997.9686418

Hocking, C. (2000). Occupational science: A stock take of accumulated insights. *Journal of Occupational Science, 7,* 58–67. http://dx.doi.org/10.1080/14427591.2000.9686466

Hocking, C. (2005). *The 2004 Francis Rutherford Lecture: Evidence from the past.* http://www.otnz.co.nz/assets/Uploads/pdfs/Awards/FRLA/FRLA-2004-ClareHocking.pdf *New Zealand Journal of Occupational Therapy, 52,* 4–16.

Hocking, C. (2009). The challenge of occupation: Describing the things people do. *Journal of Occupational Science 16,* 140–150. http://dx.doi.org/10.1080/14427591.2009.9686655

Humbert, T. K., Bess, J. L., & Mowery, A. M. (2013). Exploring women's perspectives of overcoming intimate partner violence: A phenomenological study. *Occupational Therapy in Mental Health, 29,* 246–265. http://dx.doi.org/10.1080/0164212x.2013.819465

Hvalsøe, B., & Josephsson, S. (2003). Characteristics of meaningful occupations from the perspective of mentally ill people. *Scandinavian Journal of Occupational Therapy, 10,* 61–71. http://dx.doi.org/10.1080/11038120310009489

Ivarsson, A., & Müllersdorf, M. (2009). Occupation as described by occupational therapy students in Sweden: A follow-up study. *Scandinavian Journal of Occupational Therapy, 16,* 57–64. http://dx.doi.org/10.1080/11038120802570845

Iwama, M. K. (2006). *The Kawa model: Culturally relevant occupational therapy.* Philadelphia: Churchill Livingstone/Elsevier.

Iwama, M. K. (2007). Culture and occupational therapy: Meeting the challenge of relevance in a global world. *Occupational Therapy International, 14,* 183–187. http://dx.doi.org/10.1002/oti.234

Iwama, M., Thomson, N., & MacDonald, R. (2009). The Kawa model: The power of culturally responsive occupational therapy. *Disability and Rehabilitation, 31,* 1125–1135. http://dx.doi.org/10.1080/09638280902773711

Jackson, J., Carlson, M., Mandel, D., Zemke, R., & Clark, F. (1998). Occupation in lifestyle redesign: The well elderly study occupational therapy program. *American Journal of Occupational Therapy, 52,* 326–336. http://dx.doi.org/10.5014/ajot.52.5.326

Jonasson, I., Marklund, B., & Hildingh, C. (2007). Working in a training garden: Experiences of patients with neurological damage. *Australian Occupational Therapy Journal, 54,* 266–272. http://dx.doi.org/10.1111/j.1440-1630.2007.00634.x

Kang, C. (2003). A psychospiritual integration frame of reference for occupational therapy. Part 1: Conceptual foundations. *Australian Occupational Therapy Journal, 50,* 92–103. http://dx.doi.org/10.1046/j.1440-1630.2003.00358.x

Kirsh, B. (1996). A narrative approach to addressing spirituality in occupational therapy: Exploring personal meaning and purpose. *Canadian Journal of Occupational Therapy, 63,* 55–61. http://dx.doi.org/10.1177/000841749606300107

Kroeker, P. T. (1997). Spirituality and occupational therapy in a secular culture. *Canadian Journal of Occupational Therapy, 64,* 122–126. http://dx.doi.org/10.1177/000841749706400308

Lloyd, C., & O'Connor, C. (2007). Integrating spirituality into mental health rehabilitation. *International Journal of Therapy and Rehabilitation, 14,* 168–172.

Lloyd, C., Wong, S. R., & Petchkovsky, L. (2007). Art and recovery in mental health: A qualitative investigation. *British Journal of Occupational Therapy, 70,* 207–214. http://dx.doi.org/10.1177/030802260707000505

Lorenzo, T. (2003). No African renaissance without disabled women: A communal approach to human development in Cape Town, South Africa. *Disability and Society, 18,* 759–778. http://dx.doi.org/10.1080/0968759032000119505

Luboshitzky, D. (2008). Exploring the spiritual meaning of suffering: A strategy of self-help, recovery, and hope. *Occupational Therapy in Health Care, 22,* 21–38. http://dx.doi.org/10.1080/J003v22n01_03

Luboshitzky, D., & Gaber, L. B. (2001). Holidays and celebrations as a spiritual occupation. *Australian Occupational Therapy Journal, 48,* 66–74. http://dx.doi.org/10.1046/j.1440-1630.2001.00251.x

Lyons, M., Orozovic, N., Davis, J., & Newman, J. (2002). Doing–being–becoming: Occupational experiences of persons with life-threatening illnesses. *American Journal of Occupational Therapy, 56,* 285–295. http://dx.doi.org/10.5014/ajot.56.3.285

MacGillivray, P. S., Sumsion, T., & Wicks-Nicholls, J. (2006). Critical elements of spirituality as identified by adolescent mental health clients. *Canadian Journal of Occupational Therapy, 73,* 295–302. http://dx.doi.org/10.2182/cjot.06.006

Mack, S. (2002). Where the rainbow speaks and catches the sun: An occupational therapist discovers her true colors. *Occupational Therapy in Mental Health, 17*(3–4), 43–58. http://dx.doi.org/10.1300/J004v17n03_04

Mattingly, C., & Fleming, M. (1994). *Clinical reasoning: Forms of inquiry in a therapeutic practice.* Philadelphia: F. A. Davis.

McColl, M. A. (2000). Spirit, occupation and disability. *Canadian Journal of Occupational Therapy, 67,* 217–228. http://dx.doi.org/10.1177/000841740006700403

McColl, M. A., (2011). *Spirituality and occupational therapy* (2nd ed.). Ottawa, ON: CAOT Publications.

McCuaig, M., & Frank, G. (1991). The able self: Adaptive patterns and choices in independent living for a person with cerebral palsy. *American Journal of Occupational Therapy, 45,* 224–234. http://dx.doi.org/10.5014/ajot.45.3.224

Moyers, P. A. (1997). Occupational meanings and spirituality: The quest for sobriety. *American Journal of Occupational Therapy, 51,* 207–214. http://dx.doi.org/10.5014/ajot.51.3.207

Moylan, M. M., Carey, L. B., Blackburn, R., Hayes, R., & Robinson, P. (2015). The Men's Shed: Providing biopsychosocial and spiritual support. *Journal of Religion and Health. 54,* 221–234. http://dx.doi.org/10.1007/s10943-013-9804-0

Nelson, D. (1988). Occupation: Form and performance. *American Journal of Occupational Therapy, 42,* 633–641. http://dx.doi.org/10.5014/ajot.42.10.633

Peloquin, S. M. (1997). Nationally Speaking—The spiritual depth of occupation: Making worlds and making lives. *American Journal of Occupational Therapy, 51,* 167–168. http://dx.doi.org/10.5014/ajot.51.3.167

Pentland, W., & McColl, M. A. (2011). Occupational choice. In M. A. McColl (Ed.), *Spirituality and occupational therapy* (2nd ed., pp. 141–149). Ottawa, ON: CAOT Publications.

Pereira, R. B., & Stagnitti, K. (2008). The meaning of leisure for well-elderly Italians in the Australian community: Implications for occupational therapy. *Australian Occupational Therapy Journal, 55,* 39–46. http://dx.doi.org/10.1111/j.1440-1630.2006.00653.x

Persson, D., Erlandsson, L., Eklund, M., & Iwarsson, S. (2001). Value dimensions, meaning, and complexity in human occupation—A tentative structure for analysis. *Scandinavian Journal of Occupational Therapy, 8,* 7–18. http://dx.doi.org/10.1080/11038120119727

Phelan, S., & Kinsella, E. A., (2009). Occupational identity: Engaging sociocultural perspectives. *Journal of Occupational Science, 16,* 85–91. http://dx.doi.org/10.1080/14427591.2009.9686647

Pizzi, M. A., & Briggs, R. (2004). Occupational and physical therapy in hospice: The facilitation of meaning, quality of life, and well-being. *Topics in Geriatric Rehabilitation, 20,* 120–130. http://dx.doi.org/10.1097/00013614-200404000-00007

Ramugondo, E. L. (2005). Unlocking spirituality: Play as a health-promoting occupation in the context of HIV/AIDS. In F. Kronenberg, S. A. Algado, & N. Pollard (Eds.), *Occupational therapy without borders: Learning from the spirit of survivors* (pp. 313–325). New York: Elsevier/Churchill Livingstone.

Rebeiro, K. L., Day, D., Semeniuk, B., O'Brien, M., & Wilson, B. (2001). Northern initiative for social action: An occupational-based mental health program. *American Journal of Occupational Therapy, 55,* 493–500. http://dx.doi.org/10.5014/ajot.55.5.493

Reid, D. (2010). Mundane occupations: Providing opportunity for engagement and being-in-the-world. *OT NOW, 12,* 24–26. https://www.highbeam.com/doc/1P3-2052345451.html

Romanoff, B. D., & Thompson, B. E. (2006). Meaning construction in palliative care: The use of narrative, ritual, and the expressive arts. *American Journal of Hospice and Palliative Care, 23,* 309–316. http://dx.doi.org/10.1177/1049909106290246

Rudman, D. L., & Dennhardt, S. (2008). Shaping knowledge regarding occupation: Examining the cultural underpinnings of the evolving concept of occupational identity. *Australian Occupational Therapy Journal, 55,* 153–162. http://dx.doi.org/10.1111/j.1440-1630.2007.00715.x

Sakellariou, D., & Simó-Algado S. (2006). Sexuality and occupational therapy: Exploring the link. *British Journal of Occupational Therapy, 69,* 350–356. http://dx.doi.org/10.1177/030802260606900802

Schmid, T. (2004). Meanings of creativity within occupational therapy practice. *Australian Occupational Therapy Journal, 51,* 80–88. http://dx.doi.org/10.1111/j.1440-1630.2004.00434.x

Schoessow, K. A. (2010) Shifting from compensation to participation: A model for occupational therapy in low vision. *British Journal of Occupational Therapy, 73,* 160–169. http://dx.doi.org/10.4276/030802210X12706313443947

Schulz, E. K. (2005a). The meaning of spirituality for individuals with disabilities. *Disability and Rehabilitation, 27,* 1283–1295. http://dx.doi.org/10.1080/09638280500076319

Schulz, E. K. (2005b). Spirituality and disability: An analysis of select themes. *Occupational Therapy in Health Care, 18,* 57–83. http://dx.doi.org/10.1080/J003v18n04_05

Schwarz, L., & Fleming Cottrell, R. P. (2007). *Physical and Occupational Therapy in Geriatrics, 26,* 43–61. http://dx.doi.org/10.1300/J148v26n01_04

Shearsmith-Farthing, K. (2001). The management of the altered body image: A role for occupational therapy. *British Journal of Occupational Therapy, 64,* 387–392. http://dx.doi.org/10.1177/030802260106400803

Simó-Algado, S., & Burgman, I. (2005). Occupational therapy intervention with children survivors of war. In F. Kronenberg, S. A. Algado, & N. Pollard (Eds.), *Occupational therapy without borders: Learning from the spirit of survivors* (pp. 313–325). New York: Elsevier/Churchill Livingstone.

Simó-Algado, S., Mehta, N., Kronenberg, F., Cockburn, L., & Kirsh, B. (2002). Occupational therapy intervention with children survivors of war. *Canadian Journal of Occupational Therapy, 69,* 205–218. http://dx.doi.org/10.1177/000841740206900405

Smith, S. (2008). Toward a flexible framework for understanding spirituality. *Occupational Therapy in Health Care, 22,* 39–54. http://dx.doi.org/10.1080/J003v22n01_04

Smith, S., & Suto, M. J. (2012). Religious and/or spiritual practices: Extending spiritual freedom to people with schizophrenia. *Canadian Journal of Occupational Therapy, 79,* 77–85. http://dx.doi.org/10.2182/cjot.2012.79.2.3

Smith-Gabai, H., & Ludwig, F. (2011). Observing the Jewish Sabbath: A meaningful restorative ritual for modern times. *Journal of Occupational Science, 18,* 347–355. http://dx.doi.org/10.1080/14427591.2011.595891

Stadnyk, R. L. (2011). Canadian contributions to the field of occupational science. *Journal of Occupational Science, 18,* 193–194. http://dx.doi.org/10.1080/14427591.2011.594547

Thibeault, R. (1997). A funeral for my father's mind: A therapist's attempt at grieving. *Canadian Journal of Occupational Therapy, 64,* 107–114. http://dx.doi.org/10.1177/000841749706400306

Thompson, B. E., & MacNeil, C. (2006). A phenomenological study exploring the meaning of a seminar on spirituality for occupational therapy students. *American Journal of Occupational Therapy, 60,* 531–539. http://dx.doi.org/10.5014/ajot.60.5.531

Townsend, E. A., & Polatajko, H. J. (2007). *Enabling occupation II: Advancing an occupational therapy vision for health, well-being and justice through occupation.* Ottawa, ON: CAOT Publications.

Tse, S., Lloyd, C., Petchkovsky, L., & Manaia, W. (2005). Exploration of Australian and New Zealand indigenous people's spirituality and mental health. *Australian Occupational Therapy Journal, 52,* 181–187. http://dx.doi.org/10.1111/j.1440-1630.2005.00507.x

Tzanidaki, D., & Reynolds, F. (2011). Exploring the meaning of making traditional arts and crafts among older women in Crete, using interpretative phenomenological analysis. *British Journal of Occupational Therapy, 74,* 375–382. http://dx.doi.org/10.4276/030802211X13125646370852

Unruh, A. M., & Elvin, N. (2004). In the eye of the dragon: Women's experience of breast cancer and the occupation of dragon boat racing. *Canadian Journal of Occupational Therapy, 71,* 138–149. http://dx.doi.org/10.1177/000841740407100304

Unruh, A. M., Smith, N., & Scammell, C. (2000). The occupation of gardening in life-threatening illness: A qualitative pilot project. *Canadian Journal of Occupational Therapy, 67,* 70–77. http://dx.doi.org/10.1177/000841740006700110

Urbanowski, R., & Vargo, J. (1994). Spirituality, daily practice, and the occupational performance model. *Canadian Journal of Occupational Therapy, 61,* 88–94. http://dx.doi.org/10.1177/000841749406100204

Vrkljan, B., & Miller-Polgar, J. (2001). Meaning of occupational engagement in life-threatening illness: A qualitative pilot project. *Canadian Journal of Occupational Therapy, 68,* 237–246. http://dx.doi.org/10.1177/000841740106800407

Watson, R. (2006). Being before doing: The cultural identity (essence) of occupational therapy. *Australian Occupational*

Therapy Journal, 53, 151–158. http://dx.doi.org/10.1111/j. 1440-1630.2006.00598.x

Wilcock, A. A., & Townsend, E. A. (2014). Occupational justice. In B. A. Boyt Schell, G. Gillen, & M. Scaffa (Eds.), *Willard and Spackman's occupational therapy* (12th ed., pp. 541–552). Philadelphia: Lippincott Williams & Wilkins.

Wilding, C. (2007). Spirituality as sustenance for mental health and meaningful doing: A case illustration. *Medical Journal of Australia, 186*(10), S67–S69. http://1.usa.gov/1Rmg3nA

Wilding, C., May, E., & Muir-Cochrane, E. (2005). Experience of spirituality, mental illness and occupation: A life-sustaining phenomenon. *Australian Occupational Therapy Journal, 52,* 2–9. http://dx.doi.org/10.1111/j.1440-1630.2005.00462.x

Williams, B. J. (2008). An exploratory study of older adults' perspectives of spirituality. *Occupational Therapy in Health Care, 22,* 3–19. http://dx.doi.org/10.1080/J003v22n01_02

Wilson, L. (2011). Occupational analysis and spirituality. In L. Mackenzie & G. O'Toole (Eds.), *Occupational analysis in practice* (pp. 53–65). Hoboken, NJ: Wiley-Blackwell.

World Federation of Occupational Therapists. (2012). *Definition of occupation.* Retrieved from http://www.wfot.org/aboutus/aboutoccupationaltherapy/definitionofoccupationaltherapyaspx

Zecevic, A., Magalhaes, L., Madady, M., Halliagan, M., & Reeves, A. (2010). Happy and healthy only if occupied? Perceptions of health sciences students on occupation in later life. *Australian Occupational Therapy Journal, 57,* 17–23. http://dx.doi.org/10.1111/j.1440-1630.2009.00841.x

CHAPTER 7.

SPIRITUALITY IN OCCUPATIONAL THERAPY: A CONCEPTUAL MODEL FOR PRACTICE

Tamera Keiter Humbert, MA, OTD, OTR/L

Chapter Highlights

✧ Questions to consider about spirituality and practice
✧ Spirituality in occupational therapy
✧ Occupational therapy literature related to spirituality and the therapeutic process
✧ Putting it together: Four aspects of spirituality in occupational therapy practice
✧ Thoughts on and critique of the model.

Key Terms and Concepts

✧ Cultivating spiritual practices
✧ Goal setting
✧ Honor and respect
✧ Identity formation and strength
✧ Incorporated spirituality
✧ Just-right challenge
✧ Life meaning activities
✧ Life meaning and purpose
✧ Meaningful activities
✧ Occupational integrity
✧ Occupational meaning and choice
✧ Occupations of the spirit

✧ Reframing narratives
✧ Religious beliefs
✧ Resilience
✧ Religious, faith, and spiritual practices
✧ Select occupations and routines
✧ Spiritual meaning
✧ States of being
✧ Theological beliefs
✧ Therapeutic use of self
✧ Volition
✧ Wisdom traditions

The concept of *spirituality* is complex and diverse. Occupational therapy scholars cannot agree on one definition of spirituality, they cannot even agree that spirituality is a topic that should be studied or promoted within the field of occupational therapy, and they are only starting to critique the theoretical perspectives about spirituality espoused in occupational therapy. Therefore, a legitimate question to ask is, Why should a conceptual model of spirituality for occupational therapy practice be proposed? The answer: This model gives voice to the many people who find value in the use of spirituality in practice. It is a way to continue conversations and elicit critiques so occupational therapy may expand on and nurture this aspect of life and practice.

This chapter begins with questions about spirituality in occupational therapy and readers' thoughts about and experiences with this topic. It then briefly reviews constructs related to spirituality and the individual person (or client) as represented in the occupational therapy literature. Finally, the chapter gives an overview of how occupational therapy practitioners have conceptualized the therapeutic process and spirituality. This chapter provides a cursory review of spirituality as it directly applies to practice, allowing readers to consider some fundamental ideas about spirituality and the concrete and pragmatic application of spirituality to occupational therapy.

Spirituality is a wide-ranging topic, relatively new to the occupational therapy profession, and often difficult for many occupational therapy practitioners to understand or embrace. The following phrase embodies the challenges presented by spirituality in occupational therapy practice: "Pinning jelly to the wall takes the right equipment and dedication to conquer the task" (author unknown). However, addressing spirituality's many perspectives will broaden our understanding of it and encourage continued conversations about it.

Questions to Consider About Spirituality and Practice

It is important for occupational therapy practitioners to consider several questions about spirituality and practice. The following three questions are discussed here:

1. Why should spirituality be used in practice?
2. Shouldn't spirituality be left to the professionals?
3. How do you define or describe spirituality?

Why Should Spirituality Be Used in Practice?

Spirituality is becoming more common in mainline culture today, and clients are often interested in incorporating spirituality into their daily lives, especially after a major life crisis (Heinz et al., 2010; Kang, 2003). Because the field of occupational therapy stresses being culturally responsive and providing client-centered care, practitioners need to be aware of that interest (see Chapter 1, "Addressing Spirituality in Occupational Therapy," for a more detailed outline and articulation of this viewpoint).

Should Spirituality Be Left to Chaplains?

Some occupational therapy practitioners may believe that spirituality should be the sole purview of professionals such as ministers, rabbis, priests, mullahs, shamans, humanist counselors, spiritual directors, and chaplains. In addition, according to research (albeit limited) conducted with occupational therapy students and practitioners, many practitioners are reluctant or uncertain about how to address spirituality in therapy. Reasons cited for this reluctance and uncertainty include not wanting to impose personal views on others, not wanting to confuse spirituality with religious beliefs and practices, not understanding how occupational therapy should incorporate spirituality into practice, and not knowing how to document or get reimbursed for such discussions with clients and families (Kirsh, Dawson, Antolikova, & Reynolds, 2001; Thompson & MacNeil, 2006). Nonetheless, many practitioners recognize the value and importance of spirituality in their personal and professional lives (Collins, Paul, & West-Frasier, 2001; Taylor, Mitchell, Kenan, & Tacker, 2000).

How Do You Define or Describe Spirituality?

What images come to mind when you think about spirituality? Figure 7.1 shows images of spirituality as it relates to nature, creative self-expression, seeking truth or enlightenment, and through engagement in valued occupations. If you were to offer your own images for this book, what would they be? Take a few moments to think about the application of these

Figure 7.1. Images of spirituality.

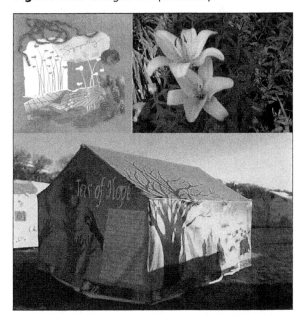

ideas to occupational therapy. How might they be considered important (or not) to the field? Continue the reflection by thinking about spirituality in occupational therapy. Does it have a place or not? If so, how would you picture that actually happening? Have you experienced spiritual moments in your life or in the observance of occupational therapy?

Spirituality in Occupational Therapy

When spirituality is used in occupational therapy, practitioners should consider how clients understand spirituality, including personal beliefs and values, and incorporate clients' perspectives about spirituality into assessment and intervention. Bouthot, Wells, and Black (2011) provided suggestions about how to understand a person's spirituality through the use of the FICA (*f*aith and belief, *i*mportance, *c*ommunity, and *a*ddress in care) Spiritual History Assessment (Puchalski, 1999). Bouthot et al. encouraged occupational therapy practitioners, at least in the medical health care environment, to ask clients questions to better understand their beliefs and faith practices.

Knowing clients' spiritual beliefs can aid in choosing the most effective therapy approaches. For example, Szafran (2011) addressed reducing pain and restoring occupational performance in the elderly. She suggested that practitioners use caution when

approaching older clients about certain contemporary therapies, such as mindfulness training, meditation, and the movement-based activities of tai chi and qigong. These activities may entail aspects of spirituality that might not fit into the spiritual values of some older people. However, Szafran valued spirituality as an occupation. She described spirituality as

> an area of occupation affecting an older person's ability to manage pain. Finding meaning and purpose in defining the quality of life is an occupation that may cause relief from suffering for some older people who encounter changes in their lives that are unplanned, including acquiring a disability, losing support systems, and moving to controlled settings such as nursing homes. (p. CE2)

In the first published book entirely related to spirituality in occupational therapy, McColl (2003) described what assumptions and motivations guided her text. Along with the historical understanding and value of spirituality as described by the Canadian Association of Occupational Therapists (2002), she wrote about the need to explore and understand realms beyond the tangible; deal with issues related to death, pain, suffering, and loss; and attend to spirituality in occupational therapy. These diverse perspectives on spirituality make it harder to pin that jelly to the wall. Additional tools are needed to make sense of spirituality in occupational therapy.

Occupational Therapy Literature Related to Spirituality and the Therapeutic Process

Review Process

Lauren Rossi and Amanda Sedlak (former graduate students at Elizabethtown College, Elizabethtown, PA) and I were interested in broadly understanding spirituality in occupational therapy—going beyond only the definitions espoused by scholars in the field. Therefore, we undertook a systematic literature review of the use of spirituality within the therapeutic process. Because of the differences in the use of the term *spirituality* in occupational therapy (see Appendix 7.A), the search included any publication written in English by an occupational therapy practitioner or researcher. The following words guided the search: *spirituality, spiritual, spirit, religious practice, religious concerns, conceptualization of spirituality,* and *application of spirituality to practice.* We also expanded the search to include *suffering, motivation, therapist development, auto-ethnography,* and *palliative care.*

The expanded search came about for two reasons. First, an article by Egan and Swedersky (2003) described *spirituality* as a concept surrounding suffering and a response to major life challenges. Egan and Swedersky identified the following four themes of how occupational therapy practitioners address spirituality in practice:

1. *Dealing with clients' religious concerns* (practitioners consider clients' use of faith in a higher power to alleviate their suffering)
2. *Addressing clients' suffering* (practitioners believe they have an obligation to meet the needs of clients in distress)
3. *Encouraging the clients' self* (practitioners work to understand the meaning and importance of clients' illnesses or injuries to alleviate suffering and attain well-being, and they discover occupations that enliven clients, or make them happy)
4. *Addressing therapist development* (practitioners reflect on their own experiences and benefits of helping clients).

Second, in exploring how others discussed this subject outside official occupational therapy documents and terminology (see Chapter 2, "Contemporary History of Spirituality and Occupational Therapy," and Chapter 3, "Definitions and Descriptions of Spirituality in Occupational Therapy Literature"), we gleaned the expanded search terms from our initial readings about spirituality and background literature relative to occupational therapy in spirituality.

A total of 88 descriptive articles and texts, published from 1991 to 2011 from the United States, Canada, Australia, Scandinavia, Thailand, and South Africa, were initially reviewed, and 59 articles were considered relevant and included in the preliminary literature review (see Appendix 7.B). We were most interested in the descriptive literature in which practitioners and researchers described specific real-life examples of spirituality used in practice.

We initially found that the literature could be placed into two categories: (1) spirituality as it related directly to the client (spirituality was typically described by the practitioner but sometimes described by both practitioner and client) and (2) spirituality as part of the therapy process.

In later analysis, we used McColl's (2003, 2011) comprehensive description of spirituality and incorporated themes from her work into the themes we initially identified. Last, additional literature from 2011 to 2015 was analyzed and incorporated into the model. The following sections highlight these various perspectives.

Personal Experiences of Spirituality

Our analysis related to personal experiences of spirituality was characterized by a description of spirituality as part of the therapy process, part of the person's daily life, or part of a major life crisis. Personal experiences of spirituality included connections with the self, others, nature, the world, or a higher power and were realized through

- Occupational meaning and choice,
- Life meaning and purpose,
- Volition and resilience,
- Religious and theological beliefs and spiritual meaning, and
- States of being (Figure 7.2).

Occupational meaning and choice

Occupational meaning and choice is experienced by a person through the selection of and engagement in occupations that hold value and importance. Meaning and choice may be articulated and understood through

- Occupational roles,
- Valued activities and rituals,
- Connection to others, and
- Occupational integrity (defined later; see Figure 7.2).

Occupational meaning is dependent on the person's personal interests, routines, and values related to choosing, performing, and engaging in select occupations. In the articles reviewed, clients found meaning through occupational activities such as baking, playing card games, writing in a journal, giving

Figure 7.2. Personal experiences of spirituality.

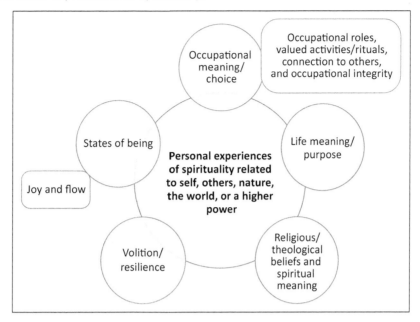

manicures, caring for hair, doing laundry, singing, making jewelry, and washing dishes (Leslie, 2006; Mathis, 1996; Strzelecki, 2009; Whitney, 2010).

For example, Bowen (2006) shared a story of an 87-year-old woman who found particular spiritual meaning through select occupations, routines, and habits when the activities brought her "loving support, the expression and demonstration of caring, interaction, gentle humor and quiet guidance" (p. 48).

Whitney (2010) found that by personally engaging in the occupation of writing, "her spirit was touched" (p. 33). She stated, "For me, writing is an action of my spirit. I have rituals, habits and a writer's lens through which rich moments of life filter into my brain and fall into imaged pages or possible novels or essays or poems" (p. 33). Thibeault (2011d) spoke about the beauty and intensity of rituals that become "ceremonies of life," particularly if they are aligned with grief and loss. In all of these examples, the chosen activities and occupations are generally identified by each person as having spiritual significance and meaning and are integrated into roles and routines.

In an example of reintroducing valued occupations and roles, Ramugondo (2005), an African occupational therapist, shared her perspective of mothers living with a diagnosis of HIV/AIDS. The mothers often saw their children, who were also HIV/AIDS positive, as a "dying being" (p. 319) and subsequently

experienced challenges identifying and connecting with their mother role and their children. However, when the activity of play was reintroduced therapeutically, the mothers could connect with their children and themselves. Through the use of play, the mother "reconnects with her own spirit since spirituality is related to one's understanding of one's role in life" (p. 319).

Although occupational therapy practitioners embrace the idea of engagement in occupations and promote that concept through therapeutic tasks, they also acknowledge that people regularly discover, choose, and engage in occupations that reflect their values and beliefs, give life meaning, and allow them to express the essence of who they are within the context of their life events (Pentland & McColl, 2011). *Occupational integrity* is "integrating into one's occupational choices what matters most" (Pentland & McColl, 2011, p. 142). It is dynamic and often significantly shifts when people are faced with a new disability, injury, or illness or when dealing with a long-term crisis. Therefore, occupational meaning and choice are not stagnant. For example, the simple act of making and enjoying a cup of coffee may shift from a mundane daily task that required little effort or thought before a devastating accident to one that brings a sense of peace and enjoyment when accomplishing the task and through the gratitude in being able to do so.

Life meaning and purpose

Life meaning and purpose reflects the underlying beliefs and assumptions about the reason for existence—for living and being part of the world. For some, thoughts about life meaning and purpose may not be conscious, attended to, articulated, or even considered until a crisis occurs (McColl, 2011). Thibeault (2011a) described people who had to deal with epidemics, extreme poverty, political injustice, violence, and the stigma and rejection related to disability. The meaning that these people gave to their suffering and life provided a deeper understanding of their mission in life and the value of life even in light of extreme challenges.

Work activities, whether paid or unpaid, may fulfill life meaning and purpose. For example, Baptiste (2011) furthered the concept of spirituality by connecting life meaning and purpose to work. She intricately intertwined her own story of how work demands and her professional career started to challenge her own sense of self and purpose. Consequently, she needed to reassess and rediscover her life work and purpose. Although many might see work as just a financial means to maintain and support life, others may find meaning, purpose, and ultimately spirituality through their work.

Volition and resilience

Volition is the intrinsic motivation to engage in and sustain valued life tasks. If volition is lost, it can be regained through extrinsically facilitated occupational therapy intervention. Whether internally or externally facilitated, it is created by accomplishing or completing activities and by gaining confidence that is developed through these successes.

For example, the occupational therapy literature includes descriptions of clients with a terminal illness or physical impairment who have increased motivation to engage in therapy after the occupational therapist and client have collaborated and identified meaningful and successful activities to engage in, such as baking pies and doing typewriter art (Doughton, 1996; Mathis, 1996). These activities, and the ability to engage in them, were explicitly linked to the client's sense of self, volition, and spirituality.

In another example, therapists working with a child with severe burns encouraged the child to replace his own wound dressing, but his initial response was expressed in aggravation and agony (Burns, 2007). Because his pain was so severe, he had little volition to take over this self-care task. After he realized that the occupational therapy team would not budge on this expectation, he began to slowly engage in the task. His increased success with the task and resulting volition eventually became evident as treatment progressed. According to Burns (2007), through the empowerment and volition gained during occupational therapy interventions, the child not only started to incorporate this self-care task into his routines, he "appeared to grow spirituality within the context of the hospital" (p. 3).

In a story depicting a community's response to great loss and grief, volition and *resilience,* or the ability of a person to persevere in extreme situations, were facilitated through engagement in occupations. In 2004, a tsunami devastated southern Thailand. Afterward, many people affected by the destruction felt unmotivated and engaged in only limited occupations as a result of a lack of physical and emotional resources. A group of occupational therapy students intervened by providing group activities, individual occupations, and social interactions. For example, through "dancing, which resulted in relaxation, the participants focused on meaningful occupations, consequently relieving boredom and depression" (Pongsaksri, 2007, p. 32). According to the author, these meaningful occupations served to provide the participants with a spiritual experience through feelings of "excitement, discovery, competence, satisfaction, pride, and awareness of an increase of self-esteem" (Pongsaksri, 2007, p. 32).

Thibeault (2011c) highlighted the concept of resilience to use volition repeatedly and steadily through a process of occupational engagement and transformation. In these examples, spirituality is dynamically associated with both volition and resilience.

Religious and theological beliefs and spiritual meaning

Spirituality might be explicitly connected to the client's religious and theological beliefs. Spiritual meaning may be intertwined with engagement in occupations as well as a personal belief in a higher power or understanding of a universal human spirit.

Religious beliefs. Religious beliefs center on trusting in a higher power to cope with an illness or crisis or connecting with something greater than ourselves. For example, Spencer (2007) wrote about a 54-year-old woman who had a stroke. The woman had conversations with God throughout her grieving process, declaring that she did not want to be confined to a wheelchair the rest of her life. As time and therapy progressed, she was able to thank God each day for her blessings and the small incremental improvements made in therapy. According to the author, through her strong faith, the woman was able to persevere with patience during her recovery. The woman commented, "I've always been a woman of faith. I don't know how people get through life, let alone a major crisis, without God and loving, supportive family and friends" (Spencer, 2007, p. 93).

In another example of spirituality through religious beliefs, a client with spastic paralysis found comfort in communicating with and having a relational understanding of God, that is, he and God communicated with each other. According to Doughton (1996), the client "credits his strength and persistence to faith and trust in God" (p. 19). He also believed that his relationship with God helped him complete select occupations. For example in the occupation of typewriter art, "God provides the pictures while the client punches the typewriter keys" (Doughton, 1996, p. 19). The client's religious faith was the foundation for his values and also gave "structure and meaning to his actions" (Doughton, 1996, p. 19).

Other authors discussed personal experiences of a health or life crisis in which they communicated with God or experienced another presence or realm. These experiences provided not only an avenue to find comfort and hope for the future but also established or reinforced religious beliefs. For example, an occupational therapist with bipolar affective disorder looked to God during manic and depressive episodes. She stated, "Surely God would find a place for me in another world because I have been a special person at one time and may be He would remember that, despite the fact that I clearly did not fit in anymore" (Hatchard & Missiuna, 2003, p. 9).

Theological beliefs.   Religious expressions may be part of the spiritual experience for some people but not for all. According to Rosenfeld (2000), "spirituality does not necessarily imply a belief in God. . . . [R]ecovery frequently requires finding one's spiritual center, [which is defined as] a connection

with God or with the human spirit, one's inner voice, the spirit of love, or valued group" (p. 17). Rosenfeld's examples of spirituality indicate that it encompasses more than the doing of occupations; it is part of a larger conceptualization, appreciation, and understanding of life, which I have labeled *theological beliefs*.

For example, Forhan (2010), an occupational therapist, addressed her theological beliefs after the stillbirth of her son. Although family members found "comfort in prayer and quiet reflection" (Forhan, 2010, p. 148), the mother spoke of her own sense of presence as she felt the baby's spirit during the funeral. According to Forhan, the baby's brother also had a spiritual connection, a "strong connection to his spirituality and a strong belief that there is life after death and that his brother is now an angel" (p. 147).

Spiritual meaning.   Pentland and McColl (2011) furthered discussion of spiritual beliefs to include the concept of *spiritual meaning,* or the way in which people make sense of the events in their lives. They stated, "For some, spiritual meaning is associated with the concept of a higher being and may conform to religions or faith traditions. For others, spiritual meaning derives from a sense of connection—with others, with nature, with the past, present, and future" (p. 147).

States of being

States of being, or the way in which people experience life in the present moment, are also attributed to spirituality within the occupational therapy literature. Although not predominant in the literature, two articles were found that equated emotional or affective responses of a person with engagement in a valued activity or in the completion of a therapeutic goal and with the person's spirituality. These responses included *joy,* or feelings of great delight, and *flow,* the experience of timelessness (see Figure 7.2).

For example, a child displayed extreme happiness and joy after independently completing an activity of daily living (Gavacs, 2009). After struggling for some time to be able to put his shirt on by himself, the child finally accomplished the task successfully. The occupational therapist stated that the child, conveying tremendous joy, began to dance after his success, calling it the "Indepen-dance"

(Gavacs, 2009, p. 32). The therapist stated, "The word *independence* will now be associated with a dance that expresses the spirit of the person, not just a task" (Gavacs, 2009, p. 32, italics added).

Nesbit (2004, 2006), an occupational therapist, described her personal journey through breast cancer treatment and recovery. During this process, she reflected on her experiences and the coping mechanisms that she used to endure and persevere through her treatments and recovery. She used valued occupational activities such as walking, engaging in music and nature, swimming, and painting. She connected with others through socialization, and she found life meaning through humor, attitudes of gratitude and grace, and solitude. The activities she engaged in frequently elicited flow, which provided her with a way to enrich her life during a time of grief and loss. With flow, the author found ordinary, everyday experiences to be spiritual, and through this spirituality, she found meaning in her life.

Conclusions: Personal spirituality review

Although authors in the reviewed occupational therapy literature may have advocated an understanding of personal spirituality through one or more of the constructs discussed, all of these constructs can be considered aspects of a larger concept of spirituality and may also be associated with occupational roles and tasks. It is important to remember that the client comes to therapy sessions with elements of his or her own being and spirituality. These authors, therefore, suggested that, within the therapy process, practitioners work to recognize these aspects of a person, attend to them, and reinforce them so that clients may find new meaning in their lives and hope for the future.

It is also important to understand that these constructs may not apply to all people. For example, some people do not acknowledge or desire to give credence to a higher power or spiritual or theological belief system. Some people may never experience a state of flow, or the other constructs mentioned, but still consider themselves spiritual. Two questions may be asked:

1. Is what we do in occupational therapy spiritual by the inherent nature of what we do, or is spirituality in occupational therapy something unique?
2. Are some therapeutic activities spiritual and others not?

Application to Practice: Occupational Therapy's Role

We reviewed occupational therapy literature that advocated particular assessment or intervention strategies and therapeutic considerations related to spirituality. The process of applying spirituality to practice includes using assessments, observations, and life narratives; providing just-right challenges during intervention and promoting hope and motivation; and thoughtfully using the following occupations: meaningful activities; life meaning activities; religious, faith, and spiritual practices; creative activities; and *occupations of the spirit*—those activities and routines that are intentionally engaged to develop or enhance spirituality (e.g., prayer, meditation, pilgrimage). Finally, encompassing the entire therapeutic process is developing and using the therapeutic use of self (see Figure 7.3).

Using assessments, observations, and life narratives

The evaluation process includes using assessments, observations, and life narratives to obtain information from clients and their significant others that will help guide and facilitate intervention. This information may include the client's personal beliefs, values, interests, and other relevant information. Many authors in the review discussed the importance of addressing spiritual components of the client's life during the initial occupational therapy evaluation.

For example, Feeney and Toth-Cohen (2008) suggested asking questions about the client's spiritual practices and religious affiliations during the initial evaluation. Examples of questions that could be asked during the initial evaluation include,

> What is your faith or belief that gives meaning to your life? What role can your beliefs play in regaining your health? Are you a part of a spiritual or religious community or group that is important to you? How would you like the [occupational therapist] to address these issues in your treatment? (Rosenfeld, 2001b, p. 6)

According to Feeney and Toth-Cohen (2008), Hettinger (1996), and Rosenfeld (2001b), asking questions about spirituality facilitates an open environment and lets clients know that the occupational therapy practitioner is available as a spiritual resource

Figure 7.3. Application to practice: Occupational therapy's role.

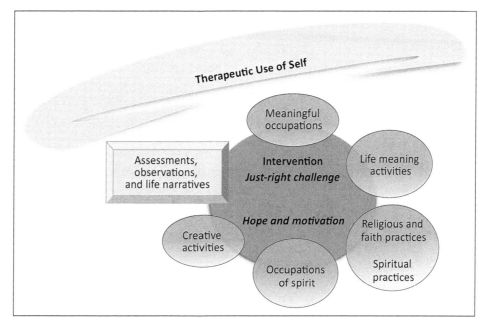

if needed. These authors noted that it is imperative for practitioners to discuss spiritual beliefs with not only the client but also the family and significant others, who may provide important insights about the client. For example, Hettinger stated that "occupational therapists talk to clients and families, find out what is important to them, and help get [the client] back to that" (p. 16). Vrkljan (2000) also suggested that occupational therapy practitioners obtain information about clients through interviews and observations and through reports from significant others.

To tap into the client's spiritual dimension, occupational therapy practitioners need to specifically pay attention to the client's personal beliefs, values, and worldviews. McColl (2011) highlighted the importance of active listening during conversations with a client to engage the client's perspective about his or her disability and issues of awareness, intimacy, trust, vulnerability, and purpose. In addition, according to Hettinger (1996), "occupational therapists should learn to listen, engage the client, find out who they are, and give respect to the essence of the individual" (p. 17).

Greven (2007) discussed the importance of the practitioner obtaining a client's life narrative during his or her initial evaluation and interview and designing and implementing meaningful interventions around this life narrative. In addition, to provide applicable experiences in therapy, it is essential for the practitioner to understand the personal meaning of an intervention activity to a client and the client's perceptions of his or her disability or illness (Rosenfeld, 2001a). Depending on these perceptions, the client's faith or beliefs may influence the treatment process (Rosenfeld, 2001b) and further shape the client's life narrative. Moreover, Burgman and King (2005) stated that for the therapeutic process to be successful, a change must occur in the client's life narrative. This change happens most often when the practitioner understands the stories of the client's life while "remaining cognizant of the power of the client's perceptions" (Burgman & King, 2005, p. 155).

Providing just-right challenges during intervention and promoting hope and motivation

After the evaluation is completed, intervention is considered. The overall arching consideration of this part of the therapy process as it is linked with spirituality is providing just-right challenges during intervention and promoting hope and motivation.

Just-right challenge. The *just-right challenge* involves the practitioner setting goals and providing treatment activities that are appropriate for the client according to the client's strengths, needs, and skill level. It is, at a preliminary level, the ability to find the intricate balance between supporting and challenging the client by using the most applicable therapeutic approach.

Goal setting, an important component of the occupational therapy process, considers the client's skills, abilities, and challenges and promotes the client's commitment to a goal by enhancing the belief that he or she will achieve the goal. Accomplishing the goal further supports the client's motivation and increases self-efficacy (Hoppes, 1997). In selecting appropriate group interventions (e.g., exercise, cooking groups) in which the same therapeutic activities are provided to all of the participants, Radomski (2000) noted, "To improve self-perceptions of efficacy, patients must be grouped according to their proficiencies and therapeutic needs rather than according to profit margin or the occupational therapist's convenience" (p. 2).

In a discussion of sensory integrative treatment and the just-right challenge, Ayres (1998) noted that if a child cannot explore his or her own potential, then the therapist must intervene by aiding, assisting, modifying, or adapting the intervention session to match the child's relative capabilities. By finding a balance between the client's limitations and abilities, the practitioner can engage the client in appropriate and meaningful occupations, facilitate accomplishment and success, improve motivation, and enhance the client's spiritual experience. The just-right challenge is supported elsewhere in the literature, emphasizing that the practitioner must be attentive to the client and learn how to intuitively assess how and when to push or assist the client during intervention (Ayres, 1998; Caracciolo, 1995; Hoppes, 1997; Radomski, 2000).

Promoting hope and motivation.   Promoting hope and motivation is a way for occupational therapy practitioners to provide optimism to and foster motivation in clients by believing in the client's abilities and providing applicable interventions. According to Bowen (1999), Hettinger (1996), and Rosenfeld (2004), practitioners need to promote an optimistic but realistic level of expectation with consumers of occupational therapy. Bowen noted hope as a vital component to the survival of a person. Moreover, Bowen stated that hope is born of the kind of faith that makes people believe that their lives serve an ultimate purpose in the scheme of things. Hafez (1998) and Hettinger (1996) espoused that to

establish hope in a client, the practitioner must help the client identify what assisted him or her in getting through a past crisis and demonstrate how that experience can influence and support current challenges.

Swarbrick and Burkhardt (2000) described hope as "the single impetus for positively changing and improving one's distressing, life threatening situation" (p. 1). When a client is hopeful, the therapy process can produce maximal benefits. According to the literature reviewed, an occupational therapy practitioner serves as an agent of change for the client by providing "positive constructive suggestions and persuasion that can be powerful motivational catalysts to realign spiritual balance" (Swarbrick & Burkhardt, 2000, p. 2). In addition, McColl (2011) highlighted the role of occupational therapy practitioners in fostering and maintaining hope by assisting clients to focus on the future in a positive way.

Thoughtfully using select occupations

As the practitioner and client work on identifying goals and approaches for reaching goals, they also carefully choose activities to implement in therapy. According to the literature reviewed, several types of activities contribute to spirituality, including

* Meaningful activities
* Life meaning activities
* Religious, faith, and spiritual practices
* Creative activities
* Occupations of the spirit.

Meaningful activities.   Meaningful activities used during occupational therapy intervention should reflect the valued occupations and roles of the client. For example, for an adolescent with an intellectual disability who had been in a catatonic state Leslie (2006) chose activities that had meaning before she entered the catatonic state. Mathis (1996) wanted to work on a client's "standing balance, endurance, upper extremity strengthening and reach" (p. 16). Therefore, she used a former valued occupation of the client, baking pecan pies, to make these goals meaningful to her. Allowing a client to choose a meaningful activity to engage in during intervention empowers the client (Strzelecki, 2009). By using activities that are meaningful to the client, practitioners may tap into his or her fundamental essence.

Practitioners may have to come to appreciate that the meaning of an activity for a client may go beyond its everyday meaning. In other words, activities may be symbolic or representative of something greater for the client than what is commonly understood. For example, Peloquin (1997) introduced the idea that self-care activities, such as hair care and grooming, can have meaning for people beyond just a routine task. A client may interpret grooming and hair care as a way to appreciate and love their body or as a way to express their essence or uniqueness. Therefore, these tasks are valuable in therapy because of the positive impact they have on the client.

Rosenfeld (2001a) and Urbanowski (1997) identified daily tasks such as brushing teeth, toileting, dressing, cooking, and grooming activities as having a spiritual and symbolic component. Cooking is not just a way to nourish the body but can also entail a spiritual activity in which inspiration and creativity is explored and experienced. Therefore, use of these daily tasks in therapy goes beyond just completing a valued role; they may foster an inspired or spiritual state of discovery or being.

Thibeault (2011a) provided a glimpse into how practitioners may recognize, bring to light, and support meaningful occupations as clients shift focus and readjust to new life experiences. Thibeault shared the story of her father who was dealing with dementia and how he moved from his past beloved roles and occupations of reading the latest governmental reforms and following the stock exchange to appreciating time spent with grandchildren in completing homework. When necessary, helping clients let go of past activities and take on different occupations can be supported in therapy. Therefore, practitioners should consider not only what the client holds as valuable and helpful in restoring or maximizing function but also what additional activities could be used in therapy to spark a spiritual or meaningful connection for the client.

Life meaning activities. **Life meaning activities** are used therapeutically to discover and make sense of current suffering, trauma, pain, and even the death process (McColl, 2011). For example, while working in a hospice setting, Trump (2001) was able to engage a client in the meaningful occupation of writing letters to her daughter to facilitate reflections about her life. As an active participant in this process, the client "had a sense of accomplishment when the task was completed and a sense of peace from knowing that her daughter would read her words" (Trump, 2001, p. 10) after she passed on. According to Trump, the occupational therapy practitioner can play a crucial role in facilitating a client's life meaning in this type of setting.

Dawson and Stern (2007) and Jung et al. (1999) further explained that occupational therapy practitioners have and continue to play diverse roles in facilitating participation in valued occupations and shaping new life meaning. Practitioners are able to recognize that the "goal [of intervention] is not that [clients] are merely performing disjointed activities but that they are doing personally meaningful occupations that will in turn define the person" (Dawson & Stern, 2007, p. 4). As the person is further defined or self-identity is expanded through the doing of activities, new life meaning may also be realized.

New life meaning can provide purpose for the future. For example, Vrkljan (2000) stated that clients must engage in activities that are meaningful and functional to successfully transition from past to future occupational performance. Moreover, practitioners can help the client create new meaning during this transition. According to Rosenfeld (2004), occupational therapy intervention may incorporate different activities and occupations into therapy to restore a sense of continuity and consequently enhance or reaffirm life meaning (Rosenfeld, 2004). In addition, Reid (2010) stated that "participation in meaningful occupations helps organize, give meaning and a sense of presence in clients, a requirement for being in the world" (p. 24).

Billock (2009) discussed ways for practitioners to facilitate meaningful occupations in the home environment through the use of special objects such as pictures, items from travels, and treasured gifts. According to Billock, the use of these objects may "support the potential for experiencing spirituality" (p. 3) by furthering the life narrative of the client and reassuring or reaffirming life meaning. In addition, using discussion and conversations, engaging in storytelling, and offering activities that support grieving may all contribute to a new or reinforced sense of life meaning (McColl, 2011).

Religious, faith, and spiritual practices. Supporting **religious, faith, and spiritual practices** of clients, families, and communities entails occupational therapy practitioners using knowledge about and skills involving these practices to facilitate clients' engagement in desired routines. Occupational therapy is relevant in addressing religious, faith, and spiritual concerns for clients and families because "religion often influences spiritual experience by providing its practitioners with occupations such as reading theological books, praying, meditating and attending religious services" (Billock, 2009, p. 3). Feeney and Toth-Cohen (2008) emphasized the importance of practitioners listening to clients' comments and observing objects in the clients' rooms to best assist clients' spiritual routines and practices during therapy. Swedberg (2001) suggested that practitioners should promote clients' roles within faith communities if they express this activity as a meaningful occupation. Through role identification and engagement in meaningful occupations pertaining to religious, faith, and spiritual practices, people are able to "grow old in spiritual peace and giving [sic] back to their communities" (Berg, 1997, p. 18).

Brémault-Phillips and Chirovsky (2011a, 2011b) provided the occupational therapy community with the concept of **cultivating spiritual practices,** or developing regular disciplines and routines that promote clients' spirituality. The **wisdom traditions,** not specific to any religious or faith community, is a collective and universal understanding that emphasizes and acknowledges the possibility for all individuals to have a deep sense of knowing truth. Select activities from the wisdom traditions may be encouraged and used to promote health and well-being, deal with crisis and suffering, and develop the self. Examples of such practices include meditating; engaging in spiritual writings, prayers, and pilgrimages; cultivating healthy life habits; having a spiritual mentor or guide; developing virtues; practicing acts of kindness and forgiveness; extending blessings to others; promoting giving and stewardship; and celebrating life.

Creative activities.   Creative activities can facilitate spiritual awareness, have a positive influence on a client's health and well-being, and provide transformational opportunities (McColl, 2011). Sadlo (2004) espoused that humans seem to have an intrinsic drive to purposefully use creative occupations to relieve symptoms such as depression. In addition, Sadlo stated that "growing discontent and spiritual disconnection may be linked with a lack of experience in making beautiful things in this age of passive occupations such as watching television" (p. 95) and that "[c]reativity is a synthesis of intellectual, emotional and spiritual intelligence, and requires integration of the performance sub-systems" (p. 95). However, Toomey (2011) suggested that creative expression involves inherent risk and can elicit feelings of vulnerability. Therefore, occupational therapy practitioners should recognize and value creative occupations (Sadlo, 2004) and honor and support both the client and the creative activity.

Occupations of the spirit.   In contrast to occupations that facilitate spirituality such as creative expression and religious or spiritual activities, occupations of the spirit entail activities that intentionally elicit spiritual awareness and practice (Kang, 2003). Although the term *occupations of the spirit* is not commonly found in the literature, it has been used to describe activities that occupational therapy practitioners use in practice (based on the client's valued goals and meaningful routines) to help clients connect with spirituality. For example, activities such as prayer, deep relaxation, meditation, imagery, chanting, and restorative yoga may not only support wellness practices but also promote spiritual experiences and personal growth (Dickenson, 2012; Farah & McColl, 2008; Hess & Ramugondo, 2014). In addition, engaging in nature and creating spaces for reflection and renewal may restore health and provide spiritual grounding (Unruh, 2011).

In the literature, occupational therapy has been viewed as relevant in the use of occupations of the spirit to guide treatment. For example, Christiansen (1997) stated, "Activities of spirit can create opportunities for meaning making, which is necessary for establishing an identity, gaining a sense of control, and connecting one's personal story or narrative to something greater than self" (p. 170). Rosenfeld (2001a) stated,

> Occupations of the spirit can foster an inspired state of spiritual function by including charitable projects, offering forgiveness, preparing traditional foods, crafting religious objects, celebrating holidays, singing hymns, practicing tai chi and yoga, meditating studying, having contact with nature, and performing tasks with clarity and purpose. (p. 20)

Morrell (1998), a chaplain, worked closely with health care workers in a home health environment, and despite the variety of professionals in that setting, most of his referrals were from occupational therapy practitioners. He determined through his experiences that not only is occupational therapy relevant but it is also imperative in addressing clients' spirituality because of the personal nature of the therapeutic activities used in practice.

Gourley (2001) noted that "virtually no difference [exists] between occupational therapy and spirituality" (p. 13). He stated that "the spiritual realm is purpose and meaning and [practitioners provide] access to it because [they] operate in there all the time. As [occupational therapists], we facilitate the purpose and meaning of life, and that's what heals patients" (p. 14). Therefore, according to Gourley's statements, the engagement of any occupation within the therapy process that brings awareness, insight, and hope to the client and that touches the client's spirit would be considered an occupation of the spirit.

Even though some practitioners may purposefully introduce activities into therapy that are inherently spiritual to the client, clinicians have a responsibility to recognize when their approaches are spiritual in nature, whether intentional or not, and respect boundaries in using such approaches (Hess & Ramugondo, 2014). For example, McColl (2011) suggested the following four questions to consider before using such activities as direct intervention tools:

1. Is the client's problem spiritual in nature?
2. Would the client be receptive to a direct spiritual intervention?
3. Is the [practitioner] equipped to offer spiritual intervention?
4. Would the workplace support it? (p. 195)

Therapeutic use of self

Surrounding the therapy process is **_therapeutic use of self_**, or the way in which occupational therapy practitioners relate to clients and their significant others, which supports practitioners' understanding of their own belief system and values and their development of cultural sensitivity and responsive care when working with clients (Taylor, 2008).

To facilitate meaningful occupational therapy, practitioners need to spend time researching and gaining knowledge about the specific culture related to their area of practice, setting, and clients' practices. According to Fox (2009), cultural sensitivity allows practitioners to provide the best intervention possible because the intervention is based on the client's belief system and values.

As practitioners become culturally sensitive and responsive to the beliefs and values of their clients, they are better able to respect differences between the client's beliefs and their own. In turn, practitioners are better able to maintain appropriate boundaries when working with clients. These boundaries are absolutely necessary during the intervention process to, for example, "effectively pursue engagement in occupations of the spirit" (Crepeau et al., 2000, p. 23).

Swarbrick and Burkhardt (2000) emphasized the importance of "being aware of one's personal spiritual beliefs that affect a client's occupations, behaviors...and coping strategies in relation to loss, injury, and illness" (p. 2). In addition, they described their understanding of how the therapeutic relationship is created. This relationship is first supported by practitioners recognizing their own belief system and values, which allows them to maintain perspective during the occupational therapy process. Then, it is the "therapists caring, intentional presence [that] fosters sharing of spiritual concerns [of clients]" (Swarbrick & Burkhardt, 2000, p. 2). Gabriel (2005) also espoused that "to fully understand spirituality as it guides our interactions with others, we must first understand and nurture spirituality in ourselves" (p. 207).

McColl (2011) further challenged practitioners to honestly assess their own comfort level with this topic of spirituality and understand personal–professional boundaries. Notwithstanding, she also encouraged practitioners to "adapt a willingness to learn from the experiences of patients and accept our own limited understanding" (p. 274). Moreover, developing attitudes of courage, justice, compassion, agency, and awareness strengthen practitioners' therapeutic use of self, and using personal transformative experiences and personal growth help develop authenticity.

Conclusions: Occupational therapy process review

Based on the literature reviewed, the occupational therapy process (assessment, intervention planning and implementation, and the practitioner's therapeutic use of self) includes a link to spirituality. Through the intentional use of activities and occupations that are considered to be spiritual by the client and the use of the occupational therapy process, which brings awareness of a person's life meaning and purpose, practitioners can tap into the spiritual world of the client. The following questions about the practitioner's role in using spirituality in the therapy process arose as a result of our literature review:

- Is it the practitioner's responsibility to attend to and incorporate spiritual or religious occupations into therapy when the client identifies the importance and meaningfulness of such occupations?
- Does the practitioner have the willingness and openness to identify and explore spiritual aspects of the therapy process with the client?
- How do practitioners best prepare to be active participants with the client in being sensitive and attentive to spirituality within the occupational therapy process?

Putting It Together: Four Aspects of Spirituality in Occupational Therapy Practice

The empirical and descriptive literature presented in this text can be synthesized into four aspects of spirituality in occupational therapy practice, which can be viewed from the client or practitioner perspective (Table 7.1). By using the perspectives of spirituality and phenomenology or meaning making (see Chapter 6, "The Meaning of Meaning: Thinking About Phenomenology and Meaning") and the information in this chapter on how practitioners can use spirituality in practice, the following four aspects of spirituality in occupational therapy become clear:

1. Honor and respect
2. Select occupations and routines
3. Identity formation and strength
4. Incorporated spirituality.

In addition, the focus on spirituality in therapy lessens as occupations become the primary focus or supporting intervention and vice versa (Figure 7.4).

The aspects of honor and respect and select occupations and routines focus predominantly on occupations, although spirituality is valued and explored within that context. Conversely, the aspects of identity formation and strength and integrated spirituality focus mostly on spirituality, but within the context of occupations.

As represented in the literature, any one of these aspects may become part of intervention or be a lens through which to view and understand client perspectives. In addition, use of any one of these aspects might be more or less important in therapy depending upon the client's values and goals and the practitioner's comfort and skill level. Moreover, because practice is fluid (i.e., it may be influenced by intervention settings, time allotment, duration of services, or the comfort of both the client and the practitioner), the use of these four aspects also needs to be fluid.

Honor and Respect

Honor and respect entails an attitude of commitment to the client (and the family or community, if applicable), recognizing the inherent spiritual qualities that both the client and the practitioner bring to the therapy process. The occupational therapy practitioner values the client and his or her experiences, which further inform practice. Going beyond the general idea of recognizing the dignity or humanity of all people, this aspect requires the practitioner to know the client and his or her desires, goals, and motivation for therapy and to respectfully incorporate the client's perspectives into the therapy process.

Although the activities and occupations addressed within the therapy process may not be overtly connected to any spiritual practice or engagement for the client, honor and respect requires that the practitioner be aware of and acknowledge the spiritual nature of occupations and the potential impact their use may have on the client. Therefore, the practitioner must use thoughtfulness and self-reflection regarding the selection and use of therapeutic interventions and occupations.

Select Occupations and Routines

Select occupations and routines offers the occupational therapy practitioner opportunities to incorporate occupations and routines deemed important

Table 7.1. Literature on the Four Aspects of Spirituality in Occupational Therapy Practice: Client and Practitioner Perspectives

Perspective	Honor and Respect	Select Occupations and Routines	Identity Formation and Strength	Incorporated Spirituality
Client	Bowen (2006) Gavacs (2009) Hannam (1997) http://bit.ly/ 1KByPWD Mathis (1996) Pereira & Stagnitti (2008) http://bit.ly/ 1W8aDfb Pongsaksri (2007) http://bit.ly/ 1oqICWB Tzanidaki & Reynolds (2011) http://bit.ly/ 1PVsGRB	Allen, Kellegrew, & Jaffe (2000) Doughton (1996) Griffith, Caron, Desrosiers, & Thibeault (2007) http://bit.ly/ 1UZ2Ksp	Burns (2007) Forhan (2010) http://bit.ly/1PMvGno Griffith et al. (2007) http://bit.ly/1UZ2Ksp Hatchard & Missiuna (2003) http://bit.ly/1nWdeOq Kronenberg et al. (2005, 2011) Ramugondo (2005) Schmid (2004) http://bit.ly/1Se5AMc Spencer (2007) http://bit.ly/20TTsRV Thibeault (2011a; 2011c) Unruh & Elvin (2004a) http://bit.ly/1Qpzqre Unruh, Smith, & Scammel (2000) http://bit.ly/23V3GEc Vrkljan & Miller-Polgar (2001) http://bit.ly/1SdZM5r	Beagan & Etowa (2011) http://bit.ly/ 1RmxJ2G Kronenberg et al. (2005, 2011) Nesbit (2004, 2006) http://bit.ly/ 1Q21aGh http://bit.ly/ 219dIiF Pentland & McColl (2011) Smith & Suto (2012) http://bit.ly/ 1JIBoWW Thibeault (2012d) Whitney (2010) Williams (2008) http://bit.ly/ 1SWxpJ5
Practitioner	Bowen (1999) Caracciolo (1995) Hettinger (1996) Hoppes (1997) Leslie (2006) Mathis (1996) Peloquin (1997) http://bit.ly/ 1mqHX4Q Radomski (2000) Rosenfeld (2001a, 2004) Strzelecki (2009) Toomey (2011) Urbanowski (1997)	Berg (1997) Billock (2009) Brémault-Phillips & Chirovsky (2011a) Feeney Toth-Cohen (2008) Swedberg (2001) Trump (2001)	Burgman & King (2005) Dawson & Stern (2007) http://bit.ly/1PReEkH Hafez (1998) Jung et al. (1999) http://bit.ly/20ZMHlg Kronenberg et al. (2005, 2011) McColl (2011) Rosenfeld (2004) Sadlo (2004) Thibeault (2011a; 2011b) Toomey (2011) Vrkljan (2000)	Brémault-Phillips & Chirovsky (2011b) Christiansen (1997) http://bit.ly/ 1PMxfBI Dickenson (2012) Kronenberg, et al. (2005, 2011) McColl (2011) Unruh (2011)

by the client, family, or community that are also considered spiritual or religious in nature. This aspect moves beyond honor and respect by intentionally addressing occupations that enhance lives and bring meaning to and further support the client, family, or community. In addition, this aspect requires the practitioner to have a level of cultural sensitivity and responsiveness to ensure that the

Figure 7.4. Four aspects of spirituality in occupational therapy practice: Converse relationship between spirituality and occupations.

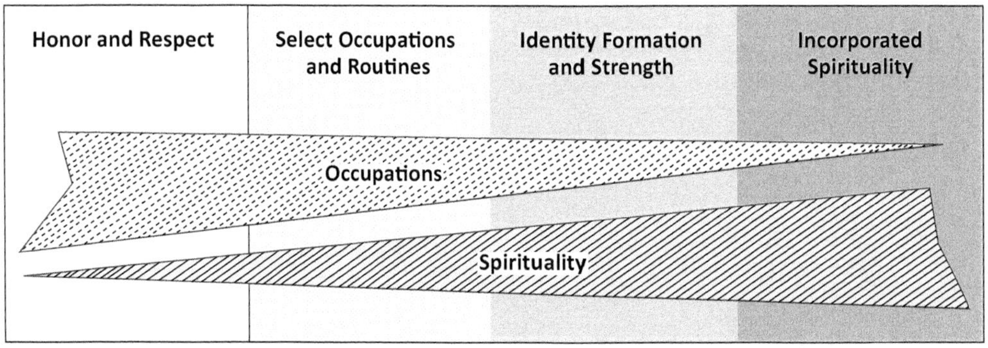

occupations used and addressed are applicable to the needs and desires of the client.

Identity Formation and Strength

Identity formation and strength promotes the use of occupations to assist in the framing or reframing of identity. The primary focus is not on the occupation, per se, but on the process of transformation, healing, and developing resiliency. However, occupations used during intervention are the means to identity formation and strength. In addition, the selection and application of occupations are based on sound clinical reasoning, and, therefore, the occupations may or may not directly embody spiritual or religious qualities. The overall goal of the client may also not explicitly involve identity formation or strength, but this aspect may be a byproduct or outcome of the therapy process. The practitioner must be attentive to such experiences and support the client as needed.

Incorporated Spirituality

Incorporated spirituality involves directly engaging in spirituality in the context of practice. It is the intersection among occupational engagement, spirituality, and meaning making or identity. During the therapy process, the client (and family and community, if applicable) and practitioner intentionally and collaboratively focus on spirituality, which is explicitly sought, engaged in, and affirmed for the client. In addition, the literature has demonstrated an expanded understanding of which occupations enhance spirituality and meaning making in particular contexts.

Thoughts on and Critique of the Model

My clinical experience as an occupational therapy practitioner and my involvement as a fieldwork supervisor, administrator, educator, and researcher has shown me that occupational therapy students and practitioners are most comfortable in using the constructs related to meaningful and valued occupations and roles within therapy (i.e., the aspect of honor and respect). They focus on trying to understand what holds significance for the client and strive to incorporate meaningful and valued activities into practice. However, many questions and considerations arise when incorporating spirituality into practice.

Is or Should Therapy Be Spiritual?

Occupational therapy practitioners need to be aware that some of the activities that they introduce into a therapy session may or may not have any significance for the client or touch the spiritual essence of the client. Is this therapy or not? In other words, does an activity need to be significant to be therapeutic? Does every therapeutic activity need to be one that is considered meaningful? Are all meaningful activities spiritual ones? Is the ultimate goal in therapy to have a spiritual experience, or do practitioners only need to be aware that therapy activities and approaches might evoke a spiritual response from the client?

Addressing Difficult Problems

Seasoned occupational therapy practitioners often pull from their professional and personal knowledge to offer hope, motivation, and new life meaning by providing new images of possibility and adding to the life narratives of clients, families, and communities (i.e., the aspect of identity formation and strength). Mattingly and Fleming (1994) described this process as **reframing narratives.** It is not uncommon for practitioners to work with clients, families, and communities who question why devastating life events are occurring and wonder how to make sense of them.

Although practitioners can provide insights into and new images of potential future life-affirming occupations to clients during the therapy process, clients who are questioning the meaning of life, suffering, experiencing pain, or facing or dealing with death and asking philosophical or theological questions can present a great challenge for many practitioners. Practitioners usually do not have the language or professional background to adequately address these questions—and often are not cognizant of how they personally make sense of such issues. Therefore, when clients and families explicitly articulate life meaning questions and wish to discuss their concerns, practitioners should refer them to other professionals, such as chaplains (see Chapter 4, "Spirituality Through the Lens of Health Care Chaplaincy," for a detailed description of the chaplain's role).

Cultural Sensitivity and Responsiveness

Occupational therapy students and practitioners may be challenged to understand different religious beliefs and practices (i.e., the aspect of select occupations and routines). To best support clients, families, and communities in the resumption of valued occupations that encompass religious, faith, or spiritual practices, practitioners must have an understanding of those practices. As mentioned earlier, developing such an understanding requires a willingness to expand the therapeutic use of self and discover and ask pertinent questions to be better informed and culturally sensitive and responsive (Muñoz, 2007).

Occupations of the Spirit

Although many occupational therapy practitioners can envision and support spirituality as part of the process of engaging clients in meaningful roles and activities, in finding new life meaning, and in expanding the understanding of self, especially through disability and crisis, the idea of occupations of the spirit (i.e., the aspect of incorporated spirituality) is especially challenging. According to the *Occupational Therapy Practice Framework: Domain and Process* (*Framework;* American Occupational Therapy Association [AOTA], 2014), practitioners engage in a host of activities or occupations, including activities of daily living, instrumental activities of daily living, rest and sleep, work, education, play, leisure, and social participation. However, occupational therapy does not yet have a category that is specifically related to spiritual occupations. This topic, sometimes uncomfortable for practitioners, raises several questions. Are there occupations specifically related to spirituality, or is spirituality embedded in the occupations already listed in the *Framework* (AOTA, 2014)? Are occupations of the spirit about being and not so much about doing? Could it encompass both? More jelly has just been added to the wall.

Practitioner Responsibility

Practitioner responsibility regarding spirituality in occupational therapy practice involves several factors for occupational therapy students and practitioners. First, they must know what they are speaking about when discussing spirituality in occupational therapy practice. This chapter, and this book, has provided ways in which spirituality has been understood by many occupational therapy clinicians and researchers as it directly applies to the therapeutic process. Multiple perspectives and aspects of spirituality have been presented, most related to individual therapy intervention and not larger community perspectives. To further the discussion about spirituality in occupational therapy practice, practitioners need to gain as much knowledge as possible about the topic and appreciate its intricacies (see, especially, Chapter 2, "Contemporary History of Spirituality and Occupational Therapy"; Chapter 3, "Definitions and Descriptions of Spirituality in Occupational Therapy Literature"; and Chapter 6, "The Meaning of Meaning: Thinking About Phenomenology and Meaning").

Second, practitioners must be self-reflective, understanding their own biases regarding spirituality and the aspects of spirituality with which they are comfortable and uncomfortable. They can start by thinking about not only their own understanding of spirituality but also their own life meaning and purpose. All of the examples provided in this chapter reflect a personal bias and a predominantly Western preference regarding spirituality. How might these perspectives change and the model expand with other ideas? In addition, they also need to develop their therapeutic use of self and challenge themselves to become more knowledgeable about others' beliefs and practices.

Third, practitioners need to further the dialogue about spirituality in occupational therapy practice and researchers need to continue to collect evidence on the use of meaningful occupations and spirituality in practice. Most of the research related to spirituality and occupational therapy that has been completed up until now is related to students' and practitioners' perspectives about spirituality. Although some qualitative research has provided preliminary insights into what is most meaningful in recovery and well-being from the client's perspective (see Chapter 1, "Addressing Spirituality in Occupational Therapy," and Chapter 3, "Definitions and Descriptions of Spirituality in Occupational Therapy Literature"), more evidence from this perspective is needed.

Summary

Occupational therapy practitioners should be attentive to their own understanding of spirituality and have an appreciation of how spirituality may be incorporated into the therapy process. Based on the literature, spirituality in occupational therapy is promoted when the practitioner honors the client and his or her own experiences and personal beliefs, incorporates valued and meaningful occupations into intervention, helps facilitate new images of hope and life purpose, and when agreeable and applicable to both the client and the practitioner, incorporates and promotes spiritual practices into daily routines.

References

Allen, J. M., Kellegrew, D. H., & Jaffe, D. (2000). The experience of pet ownership as a meaningful occupation. *Canadian Journal of Occupational Therapy 67,* 271–278. http://dx.doi.org/10.1177/000841740006700409

American Occupational Therapy Association. (2014). The Occupational therapy practice framework: Domain and process (3rd ed.). *American Journal of Occupational Therapy, 68*(Suppl. 1), S1–S48. http://dx.doi.org/10.5014/ajot.2014.682006

Ayres, A. J. (1998). The art of therapy. *Sensory Integration Special Interest Section Quarterly, 21*(4), 1–3, 6.

Baptiste, S. (2011). Work: Understanding spirituality and work. In M. A. McColl (Ed.), *Spirituality and occupational therapy* (2nd ed., pp. 241–248). Ottawa, ON: CAOT Publications.

Beagan, B. L, & Etowa, J. B. (2011). The meaning and functions of occupations related to spirituality for African Nova Scotian women. *Journal of Occupational Science 18,* 277–290. http://dx.doi.org/10.1080/14427591.2011.594548

Berg, J. (1997). Aging as in "sage-ing." *OT Week, 11*(50), 18.

Billock, C. (2009). Integrating spirituality into home health occupational therapy practice. *Home and Community Health Special Interest Section Quarterly, 16*(1), 1–4.

Bouthot, J., Wells, T., & Black, R. M. (2011). Spirituality in practice: Using the FICA Spiritual History Assessment. *OT Practice, 16,* 13–16.

Bowen, J. E. (1999). Health promotion in the new millennium: Opening the lens—adjusting the focus. *OT Practice, 4*(12), 14–18.

Bowen, J. E. (2006). Reflections from the heart: The healing-within relationship. *OT Practice, 11*(1), 48.

Brémault-Phillips, S., & Chirovsky, A. (2011a). Spiritual practices. In M. A. McColl (Ed.), *Spirituality and occupational therapy* (2nd ed., pp. 183–192). Ottawa, ON: CAOT Publications.

Brémault-Phillips, S., & Chirovsky, A. (2011b). The spiritual path. In M. A. McColl (Ed.), *Spirituality and occupational therapy* (2nd ed., pp. 151–158). Ottawa, ON: CAOT Publications.

Burgman, I., & King, A. (2005). The presence of child spirituality. In F. Kronenberg, S. A. Algado, & N. Pollard (Eds.), *Occupational therapy without borders: Learning from the spirit of survivors* (pp. 153–165). New York: Elsevier Churchill Livingstone.

Burns, J. (2007). OT leads the way: A child's triumph in war-torn Iraq. *OT Practice, 12*(1), 7–9.

Canadian Association of Occupational Therapists. (2002). *Enabling occupation: An occupational therapy perspective* (rev. ed.). Ottawa, ON: CAOT Publications.

Caracciolo, R. (1995). Is there something missing? *OT Week, 9*(50), 13.

Christiansen, C. (1997). Acknowledging a spiritual dimension in occupational therapy practice. *American Journal of Occupational Therapy, 51,* 169–172. http://dx.doi.org/10.5014/ajot.51.3.169

Collins, J. S., Paul, S., & West-Frasier, J. (2001). The utilization of spirituality in occupational therapy: Beliefs, practices, and perceived barriers. *Occupational Therapy in Health Care, 14,* 73–92. http://dx.doi.org/10.1080/J003v14n03_05.

Crepeau, E., James, A. B., Spear, P. S., Francoeur, M., Garren, K., Stewart-Whipple, J., & Rosenfeld, M. S. (2000). Letters: The spirituality discussion (continued). *OT Practice, 5*(15), 23.

Dawson, D. R., & Stern, B. (2007). Reflections on facilitating older adult's participation in valued occupations. *OT NOW, 9*(5), 3–5. http://www.caot.ca/otnow/Sept%2007/reflections.pdf

Dickenson, J. (2012). A spiritual journey—A personal perspective. In M. A. McColl (Ed.), *Spirituality and occupational therapy* (2nd ed., pp. 259–268). Ottawa, ON: CAOT Publications.

Doughton, K. J. (1996). Unlocking your client's hidden talents. *OT Week, 10*(26), 18–19.

Egan, M., & Swedersky, J. (2003). Spirituality as experienced by occupational therapists in practice. *American Journal of Occupational Therapy, 57*, 525–533. http://dx.doi.org/10.5014/ajot.57.5.525

Farah, J., & McColl, M. A. (2008). Exploring prayer as a spiritual modality. *Canadian Journal of Occupational Therapy, 75*, 5–13. http://dx.doi.org/10.1177/000841740807500103

Feeney, L., & Toth-Cohen, S. (2008). Addressing spirituality for clients with physical disabilities. *OT Practice, 13*(4), 16–20.

Forhan, M. (2010). Doing, being, and becoming: A family's journey through perinatal loss. *American Journal of Occupational Therapy, 64*, 142–151. http://dx.doi.org/10.5014/ajot.64.1.142

Fox, L. (2009). Native American spirituality: A truly holistic perspective. *Home and Community Health Special Interest Section Quarterly, 16*(1), 1–4.

Gabriel, L. (2005). Reflections on spirituality: Implications for ethics education. In R. Purtilo, G. Jensen, & C. Royeen (Eds.), *Educating for moral action: A sourcebook in health and rehabilitation ethics* (pp. 203–214). Philadelphia: F. A. Davis.

Gavacs, M. (2009). Reflections from the heart: The dance of independence. *OT Practice, 15*(10), 32.

Gourley, M. (2001). The spiritual realm of occupational therapy. *OT Practice, 6*(8), 13–14.

Greven, C. (2007). Reflections from the heart: Occupations and the elderly. *OT Practice, 12*(14), 40.

Griffith, J., Caron, C. D., Desrosiers, J., & Thibeault, R. (2007). Defining spirituality and giving meaning to occupation: The perspective of community-dwelling older adults and autonomy loss. *Canadian Journal of Occupational Therapy, 74*, 78–90. http://dx.doi.org/10.2182/cjot.06.0016

Hafez, A. (1998). OT and spirituality (continued). *OT Practice, 3*(6), 58–59.

Hannam, D. (1997). More than a cup of tea: Meaning construction in an everyday occupation. *Journal of Occupational Science, 4*, 69–74. http://dx.doi.org/10.1080/14427591.1997.9686423

Hatchard, K., & Missiuna, C. (2003). An occupational therapist's journey through bipolar affective disorder. *Occupational Therapy in Mental Health, 19*, 1–17. http://dx.doi.org/10.1300/J004v19n02_01

Heinz, A. J., Disney, E. R., Epstein, D. H., Glezen, L. A., Clark, P. I., & Preston, K. L. (2010). Pilot study on spirituality: A focus-group study on spirituality and substance-user treatment. *Substance Use and Misuse, 45*, 134–153. http://dx.doi.org/10.3109/10826080903035130

Hess, K. Y., & Ramugondo, E. (2014). Clinical reasoning used by occupational therapists to determine the nature of spiritual occupations in relation to psychiatric pathology. *British Journal of Occupational Therapy, 77*, 234–242. http://dx.doi.org/10.4276/030802214x13990455043449

Hettinger, J. (1996). Bringing spirituality into practice. *OT Week, 10*(24), 16–18.

Hoppes, S. (1997). Motivating clients through goal setting. *OT Practice, 2*(6), 22–27.

Houston, H., Dickerson, A. (2010, September). End-of-life care: A volunteer's experience. *OT Practice, 15*(16), 16–19.

Jung, B., Salvatori, P., Missiuna, C., Wilkins, S., Stewart, D., & Law, M. (1999). The McMaster lens for occupational therapists: Bringing theory and practice into focus. *OT NOW, 10*(2), 16–19.

Kang, C. (2003). A psychospiritual integration frame of reference of occupational therapy. Part 1: Conceptual foundations. *Australian Occupational Therapy Journal, 50*, 92–103. http://dx.doi.org/10.1046/j.1440-1630.2003.00358.x

Kirsh, B., Dawson, D., Antolikova, S., & Reynolds, L. (2001). Developing awareness of spirituality in occupational therapy students: Are our curricula up to the task? *Occupational Therapy International, 8*, 119–125. http://dx.doi.org/10.1002/oti.138

Kronenberg, F., Algado, S. A., & Pollard, N. (2005). *Occupational therapy without borders: Learning from the spirit of survivors.* London: Elsevier/Churchill Livingstone.

Kronenberg, F., Pollard, N., & Sakellariou, D. (Eds.). (2011). *Occupational therapies without borders: Towards an ecology of occupation-based practices* (Vol. 2). London: Elsevier/Churchill Livingstone.

Leslie, C. A. (2006). Reflections from the heart: Life's lessons. *OT Practice, 11*(6), 44.

Mathis, T. K. (1996). The magic in a pecan pie. *OT Week, 10*(25), 16.

Mattingly, C., & Fleming, M. (1994). *Clinical reasoning: Forms of inquiry in a therapeutic practice.* Philadelphia: F. A. Davis.

McColl, M. A. (2003). *Spirituality and occupational therapy.* Ottawa, ON: CAOT Publications.

McColl, M. A. (2011). *Spirituality and occupational therapy* (2nd ed.). Ottawa, ON: CAOT Publications.

Morrell, R. (1998). Home health care and the chaplain. *Home and Community Health Special Interest Section Quarterly, 5,* 3.

Muñoz, J. (2007). Culturally responsive caring in occupational therapy. *Occupational Therapy International, 14,* 256–280. http://dx.doi.org/10.1002/oti.238

Nesbit, S. G. (2004). My breast cancer: An occupational therapist's perspective. *Occupational Therapy in Mental Health, 20,* 51–67. http://dx.doi.org/10.1300/J004v20n02_03

Nesbit, S. G. (2006). Using creativity to experience flow on my journey with breast cancer. *Occupational Therapy in Mental Health, 22,* 61–79. http://dx.doi.org/10.1300/J004v22n02_03

Peloquin, S. M. (1997). The spiritual depth of occupation: Making worlds and making lives. *American Journal of Occupational Therapy, 51,* 167–168. http://dx.doi.org/10.5014/ajot.51.3.167

Pentland, W., & McColl, M. A. (2011). Occupational choice. In M. A. McColl (Ed.), *Spirituality and occupational therapy* (2nd ed., pp. 141–149). Ottawa, ON: CAOT Publications.

Pereira, R. B., & Stagnitti, K. (2008). The meaning of leisure for well elderly Italians in the Australian community: Implications for occupational therapy. *Australian Occupational Therapy Journal, 55,* 39–46. http://dx.doi.org/10.1111/j.1440-1630.2006.00653.x

Pongsaksri, M. (2007). Occupational therapy eases the suffering of tsunami victims. *World Federation of Occupational Therapists Bulletin, 55,* 30–33. http://dx.doi.org/10.1179/otb.2007.55.1.005

Puchalski, C. (1999). *FICA Spiritual History Tool.* Washington, DC: George Washington Institute for Spirituality and Health.

Radomski, M. V. (2000). Self-efficacy: Improving occupational therapy outcomes by helping patients say "I can." *Physical Disabilities Special Interest Section Quarterly, 23*(1), 1–3.

Ramugondo, E. L. (2005). Unlocking spirituality: Play as a health-promoting occupation in the context of HIV/AIDS. In F. Kronenberg, S. A. Algado, & N. Pollard (Eds.), *Occupational therapy without borders: Learning from the spirit of survivors* (pp. 313–325). New York: Elsevier/Churchill Livingstone.

Reid, D. (2010). Mundane occupations: Providing opportunity for engagement and being-in-the-world. *OT NOW, 12*(2), 24–26.

Rosenfeld, M. S. (2000). Spiritual agent modalities for occupational therapy practice. *OT Practice, 5*(2), 17–21.

Rosenfeld, M. S. (2001a). Exploring spiritual contexts for care. *OT Practice, 6*(11), 18–25.

Rosenfeld, M. S. (2001b). Spirituality, motivation, and performance. *OT NOW, 3*(6), 1–10.

Rosenfeld, M. S. (2004). Motivating elders with depression in SNFs. *OT Practice, 9*(11), 21–28.

Sadlo, G. (2004). Creativity and occupation. In M. Molineux (Ed.), *Occupation for occupational therapists* (pp. 90–100). Malden, MA: Blackwell.

Schmid, T. (2004). Meanings of creativity within occupational therapy. *Australian Occupational Therapy Journal, 51,* 80–88. http://dx.doi.org/10.1111/j.1440-1630.2004.00434.x

Smith, S., & Suto, M. J. (2012). Religious and/or spiritual practices: Extending spiritual freedom to people with schizophrenia. *Canadian Journal of Occupational Therapy, 79,* 77–85. http://dx.doi.org/10.2182/cjot.2012.79.2.3

Spencer, K. (2007) A whole new world. *Topics in Stroke Rehabilitation, 14,* 93–96. http://dx.doi.org/10.1310/tsr1404-93

Strzelecki, M. V. (2009). Careers: Luck of the draw. *OT Practice, 14*(1), 7–8.

Swarbrick, P., & Burkhardt, A. (2000). Spiritual health: Implications for the occupational therapy process. *Mental Health Special Interest Section Quarterly, 23*(2), 1–3.

Swedberg, L. (2001). Facilitating accessibility and participation in faith communities. *OT Practice, 6*(9), CE1–CE8.

Szafran, S. H. (2011). Physical, mental and spiritual approaches to managing pain in older clients. *OT Practice, 16*(3), CE1–CE8.

Taylor, E., Mitchell, J. E., Kenan, S., & Tacker, R. (2000). Attitudes of occupational therapists toward spirituality in practice. *American Journal of Occupational Therapy, 54,* 421–427. http://dx.doi.org/10.5014/ajot.54.4.421

Taylor, R. R. (2008). *The intentional relationship: Occupational therapy and the use of self.* Philadelphia: F.A. Davis.

Thibeault, R. (2011a). Occupational gifts. In M. A. McColl (Ed.), *Spirituality and occupational therapy* (2nd ed., pp. 111–120). Ottawa, ON: CAOT Publications.

Thibeault, R. (2011b). Occupational therapy values. In M. A. McColl (Ed.), *Spirituality and occupational therapy* (2nd ed., pp. 103–110). Ottawa, ON: CAOT Publications.

Thibeault, R. (2011c). Resilience and maturity. In M. A. McColl (Ed.), *Spirituality and occupational therapy* (2nd ed., pp. 121–130). Ottawa, ON: CAOT Publications.

Thibeault, R. (2011d). Ritual: Ceremonies of life. In M. A. McColl (Ed.), *Spirituality and occupational therapy* (2nd ed., pp. 217– 222). Ottawa, ON: CAOT Publications.

Thompson, B. E., & MacNeil, C. (2006). A phenomenological study exploring the meaning of a seminar on spirituality for occupational therapy students. *American Journal of Occupational Therapy, 60,* 531–539. http://dx.doi.org/10.5014/ajot.60.5.531

Toomey, M. (2011). Creativity: Spirituality through the visual arts. In M. A. McColl (Ed.), *Spirituality and occupational therapy* (2nd ed., pp. 233–240). Ottawa, ON: CAOT Publications.

Trump, S. M., (2001). Occupational therapy and hospice: A natural fit. *OT Practice, 6*(20), 7–8, 10–11.

Tzanidaki, D., & Reynolds, F. (2011). Exploring the meaning of making traditional arts and crafts among older women in Crete, using interpretative phenomenological analysis. *British*

Journal of Occupational Therapy 74(8), 375–382. http://dx. doi.org/10.4276/030802211X13125646370852

Unruh, A. (2011). Appreciation of nature: Restorative occupations. In M. A. McColl (Ed.), *Spirituality and occupational therapy* (2nd ed., pp. 249–256). Ottawa, ON: CAOT Publications.

Unruh, A. M., & Elvin, N. (2004a). In the eye of the dragon: Women's experience of breast cancer and the occupation of dragon boat racing. *Canadian Journal of Occupational Therapy, 71,* 138–149. http://dx.doi.org/10.1177/000841740 407100304

Unruh, A. M., Versnel, J., & Kerr, N. (2004b). Spirituality in the context of occupation: A theory to practice application. In M. Molineux (Ed.). *Occupation for occupational therapists* (pp. 32–45). Malden, MA: Blackwell.

Unruh, A. M., Smith, N., & Scammel, C. (2000). The occupation of gardening in life-threatening illness: A qualitative pilot project. *Canadian Journal of Occupational Therapy,* 67, 70–77. http://dx.doi.org/10.1177/00084174000670 0110

Urbanowski, R. (1997). Spirituality in everyday practice. *OT Practice, 2*(12), 18–23.

Vrkljan, B. H. (2000). The role of spirituality in occupational therapy practice. *OT NOW, 2,* 1–5.

Vrkljan, B., & Miller-Polgar, J. (2001). Meaning of occupational engagement in life-threatening illness: A qualitative pilot project. *Canadian Journal of Occupational Therapy,* 68, 237–246. http://dx.doi.org/10.1177/000841740106 800407

Whitney, R. (2010). Reflections from the heart: The spirit catches me and I write it down. *OT Practice, 15*(16), 33.

Williams, B. J. (2008). An exploratory study of older adults' perspectives of spirituality. *Occupational Therapy in Health Care, 22(*1), 2008, 3-19. http://dx.doi.org/10.1080/J003v 22n01_02

Appendix 7.A. Terminology and Language of Spirituality

Depending on the author's country of origin, use of language varied related to spirituality in occupational therapy in the literature. For example, Canadian authors used the term *spirituality* explicitly when discussing the topic. We hypothesized that this term was used more often because both the Canadian Model of Occupational Performance (Canadian Association of Occupational Therapists [CAOT], 2002) and the Canadian Model of Occupational Performance and Engagement (CAOT, 2007) use the word *spirituality* to describe the central being of the client.

Authors from the United States were less likely to use the term *spirituality* in their work, which may be due to a lack of theoretical frameworks that explicitly include the term as formal language. Much of the terminology used by these authors when speaking about spirituality was congruent with the occupational therapy frame of reference, the Model of Human Occupation (MOHO; Kielhofner, 2008). For example, Burkhardt (1997) used the term *habits* when discussing how spiritual activities can be incorporated into a person's daily routine. Houston and Dickerson (2010) used the terms *volition, habituation, performance capacity,* and *environment* as related to a described spiritual intervention with a client.

Doughton (1996) also used the term *volition* and further described the use of *throughput, positive feedback,* and *valued goals* as they related to motivation and spiritual experiences. In addition, Burns (2007) discussed the incorporation of an *activities of daily living routine* into the client's daily life to increase his intrinsic motivation to re-establish his will to live and engage life. Bowen (2006) used the terms *occupation, routines,* and *habits* to describe the added structure and subsequent meaning to the client's daily life. Although these authors discussed different components of MOHO, each also related these terms to spirituality and the incorporation of spirituality into the therapy process.

References

Bowen, J. E. (2006). Reflections from the heart: The healing-within relationship. *OT Practice, 11*(1), 48.

Burkhardt, A. (1997). Occupational therapy and wellness. *OT Practice, 2,* 28–31.

Burns, J. (2007). OT leads the way: A child's triumph in war-torn Iraq. *OT Practice, 12*(1), 7–9.

Canadian Association of Occupational Therapists. (2002). *Enabling occupation: An occupational therapy perspective* (Rev. ed.). Ottawa, ON: CAOT Publications.

Canadian Association of Occupational Therapists. (2007). *Enabling occupation II: Advancing an occupational therapy vision for health, well-being and justice through occupation.* Ottawa, ON: CAOT Publications.

Doughton, K. J. (1996). Unlocking your client's hidden talents. *OT Week, 10*(26), 18–19.

Houston, H., & Dickerson, A. (2010). End-of-life care: A volunteer's experience. *OT Practice, 15*(16), 16–19.

Kielhofner, G. (2008). *Model of Human Occupation: Theory and application* (4th ed.). Baltimore: Lippincott Williams & Wilkins.

Appendix 7.B. Themes of Experience of Spirituality

Initial themes and references in the systematic literature review related to spirituality in occupational therapy

Personal Experiences: Spirituality as ...	Citation
Volition	Burns, J. (2007). OT leads the way: A child's triumph in war-torn Iraq. *OT Practice, 12*(1), 7–9
	Doughton, K. J. (1996). Unlocking your client's hidden talents. *OT Week, 10*(26), 18–19.
	Houston, H., Dickerson, A. (2010). End-of-life care: A volunteer's experience. *OT Practice, 15*(16), 16–19.
	Mathis, T. K. (1996). The magic in a pecan pie. *OT Week, 10*(25), 16.
	Pongsaskri, M. (2007). Occupational therapy eases the suffering of tsunami victims. *WFOT Bulletin, 55*, 30–33. http://bit.ly/1oqlCWB
Meaning	Bowen, J. E. (2006). Reflections from the heart: The healing-within relationship. *OT Practice, 11*(1), 48.
	Gourley, M. (2001). The spiritual realm of occupational therapy. *OT Practice, 6*(8), 13–14.
	Leslie, C. A. (2006). Reflections from the heart: Life's lessons. *OT Practice, 11*(6), 44.
	Mathis, T. K. (1996). The magic in a pecan pie. *OT Week,10*(25), 16.
	Strzelecki, M. V. (2009). Careers: Luck of the draw. *OT Practice,14*(1), 7–8
	Whitney, R. (2010). Reflections from the heart: The spirit catches me and I write it down. *OT Practice, 15*(16), 33.
Religion	Doughton, K. J. (1996). Unlocking your client's hidden talents. *OT Week, 10*(26), 18–19.
	Forhan, M. (2010). Doing, being, and becoming: A family's journey through perinatal loss. *American Journal of Occupational Therapy, 64*, 142–151. http://bit.ly/1PMvGno
	Hatchard, K., & Missiuna, C. (2003). An occupational therapist's journey through bipolar affective disorder. *Occupational Therapy in Mental Health, 19*(2), 1–17. http://bit.ly/1nWdeOq
	Morrell, R. (1998). Home health care and the chaplain. *Home & Community Health Special Interest Section Quarterly, 5*(4), 3.
	Spencer, K. (2007). A whole new world. *Topics in Stroke Rehabilitation, 14*(4), 93–96. http://bit.ly/20TTsRV
Joy	Gavacs, M. (2009). Reflections from the heart: The dance of independence. *OT Practice, 15*(10), 32.
Flow	Nesbit, S. G. (2006). Using creativity to experience flow on my journey with breast cancer. *Occupational Therapy in Mental Health, 22*(2), 61–79. http://bit.ly/219dIiF

Application to Practice: Occupational Therapy Practitioner's Role	Citation
Faith and Religion	Billock, C. (2009). Integrating spirituality into home health occupational therapy practice. *Home and Community Health Special Interest Section Quarterly, 16*(1), 1–4.

(Continued)

Appendix 7.B. Themes of Experience of Spirituality *(Cont.)*

Application to Practice: Occupational Therapy Practitioner's Role	Citation
	Feeney, L., & Toth-Cohen, S. (2008). Addressing spirituality for clients with physical disabilities. *OT Practice,* 13(4), 16–20.
	Fox, L. (2009). Native American spirituality: A truly holistic perspective. *Home and Community Health Special Interest Section Quarterly, 16*(1), 1–4.
	Greven, C. (2007). Reflections from the heart: Occupations and the elderly. *OT Practice,* 12(14), 40.
	Morrell, R. (1998). Home health care and the chaplain. *Home & Community Health Special Interest Section Quarterly, 5*(4), 3.
	McCormack, G. L. (1997). What is nontraditional practice? *OT Practice,* 2(2), 17–20.
	Rosenfeld, M. S. (2000). Spiritual agent modalities for occupational therapy practice. *OT Practice, 5*(2), 17–21.
	Rosenfeld, M. S. (2001a). Exploring spiritual contexts for care. *OT Practice,* 6(11), 18–25.
	Rosenfeld, M. S. (2001b). Spirituality, motivation, and performance. *OT NOW, 3*(6), 1–10.
	Trump, S. M., (2001). Occupational therapy and hospice: A natural fit. *OT Practice, 6*(20), 7–8, 10–11.
Just-Right Challenge	Ayres, A. J. (1998). The art of therapy. *Sensory Integration Special Interest Section Quarterly, 21*(4), 1–3, 6.
	Caracciolo, R. (1995). Is there something missing? *OT Week, 9*(50), 13.
	Hoppes, S. (1997). Motivating clients through goal setting. *OT Practice,* 2(6), 22–27.
	Radomski, M. V. (2000). Self-efficacy: Improving occupational therapy outcomes by helping patients say "I can." *Physical Disabilities Special Interest Section Quarterly, 23*(1), 1–3.
Life Narrative	Burgman, I., & King, A. (2005). The presence of child spirituality. In F. Kronenberg (Ed.), *Occupational therapy without borders: Learning from the spirit of survivors* (153–165). New York: Elsevier/Churchill Livingstone.
	Feeney, L. & Toth-Cohen, S. (2008). Addressing spirituality for clients with physical disabilities. *OT Practice, 13*(4), 16–20.
	Greven, C. (2007). Reflections from the heart: Occupations and the elderly. *OT Practice, 12*(14), 40.
	Hettinger, J. (1996). Bringing spirituality into practice. *OT Week, 10*(24), 16–18.
	Rosenfeld, M. S. (2001). Exploring spiritual contexts for care. *OT Practice, 6*(11), 18–25.
	Rosenfeld, M. S. (2004). Motivating elders with depression in SNFs. *OT Practice,* 21–28.
	Rosenfeld, M. S. (2001). Spirituality, motivation, and performance. *OT NOW,* 1–10.
	Vrkljan, B. H. (2000). The role of spirituality in occupational therapy practice. *OT NOW, 2,* 1–5.
Hope/Motivation	Billock, C. (2009). Integrating spirituality into home health occupational therapy practice. *Home and Community Health Special Interest Section Quarterly, 16*(1), 3–4.

Appendix 7.B. Themes of Experience of Spirituality *(Cont.)*

Application to Practice: Occupational Therapy Practitioner's Role	Citation
	Bowen, J. E. (1999). Health promotion in the new millennium: Opening the lens-adjusting the focus. *OT Practice,4*(12), 14–18.
	Hafez, A. (1998). OT and spirituality (continued). *OT Practice, 3*(6), 58–59.
	Hettinger, J. (1996). Bringing spirituality into practice. *OT Week, 10*(24), 16–18.
	Hoppes, S. (1997). Motivating clients through goal setting. *OT Practice, 2*(6), 22–27.
	Rosenfeld, M. S. (2004). Motivating elders with depression in SNFs. *OT Practice, 9*(11), 21–28.
	Swarbrick, P., & Burkhardt, A. (2000). Spiritual health: Implications for the occupational therapy process. *Mental Health Special Interest Section Quarterly, 23*(2), 1–3.
Therapeutic Use of Self	Burgman, I., & King, A. (2005). The presence of child spirituality. In F. Kronenberg (Ed.), *Occupational therapy without borders: Learning from the spirit of survivors* (pp. 153–165). New York: Elsevier/Churchill Livingstone.
	Crepeau, E., James, A. B., Spear, P. S., Francoeur, M., Garren, K., Stewart-Whipple, J., & Rosenfeld, M. S. (2000). Letters: The spirituality discussion (continued). *OT Practice, 5*(15), 23.
	Fox, L. (2009). Native American spirituality: A truly holistic perspective. *Home and Community Special Interest Section Quarterly, 16*(1), 1–2.
	Gabriel, L. (2005). Reflections on Spirituality: Implications for ethics education. In R. Purtilo, G. Jensen, & C. Royeen (Eds.), *Educating for moral action: A sourcebook in health and rehabilitation ethics* (pp. 203–214). Philadelphia: F. A. Davis.
	Hafez, A. (1998). OT and spirituality (continued). *OT Practice, 3*(6), 58–59.
	Moses, M. D. (1997). Viewpoints: Therapeutic use of self: How can we maintain it? *OT Week, 11*(1), 50.
	Swarbrick, P., & Burkhardt, A. (2000). Spiritual health: Implications for the occupational therapy process. *Mental Health Special Interest Section Quarterly, 23*(2), 1–3.
	Trump, S. M. (2001). Occupational therapy and hospice: A natural fit. *OT Practice, 6*(20), 7–8, 10–11.
Creative Occupation	Sadlo, G. (2004). Creativity and occupation. In Molineux, M. (Ed.). *Occupation for occupational therapists* (90–100). Malden, MA: Blackwell Publishing.
Meaning: Occupational Role	Ayres, A. J. (1998). The art of therapy. *Sensory Integration Special Interest Quarterly, 21*(4), 1–3, 6.
	Berg, J. (1997). Aging as in "sage-ing". *OT Week, 11*(50), 18.
	Bowen-Irish, T. (2005). Here I sit. *OT Practice, 10*(3), 21–22.
	Swedberg, L. (2001). Facilitating accessibility and participation in faith communities. *OT Practice, 6*(9), CE1–CE8.
Meaning: Life Meaning	Trump, S. M. (2001). Occupational therapy and hospice: A natural fit. *OT Practice, 6*(20), 7–8, 10–11.

(Continued)

Appendix 7.B. Themes of Experience of Spirituality *(Cont.)*

Application to Practice: Occupational Therapy Practitioner's Role	Citation/Link
	Christiansen, C. (1997). Acknowledging a spiritual dimension in occupational therapy practice. *American Journal of Occupational Therapy, 51*(3), 169–172. http://bit.ly/1PMxfBI
	Crepeau, E., James, A. B., Spear, P. S., Francoeur, M., Garren, K., Stewart-Whipple, J., & Rosenfeld, M. S. (2000). Letters: The spirituality discussion (continued). *OT Practice, 5*(15), 23.
Meaning: Activities of Value	Burgman, I., & King, A. (2005). The presence of child spirituality. In F. Kronenberg (Ed.), *Occupational therapy without borders: Learning from the spirit of survivors* (pp. 153–165). New York: Elsevier/Churchill Livingstone.
	Dawson, D. R., & Stern, B. (2007). Reflections on facilitating older adult's participation in valued occupations. *OT NOW, 9*(5), 3–5. http://bit.ly/1PReEkH
	Feeney, L., & Toth-Cohen, S. (2008). Addressing spirituality for clients with physical disabilities. *OT Practice, 13*(4), 16–20.
	Jung, B., Salvatori, P., Missiuna, C., Wilkins, S., Stewart, D., & Law, M. (1999). The McMaster lens for occupational therapists: Bringing theory and practice into focus. *OT NOW, 10*(2), 16–19. http://bit.ly/20ZMHlg
	Larson, K. O. (1998). OT and spirituality. *OT Practice, 3*(3), 56–57.
	Peloquin, S. M. (1997). The spiritual depth of occupation: Making worlds and making lives. *American Journal of Occupational Therapy, 51*(3), 167–168. http://bit.ly/1mqHX4Q
	Reid, D. (2010). Mundane occupations: Providing opportunity for engagement and being-in-the-world. *OT NOW, 12*(2), 24–26.
	Rosenfeld, M. S. (2001). Exploring a spiritual context for care. *OT Practice, 6*(11), 18–24.
	Rosenfeld, M.S. (2001). Spirituality, motivation, and performance. *OT NOW, 3*(6), 1–10.
	Strzelecki, M. V. (2006). An OT approach to clients with cancer. *OT Practice, 11*(15), 7–8.
	Unruh, A. M., Versnel, J., & Kerr, N. (2004b). Spirituality in the context of occupation: A theory to practice application. In M. Molineux (Ed.). *Occupation for occupational therapists* (pp. 32–45). Malden, MA: Blackwell.
	Urbanowski, R. (1997). Spirituality in everyday practice. *OT Practice, 2*(12), 18–23.
	Vrkljan, B. H. (2000). Put it to practice: The role of spirituality in occupational therapy practice. *OT NOW, 2*(2), 1–5.
Meaning: Context	Billock, C. (2009). Integrating spirituality into home health occupational therapy practice. *Home and Community Health Special Interest Section Quarterly, 16*(1), 2–4.
	Larson, K. O. (1998). OT and spirituality. *OT Practice, 3*(3), 56–57.
	Rosenfeld, M. S. (2004). Motivating elders with depression in SNFs. *OT Practice, 9*(11), 21–28.
	Trump, S. M., (2001). Occupational therapy and hospice: A natural fit. *OT Practice, 6*(20), 7–8, 10–11.
Meaning: Connection to Others	Ramugondo, E. L. (2005). Unlocking spirituality: Play as a health-promoting occupation in the context of HIV/AIDS. In F. Kronenberg (Ed.), *Occupational therapy without borders: Learning from the spirit of survivors* (pp. 313–325). New York: Elsevier/Churchill Livingstone.

CHAPTER 8.

FACILITATING THERAPEUTIC USE OF SELF TO INTEGRATE SPIRITUALITY INTO OCCUPATIONAL THERAPY PRACTICE

Tamera Keiter Humbert, MA, DEd, OTR/L

Chapter Highlights

◇ Therapeutic relationship
◇ Professional development and therapeutic use of self
◇ History of therapeutic use of self
◇ Connection between therapeutic relationship and therapeutic use of self
◇ Expectations for and intention of therapeutic use of self
◇ Practitioner characteristics
◇ Client desires and expectations
◇ Developing therapeutic use of self to integrate spirituality into practice.

Key Terms and Concepts

◇ Active listening
◇ Being present
◇ Client-centered approach
◇ Collaborative approach
◇ Compassionate listening
◇ Compassionate sharing
◇ Cultural effectiveness
◇ Empathy
◇ Intentional listening
◇ Intentional Relationship Model
◇ Interactional reasoning
◇ Intuition
◇ Journeying with clients

◇ Life balance
◇ Mindfulness
◇ Occupational integrity
◇ Open-mindedness
◇ Openness
◇ Professional development
◇ Self-awareness
◇ Self-disclosure
◇ Therapeutic relationship
◇ Therapeutic use of self
◇ Transformation
◇ Transformational Model of Rehabilitation
◇ Vulnerability

The integration of spirituality into occupational therapy practice is a dynamic process between practitioners and clients.[1] What practitioners have to offer in addressing spirituality or being sensitive to spirituality with clients reflects their own lived experiences and how they have made personal sense, or meaning, of those experiences. This internal knowing, or spirituality, influences and shapes how practitioners engage others in the therapeutic relationship.

This chapter provides an opportunity for students and practitioners to assess their own understanding of the use of spirituality in the occupational therapy process and explore the possibility of expanding their comfort in discussing spirituality as part of the therapeutic relationship. It provides a brief background on and general concepts related to the therapeutic relationship and the therapeutic use of self. It then expands upon these ideas by discussing how they relate to the integration of spirituality into practice through three major paths: (1) expectations for or intention of therapeutic use of self, (2) practitioner characteristics, and (3) client desires and expectations. The chapter concludes with a discussion of developing the therapeutic use of self to integrate spirituality into practice.

Therapeutic Relationship

The ***therapeutic relationship*** is the intricate partnering between practitioner and client that facilitates the occupational therapy process (Taylor, 2008). It is complex and individualized because each client comes to the therapy process with varying desires, goals, and levels of comfort in the therapeutic relationship. For the practitioner, meeting the client where he or she is and establishing a therapeutic and helpful relationship can be challenging, especially when spirituality is added to the mix (Bray, Egan, & Beagan, 2012). In addition, the practitioner–client relationship may be compromised if the practitioner and client have difficulty relating to one another, especially when spiritual or religious values are not compatible (Schulz, 2004).

Professional Development and Therapeutic Use of Self

Professional development is the process of expanding skills and attitudes toward knowledge, reflection, self-awareness, and insights relative to the professional role. The ***therapeutic use of self*** involves occupational therapy practitioners making intentional decisions that facilitate their active engagement with clients in the therapeutic relationship. Professional development is a lifelong process and often correlates with practitioners' personal and professional strengths and challenges. Moreover, having available resources (e.g., mentoring from experienced practitioners, written material related to the topic) and the willingness to explore these challenges expands practitioners' understanding and use of spirituality in practice.

Occupational therapy practitioners are often faced with the trials of life events, through personal experiences or through clients' life transitions, and need to be prepared to make sense of those experiences. Professional development

> implies that education of healers and therapists might entail more than the accumulation and classification of external facts and knowledge of technical procedures. It might also involve the search for and cultivation of wisdom and virtue, for a spiritual measure by which to make good judgments about the treatment of clients. (Kroeker, 1997, p. 126)

Therefore, professional development is connected with the therapeutic relationship and has also been linked with spirituality (Smith, 2008).

As practitioners reflect on and make sense of pain, suffering, and death, they need to begin to assess their own understanding of how best to address such significant difficulties and loss, and what skills may be needed to do so within the therapy process. Reflection on and self-awareness of one's attitudes and the needed skills prompt the practitioner to take inventory of which aspects of the therapeutic relationship need to be emphasized and which aspects need to be further developed.

---

[1]The term *client* can also include the family and the community.

History of Therapeutic Use of Self

The occupational therapy literature has reported on the concept of therapeutic use of self for decades, but its conceptualization has evolved. The term *therapeutic use of self*, first attributed to psychiatrist Jerome Frank (1958), was initially described as the way the therapist (i.e., practitioner) improves and matures the self to develop a more complex and expansive approach to others, so the therapist can effectively use various approaches during therapy. Frank's idea of therapeutic use of self was primarily focused on the practitioner's psychosocial development to provide better therapeutic results. Frank emphasized that the practitioner projects an image to the client within the therapy session that facilitates the client's success, which the client then carries to other aspects of his or her life.

Frank's (1958) articulation of the therapeutic use of self implied that the client was lacking in some quality that enabled him or her to be successful in completing occupations, and if the practitioner were to emulate and project that quality onto the client, the client could embrace that quality and improve his or her ability to engage in occupations. According to Frank, there was a clear recognition that the therapeutic relationship was an important aspect of the therapy process and that practitioners should use their own personality and qualities to achieve success. He wrote,

> My own belief is that most of us have enough innate healing potentialities, and are well enough organized to be able to present an acting self to the patient which enables him to achieve a better integration of himself. If we do not keep our therapeutic role distinct from the rest of ourselves, we run the risk of impeding our therapeutic efficacy in several ways. . . . the therapeutic role of the occupational therapist is confined to trying to bring about modifications in the acting self of the patient. [The therapist] tries to help the patient modify his expectancies in a limited area of his functioning—the task he is doing—in the hope that the self-confidence thus gained will generalize to other areas of the patient's life. (pp. 222–223)

Throughout the past several decades, the term *therapeutic use of self* has been used in the literature, but its definition has expanded to include a more dynamic therapeutic relationship. It has progressed from an approach in which only the practitioner directs and influences the therapeutic relationship with the client to a collaborative and affirming approach that acknowledges the value of the client's life experiences and perspectives and the ability of the client to also influence and change the practitioner's perspectives through the therapeutic relationship.

Connection Between Therapeutic Relationship and Therapeutic Use of Self

The connecting theme in the professional evolution of the therapeutic use of self and the therapeutic relationship is that both involve the intentional process of engaging with a client to promote effective intervention and helpful relationships. Although the overall intention to use the therapeutic use of self and the therapeutic relationship in the therapeutic process to achieve therapeutic goals remains the same, how these concepts have been understood have changed over the past five decades (Table 8.1). The evolving descriptions have maintained the assumption that practitioners need to be aware of their own personal skills and abilities, biases, and developmental strengths and needs because these factors influence the quality and dynamic of the therapeutic relationship.

According to the *Occupational Therapy Practice Framework: Domain and Process* (American Occupational Therapy Association [AOTA], 2014), the therapeutic use of self and the therapeutic relationship are understood as parts of the clinical reasoning process in which information and perspectives about the client become part of the therapy dynamic. The *Framework* defines *therapeutic use of self* as "an integral part of the occupational therapy process . . . [that] allows occupational therapy practitioners to develop and manage their therapeutic relationship with clients by using narrative and clinical reasoning; empathy; and a client-centered, collaborative approach to service delivery" (AOTA, 2014, p. S12).

Table 8.1. Descriptions of Therapeutic Use of Self and Therapeutic Relationship in Select Editions of *Willard and Spackman's Occupational Therapy*

Edition/Author	Description
4th (Walker, 1971)	"The more effective therapists believe in what they do. They have a purpose in living" (p. 523).
	"Essential in a therapeutic environment is a therapist who possesses the basic attitude that he is a worthwhile person, a person who has a purpose he believes in and a job to do that he feels is important. When the therapist believes in himself, he believes in others" (p. 524).
7th (Hopkins & Tiffany, 1988)	"The therapist in a treatment setting is, by definition, a helper. The roles a therapist assumes may vary. The therapist may legitimately be a teacher or a facilitator who brings knowledge and skills to the client's unique situation. The most important prerequisite to being an effective helper is self-knowledge: the helper needs to be aware of his/her own needs, perceptual biases, and capabilities" (p. 108).
7th (Schwartzberg, 1988)	"A therapeutic relationship is a developmental process. The therapist needs to determine how much support and gratification are necessary to sustain the patient's health and well-being. This varies depending on the nature and phase of the therapeutic relationship" (p. 385).
8th (Schwartzberg, 1993)	"The therapist's use of self is critical to engaging the patient in occupational therapy. Three ingredients are essential to establishing a therapeutic relationship: understanding, neutrality, sometimes called *empathy,* and caring" (p. 269, *italics added*).
10th (Peloquin, 2003)	"The art of the profession's practice, like most art, is a process of making connections, evoking responses, and finding shared meaning" (p. 157).
	"One who masters the art of practice perceives and responds to the individual seeking therapy as a whole person, indivisible into parts or subsystems" (p.158).
11th (Price, 2009)	"The therapeutic relationship is the central aspect of the therapeutic process of occupational therapy and one catalyst for change" (p. 328). "Therapists use themselves as therapeutic agents when they shift their role such as director, coach, supporter, and follower, fluidly responding and using multiple strategies" (p. 336).
	"Establishing a collaborative relationship requires that clients be willing to actively engage as partners in the therapy process and that therapists be willing to offer and finely adjust therapy activities on the basis of the client's priorities and a careful reading of their desires, motives, and experiences of therapy" (p. 332).
12th (Taylor, 2013)	"One of the most common terms used to refer to therapist–client interactions is the therapeutic relationship. Literature and dialogue about the therapeutic relationship commonly address topics such as rapport building, communication, conflict resolution, emotional sharing, collaboration, and partnership between therapists and clients. Therapeutic use of self is a popular term used in occupational therapy to refer to the therapist's deliberate efforts to enhance their interactions with clients" (p. 426).

Expectations for and Intention of Therapeutic Use of Self

There is an expectation in the occupational therapy literature that practitioners be aware of and develop therapeutic use of self. However, how therapeutic use of self is actually understood and demonstrated within intervention varies. The focus of practitioners within the therapeutic relationship shapes how the therapeutic process is constructed and how it will unfold. What practitioners attend to is indicative of how they understand, value, and uphold their role in the therapeutic process. This focus has evolved from maximizing the therapeutic relationship and using a client-centered approach to journeying with clients, which includes spirituality in the therapeutic relationship. Journeying with clients involves intentionally focusing on the lived experiences of the client and incorporating them into therapy; being open to a deeper understanding of the client; and attending to meaning making, purpose, connectivity, and life choices.

Maximizing the Therapeutic Relationship

In the initial conceptualization of the therapeutic use of self, the expectations for and intention of the therapeutic use of self were to maximize the therapeutic relationship. This approach centers on the idea that the practitioner is more than a supplier of therapeutic activities, occupations, or modalities. The practitioner is also part of the therapy mix, in which his or her actions, comments, and approaches influence the client, facilitating the achievement of therapeutic goals.

Interactional reasoning, the type of clinical reasoning used by practitioners that focuses on maximizing the therapeutic relationship through verbal and nonverbal therapeutic approaches, was thus promoted to strengthen the therapeutic relationship. In addition, various roles were suggested for the practitioner to assume to facilitate therapeutic goals (Boyt Schell & Schell, 2008; Cole, 2005; Mattingly & Fleming, 1994). The assumption behind this approach is that the practitioner is the expert and has skills, knowledge, and insights that are valuable in the therapeutic process. This approach is still recognized in the current literature (Boyt Schell & Schell, 2008); however, the expectations for and intention of the therapeutic use of self has expanded beyond this approach.

Using a Client-Centered Approach

The power dynamics and focus of the therapeutic relationship have evolved from the practitioner fully directing the therapeutic assessment and intervention to the client having more input and decisions about the intervention (Townsend, 2003) in a collaborative, *client-centered approach.* The *Framework* (AOTA, 2014) describes the *collaborative*

approach as honoring contributions of clients and practitioners throughout the therapeutic process:

> Through the use of interpersonal communication skills, occupational therapy practitioners shift the power of the relationship to allow clients more control in decision making and problem solving, which is essential to effective intervention. Clients bring to the occupational therapy process their knowledge about their life experiences and their hopes and dreams for the future. They identify and share their needs and priorities. Occupational therapy practitioners bring their knowledge about how engagement in occupation affects health, well-being, and participation; they use this information, coupled with theoretical perspectives and clinical reasoning, to critically observe, analyze, describe, and interpret human performance. Practitioners and clients, together with caregivers, family members, community members, and other stakeholders (as appropriate), identify and prioritize the focus of the intervention plan. (p. S12)

However, even in the collaborative approach, the practitioner is usually the primary person directing or facilitating the therapeutic process and the one with expert knowledge and experience about the therapeutic process (Price, 2009; Townsend, 2003). Although the practitioner brings empathy to the therapeutic relationship to better understand client perspectives, his or her role still remains fairly dominant. In addition, although the client-centered approach helps in the formulation of intervention goals and strategies (Taylor & Van Puymbroeck, 2013), the therapeutic relationship and exchange are often connected to and potentially restricted by decision making and problem solving (AOTA, 2014; Price, 2009).

Therefore, the therapeutic relationship centers on the practitioner seeking advice or information from the client to address the client's needs and concerns. There is little recognition that the client may have another role in the therapeutic relationship, which is to provide insights into a life not known or understood by the practitioner.

Journeying With Clients

An approach to the therapeutic use of self associated with spirituality is beginning to emerge in the literature, in particular, in areas in which suffering is attended to as part of the therapeutic process. The phrase *journeying with clients* is used to represent a change in the therapeutic relationship from practitioner as expert to practitioner who learns about and enters the client's world. This approach requires the practitioner to acknowledge the often unknown course of events that the client experiences during major life challenges (e.g., dealing with the aftermath of a stroke) and to join the client in that unknown.

In addition, this approach offers the possibility of the practitioner delivering more responsive care by allowing daily events and therapeutic responses to them to unfold naturally. More specifically, the practitioner does not establish intervention goals and strategies for the client and then just apply them in therapy sessions but instead addresses what is most important to the client at any specific moment. The therapy session is directed by the client's present needs, and the approaches used to address those needs are discussed and explored collaboratively with the client.

Journeying with clients recognizes the personal and deep meaning that clients bring to major life events and requires practitioners not only to walk alongside clients during their journey by engaging in the co-creation of occupations and rituals but also live with and learn from clients through their journey (Beagan & Kumas-Tan, 2005; Collins, 2007; Luboshitzky, 2008; Romanoff & Thompson, 2006).

According to Luboshitzky (2008),

> occupational therapy practitioners must acknowledge [their] responsibility to accompany clients in their journey through suffering and pain and accept it not as a misfortune, causing feelings of hopelessness and helplessness, but as an empowering experience necessary for personal and universal development and growth. (p. 365)

In the context of the therapeutic use of self, in this approach, spirituality is understood as the connection between the practitioner and client and the act of practitioners journeying with clients. Moreover, the focus on spirituality within the construct of the therapeutic use of self implies intentional acknowledgment of the potential connectivity among all people associated with the therapeutic journey and a desire to be open to such connectivity. This connectivity is elucidated in Schulz's (2004) definition

of *spirituality:* "experiencing a meaningful connection to our core self, other humans, the world, and a greater power as expressed through our reflections, narratives and actions" (p. 72).

Practitioner Characteristics

The occupational therapy literature has identified the following practitioner characteristics as essential for integrating spirituality into practice:

- Empathy
- Active listening
- Compassionate listening
- Openness
- Compassionate sharing
- Being present
- Intentional listening.

Not only are these characteristics valuable and necessary when attending to the spiritual aspects of the therapeutic process, they also suggest a new paradigm in how practitioners understand boundaries within the therapeutic relationship regarding what they say and do. Although ethical boundaries are recognized in all therapeutic relationships (AOTA, 2014), the literature has indicated a shift in therapeutic relationships, in and outside the occupational therapy profession, in support of a more dynamic relationship between practitioner and client, particularly in the collaborative and client-centered approach (Provencher & Keyes, 2011; Young, 2010).

Moreover, the literature related to spirituality and therapeutic use of self has shifted further, considering not only the potential for practitioner and client *vulnerability* (i.e., shared openness about personal beliefs and perspectives) but also reciprocal personal and professional growth between client and practitioner within the therapeutic relationship (Gee & Loewenthal, 2013; Kirsh, 2011).

For example, consider a practitioner working in end-of-life care with a client and family discussing goals and desires for therapy. As part of the conversation, the client begins to share her concerns about prolonging life and expresses a desire to allow death to occur, ending life with dignity and quality.

Although this conversation might be complex and challenging for everyone involved, it entails willingness from both the client and the practitioner to enter into that conversation with openness and to honestly acknowledge that the conversation is difficult. The practitioner's life experiences (personal and professional) may or may not have adequately prepared the practitioner to know how best to respond to the client or know what to expect for the client. There is an appreciation that the practitioner brings professional and personal knowledge and experience to the relationship but is also open to being transformed by the therapeutic process.

Empathy

According to the *Framework* (AOTA, 2014), *empathy* "is the emotional exchange between occupational therapy practitioners and clients that allows more open communication, ensuring that practitioners connect with clients at an emotional level to assist them with their current life situation" (p. S12). The empathetic practitioner respects the anxiety and angst often felt and expressed by the client and significant others in light of a major life event or transition. For example, as a client comes to terms with a devastating accident resulting in multiple occupational challenges, empathy allows the practitioner to understand the level of concern and emotional turmoil and engage in conversation with the client about his or her struggles.

Active Listening

Active listening, the ability to truly hear, or understand, what the client is sharing related to his or her life and present circumstances, is necessary to cultivate empathy. It entails the practitioner putting aside their own biases, being present with and for the client, and showing and offering dignity (Pizzi & Briggs, 2004; Thibeault, 1997, 2011).

Active listening may also encompass the use of narratives and storytelling so that the practitioner has the ability to use narrative reasoning to comprehend and make sense of the client's perspectives about life and purpose (Boyt Schell & Schell, 2008; Howard & Howard, 1997; Kirsh, 1996, 2011; Mattingly & Fleming, 1994).

Compassionate Listening

Beyond empathy and active listening, authors have proposed developing and using compassionate listening

in practice, particularly as the practitioner attends to the area of spirituality. *Compassionate listening* is the ability to hold, acknowledge, and honor what the client views as life affirming and hopeful and broach conversations to elucidate these perspectives. It is more than just active listening. Unruh, Versnel, and Kerr (2004) described the need for compassionate listening:

> Because client-centered collaboration is central to occupational therapy intervention, occupational therapists talk with the client about what occupations give life meaning. Such discussions may include talking with the client about spirituality and then listening with sensitivity, with compassion, and without hurry to spiritual needs and concerns. (p. 37)

The ability to engage in conversations about life meaning, purpose, and hope requires compassionate listening and the willingness to honor the spiritual journey the person may be on or how their spiritual journey is being challenged as a result of their life circumstances.

Openness

Openness is the willingness and ability to initiate conversations and allow people to share what is most important to them, even when the topics are challenging. Kroeker (1997) identified the need for practitioners to demonstrate "openness and plurality, respect for difference and shared exploration of the meaning of reality" (p. 125). In addressing topics such as suffering, loss, grief, and death in occupational therapy, openness may involve discussing and inviting conversation about spirituality. The way practitioners understand and approach these topics reflects their therapeutic use of self (Fine, 1991; Luboshitzky, 2008; Pollard, 2006; Simó-Algado & Burgman, 2005).

Moreover, because practitioners may frequently need to address these concerns in practice, they need to learn to openly "live them" with their clients. For example, according to Pollard (2006), occupations are grounded in relationships and dying is considered an occupation. Therefore, in working with a dying client, practitioners must engage in a relationship with that client and the client's significant others and personally acknowledge their own views about life and death while affirming the client's views and the practitioner–client relationship. Practitioners attending to spirituality need to respectfully and openly broach such conversations and ways of being with those they journey with.

Compassionate Sharing

Beyond listening and showing empathy and openness, practitioners might be asked to share their own perspectives about loss, grief, purpose, and hope. *Compassionate sharing* entails practitioners sharing insights and personal and professional experiences with clients, responding with great care to their expressed concerns.

Journeying with clients during life challenges involves practitioners and clients having conversations to facilitate clients' thoughts and perspectives about the present and the future (Tse, Lloyd, Petchkovsky, & Manaia, 2005; Williams, 2008). Within this collaborative and dynamic therapeutic process, practitioners support such conversation but also provide practical images of meaning, purpose, and hope that are then reflected in the practitioner's and client's shared creation of and engagement in occupations and daily rituals (Tse et al., 2005; Williams, 2008). It is important for practitioners to offer realistic and applicable images in the midst of the client's suffering, loss, and grief.

In addition, according to Romanoff and Thompson (2006), "[i]t is important to note that the design and enactment of rituals is a co-creation of the patient and practitioner and not a stock exercise" (p. 313). Clients often ask, 'What does my future look like?' or 'Will I get better?' The practitioner must be able to sensitively balance possible future scenarios with the client's desire and hope for complete healing.

Being Present

Another characteristic of the therapeutic use of self in the literature on spirituality is the practitioner's ability to relinquish preconceived notions of what is best for the client and the notion of an expert professional role and consider a mutually shared therapeutic relationship by *being present*, or being fully aware and attentive in the present moment to the client's needs, strengths, and desires. When

the practitioner is being present with the client, the therapeutic relationship is able to develop and grow (Collins, 1998, 2007). Moreover, Romanoff and Thompson (2006) stated that

> [t]he ability to be present to a suffering patient, the willingness to simply listen, is in itself restorative. The goal is not to analyze or change the story the patient tells. Rather, the goal is to enter into a relationship to hear and to honor the story the patient tells as many times as the patient needs to tell it. There is nothing that needs to be "fixed." It is the intersubjective telling of the story in the presence of an empathetic witness that fosters healing. (p. 311)

Before practitioners initiate conversation or offer images of hope, they may be asked to only attend to and share in the immediate, and often poignant, needs of a client just after a traumatic event, honoring and supporting the client's responses to the life event. Greenberg (2003) described this practitioner role of being present in her account of life as a practitioner and resident of New York after 9/11. This "spiritual spontaneity," or "readiness to respond spiritually to the unexpected" (Greenberg, 2003, p. 162), entails learning humility and reverence, being open to new perspectives, having shared community discourse, listening deeply to others, cultivating reflection, and pondering life questions.

Intentional Listening

Intentional listening is the ability of practitioners to perceive the client's perspectives and honor these perspectives throughout the therapy process. In addition, practitioners and clients may have divergent perspectives, which may cause the practitioner to question or explore his or her personal perspectives. Practitioners must recognize that this situation can lead to a relationship in which practitioner and client both contribute to each other's growth and well-being.

In their description of intentional listening, Romanoff and Thompson (2006) suggest that the practitioner should have a willingness, and maybe even a desire, to be part of a personally transformative therapeutic relationship: "If the listener sets aside his or her own experiences for the narrator, then there is an opportunity for mutual learning and transformation" (p. 312).

Client Desires and Expectations

The empirical occupational therapy literature on client desires and expectations related to the therapeutic relationship is limited. Nevertheless, clients have identified the therapeutic relationship as critical to the intervention outcome (Cole & McLean, 2003; Palmadottir, 2003).

It is important to understand that the expectations for therapy often vary between practitioners and clients. Practitioners tend to assess the quality of the therapeutic relationship on the outcome of the therapy process, or how well the client achieved the goals of therapy (Bachelor, 2011; Ward, Linville, & Rosen, 2007). These goals are often assessed by changes in the client's actions, behaviors, and attitudes. Clients, on the other hand, tend to assess the effectiveness of the therapy process, or the outcome, on how helpful the practitioner was during the process (Bachelor, 2011; Ward et al., 2007). These differences reflect the varying perspectives and beliefs about the function of the therapeutic process and client and practitioner roles within the therapeutic relationship. In this section, research outside the field (primarily associated with psychotherapy) was used to explore clients' desires and expectations for the therapeutic relationship.

Clients have identified the therapeutic relationship as one in which some connection or bond exists between the practitioner and client. This connection is strengthened through openness between the client and practitioner and the ability of the practitioner to listen to the client. Clients must feel safe to disclose what is most important to them and to share their feelings when they are most vulnerable (Audet & Everall, 2010; Ward et al., 2007).

Practitioners must also embody trust and respect for clients during these intimate exchanges (Palmadottir, 2003). Terms used by clients to describe helpful therapeutic relationships include *openness, empathy, care,* and *alliance* (Duff & Bedi, 2010; Green et al., 2008; Shattell, Starr, & Thomas, 2007; Steffen, 2013). Primary characteristics of good therapeutic relationships include practitioner self-disclosure; collaboration; and hope, being present, and positivity. In addition, some clients have expressed a desire for spirituality in the therapeutic relationship.

Self-Disclosure

Self-disclosure, or providing personal information about oneself, is seen by some clients as helpful in establishing the therapeutic relationship. Practitioners who share information about themselves that is select and timely help clients see them as real (i.e., individuals with their own personal challenges), vulnerable, and authentic, or honest (Audet & Everall, 2010). For many clients, practitioner self-disclosure helps establish the power dynamics of the professional relationship and may encourage greater sharing and openness by the client (Audet & Everall, 2010).

Collaboration

A collaborative work relationship is identified by clients as helpful in the therapeutic process. This relationship affirms the client's perspective of his or her strengths and needs, which helps in the development of clear, progressive goals (Palmadottir, 2003). Moreover, the client not only understands the goals but also believes the goals capture what he or she truly desires (Bachelor, 2011). Collaboration may not always be equal regarding who establishes the goals, but it involves both the practitioner and client working toward goals that are important and meaningful to the client.

Hope, Being Present, and Positivity

Good therapeutic relationships involve the client feeling that hope is being offered through the therapy process. Providing images of hope offers the client different perspectives and consequently something to hold onto and work toward (Gee & Loewenthal, 2013; Ward et al., 2007). In the occupational therapy literature, hope is often represented tangibly as the ability to engage in valued occupations and build a new, albeit potentially different, future (Palmadottir, 2003). In addition, clients have identified the practitioner being present with the client during traumatic life events and offering unconditional and positive regard during the therapy process as important (Gee & Loewenthal, 2013).

Spirituality

Some preliminary literature has suggested that clients desire spirituality in the therapeutic relationship and that the ability and willingness of practitioners to engage in spirituality in practice is just as important to clients as the practitioner characteristics of empathy, compassion, and care (Gockel, 2011). In addition, some clients want practitioners to be open to spiritual aspects of healing and transformation.

Some practitioners may not address spirituality in the therapy process or use the language of spirituality to describe therapy. However, being willing to consider spirituality as a life course or journey is frequently helpful to clients. In addition, being present in the moment (Grepmair, Mitterlehner, Loew, & Nickel, 2007), attending to the client's spirit, and embodying love for the client have been identified by clients as meaningful in the therapeutic relationship (Richards & Bergin, 2005).

Moreover, practitioners should be aware that language commonly used in practice that may not be considered spiritual can have spiritual connotations. For example, hope can be seen as an aspect of spirituality in the therapy process because it places the client's life event into a larger world and life view schematic (Gockel, 2011). The concepts of *intuition* (i.e., a way of knowing beyond rationale thought) and *mindfulness* (i.e., being fully present in the moment) suggest a response to the client that is not based primarily on theoretical constructs or techniques (Audet & Everall, 2010; Gockel, 2011).

Developing Therapeutic Use of Self

No matter what approach is taken when engaging the therapeutic use of self, there is an understanding in the profession that it needs to be developed; it is not inherent. Some practitioners may possess natural qualities that contribute to the therapeutic process, such as compassion, empathetic listening, and openness to other perspectives, but how they use such qualities in a therapeutic manner depends on the development of personal and professional attributes and values. Contributors to this development include

- Respectful mentoring relationships;
- Acquisition of knowledge, self-awareness, and skills; and

- Ability to use reflection constructively (Boyt Schell & Schell, 2008).

This section discusses practitioners' emotional factors, self-awareness, personal transformation, cultural effectiveness, open-mindedness, and occupational integrity.

Intentional Relationship Model

One example of professional development that highlights practitioners' responses and reactions within the therapeutic use of self is the ***Intentional Relationship Model*** (Taylor, 2008). This approach addresses practitioners' ability to determine what emotional factors influence or contribute to the therapeutic relationship and assess them (Taylor, 2008). The assumption behind this model is the recognition that practitioners' personal emotional makeup and relational dynamics affect how they respond to clients throughout the therapeutic process. Practitioners' ability to be self-aware and to self-monitor these factors increases their ability to modify them if needed and intentionally choose to respond to clients in a helpful therapeutic manner (Smith & Taylor, 2010).

Self-Awareness

Self-awareness is the ability to know and understand one's own perspectives and skills. Authors who address spirituality in occupational therapy have provided insights into the development of self-awareness to maximize the qualities suggested for a dynamic therapeutic approach and foster the integration of spirituality into practice. This development pushes practitioners to strive to understand topics associated with spirituality, stretch personal levels of comfort in considering these topics and articulating them to others, and consider different ways to approach and conduct therapy. According to Pizzi and Briggs (2004), "the willingness to engage in spiritual discussion is likely to depend on the therapist's own personal comfort with spirituality as well as the nature of the client's spirituality" (p. 37).

Proponents of spirituality ask practitioners to be aware of and develop skills to self-assess and monitor their personal judgments, biases, values, beliefs, and emotional responses (Pizzi & Briggs, 2004; Taylor & Van Puymbroeck, 2013) and cultivate a practice that allows them to be present with clients, especially during challenging or emotional times (Pizzi & Briggs, 2004; Spector, 1996; Wilson, 2011).

Practitioners also need to be aware of their personal perspectives of pain and suffering (Hayward & Taylor, 2011; Luboshitzky, 2008) and adversity and resilience (Fine, 1991; Thibeault, 2011; Wilson, 2010, 2011) and assess how these perspectives may influence their practice decisions (Hayward & Taylor, 2011; Hooper, 1997; Low, 1997). For example, some practitioners may have to expand their comfort level with pain and suffering to accompany clients through their difficulties. According to Luboshitzky (2008), the process of self-discovery and wrestling with the concepts associated with pain and suffering is unique to each person:

> As therapists, we must realize that changing our own attitudes towards suffering can enable us to better help clients in exploring meaning in their suffering and thus their everyday life occupations as well. This process entails an attempt to accomplish the following objectives: to explore the purpose of one's suffering in relation to the unique meaning of one's life; to realize that the search for meaning is an individual task which each person must do alone; and to understand that even though one is not always able to change one's situation, one can always change one's attitude towards it. (p. 30)

Practitioners need to develop and be aware of their own worldview, including perspectives of spirituality. According to Unruh, Versnel, and Kerr (2002), developing a worldview entails exploring personal and subjective spiritual questions about the origin, purpose, meaning, and form of human life. This development involves being cognizant of not only one's personal views but also other perspectives to appreciate the diversity of thinking and be less likely to make assumptions about others' beliefs or project beliefs onto others (Bray et al., 2012; Hooper, 1997; Kang, 2003; Low, 1997; Smith, 2008; Wilson, 2010).

Transformational Model of Rehabilitation

Forster, Fardella, and McColl (2011) proposed the use and integration of the *Transformational Model of Rehabilitation* into practice to assist in dealing with burnout, compassion fatigue, and moral stress.

This model introduces the use of personal transformation, for both client and practitioner. *Transformation* is an attitude and approach that recognizes the importance of personal growth through relationships and through the therapeutic process, with the outcome being maturity for the practitioner.

Cultural Effectiveness

Cultural effectiveness is the ability of practitioners to acknowledge and respond to the cultural contexts of clients to provide effective therapeutic interventions. Practitioners must continually develop cultural sensitivity and responsiveness, particularly as they relate to spirituality or religious life. Having a deeper appreciation for and understanding of clients' beliefs, practices, and rituals may enhance the development of clients' desired goals in the therapy process (Brémault-Phillips & Chirovsky, 2011; Farah & McColl, 2008, 2011; Muñoz, 2007).

Cultural sensitivity and responsiveness include acknowledgment by practitioners that they cannot be fully aware of all cultural, religious, or spiritual differences. Instead, they need to learn more about principles of culture; develop respect for others' beliefs and rituals; and recognize when they need additional information, mentoring, and support, particularly when working with clients who are dealing with spiritual and religious concerns.

Open-Mindedness

Open-mindedness involves practitioners expanding their appreciation of and willingness to learn from their own and clients' life events. They should recognize the wisdom gained by clients as they experience life events, particularly when practitioners have limited experiences in such life events (Collins, 1998, 2007; Kirsh, 2011; Spector, 1996; Thibeault, 2011). Practitioners will inevitably need to deal with issues relative to significant loss, grief, and death while providing therapeutic intervention. These moments can be overwhelming and confusing for practitioners, possibly even causing them to question their own beliefs and values.

To cultivate open-mindedness, practitioners must care for themselves and their clients during crisis or attend to the emotional and spiritual impact that might occur with loss and death (Donohue, 2003; Forster et al., 2011; Thibeault, 2011) and be open to experiencing occupational gifts through their own and and their clients' meaning making and healing (Kirsh, 2011; Thibeault, 2011). In addition, to encourage open-mindedness, practitioners must develop their own spirituality, search for their own meaning beyond crisis and suffering (Hasselkus, 2002; Simó-Algado & Burgman, 2005), and regularly engage in restorative occupations (Unruh, 2011). The practices of seeking meaning and caring for one's mental, physical, and spiritual health give practitioners skills and perspectives to engage clients when they are suffering and to offer hope.

Occupational Integrity

Occupational integrity is the subjective experience of occupation that lies within the context of cultural, political, moral, social, and spiritual influences and engaging in the occupations that one holds as significant and valued. When conflict exists within the multiple contexts in which one lives, further analysis and assessment of personal values is required. Individuals who experience conflict between their chosen and engaged occupations and what others or society expects (e.g., living with a partner, working in a particular job, getting a divorce) must decide which occupations and roles they will uphold. Chosen occupations and roles may be or may not align with someone's personal choices and values.

Life balance is then considered the extent to which a person lives in integrity with his or her values, strengths, and meaning (Pentland & McColl, 2008; Simó-Algado & Burgman, 2005). Professional development is the process by which practitioners come to know and embrace their values, live in integrity, and find life balance. They honor this same process on which clients embark.

Summary

The term *therapeutic use of self* has evolved throughout the history of occupational therapy but has always been associated with a professional relationship between practitioner and client. How the success of this relationship is measured may vary between practitioner and client; however, it has been regarded as important and valuable to both. Practitioner characteristics such as empathy, active listening, and compassionate listening are often associated with the therapeutic use of self and the therapeutic relationship, and these characteristics are expressly valued by clients. Within the therapeutic process, practitioner self-disclosure, collaboration, and offering hope may also further the relationship. A collaborative relationship that involves journeying with clients entails the practitioner and client co-creating new images and learning and growing together within the relationship. This approach is offered as an alternative to a more autocratic style of relationship.

The focus of spirituality and a therapeutic alliance further suggests a need for practitioners to be open to what spiritual practices and beliefs clients bring to intervention. This openness requires practitioners to explore and expand their perspectives about worldviews and spiritual practices. In addition, practitioners who desire to engage in and embrace spirituality within the therapy process need to be aware of their own beliefs and practices and appreciate how they might influence, and potentially constrict, the therapeutic relationship. Facilitating intuition and mindfulness when engaged in the therapy process may enable greater potential to being present with clients during a crisis. Practitioners who attend to their own spiritual nature and healing are move to higher levels of being and becoming. Professional development is an ongoing and lifelong process in which wisdom and awareness is cultivated, embodied, and brought to the therapeutic process.

References

American Occupational Therapy Association. (2014). Occupational therapy practice framework: Domain and process (3rd ed.). *American Journal of Occupational Therapy, 68* (Suppl. 1), S1–S48. http://dx.doi.org/10.5014/ajot.2014.683005

Audet, C. T., & Everall, R. D. (2010). Therapist self-disclosure and the therapeutic relationship: A phenomenological study from the client perspective. *British Journal of Guidance and Counselling, 38,* 327–342.

Bachelor, A. (2011). Clients' and therapists' views of the therapeutic alliance: Similarities, differences and relationship to therapy outcome. *Clinical Psychology and Psychotherapy, 20,* 118–125. http://dx.doi.org/10.1002/cpp.792

Beagan, B., & Kumas-Tan, Z. (2005). Witnessing spirituality in practice. *British Journal of Occupational Therapy, 68,* 17–28. http://dx.doi.org/10.1177/030802260506800104

Boyt Schell, B. A., & Schell, J. (2008). *Clinical and professional reasoning in occupational therapy.* Philadelphia: Lippincott Williams & Wilkins.

Bray, K. E., Egan, M. Y., & Beagan, B. L. (2012). The practice experience of evangelical Christian occupational therapists. *Canadian Journal of Occupational Therapy, 79,* 285–292. http://dx.doi.org/10.2182/cjot.2012.79.5.4

Brémault-Phillips, S., & Chirovsky, A. (2011). The spiritual path. In M. A. McColl (Ed.), *Spirituality and occupational therapy* (2nd ed., pp. 151–158). Ottawa, ON: CAOT Publications.

Cole, B., & McLean, V. (2003). Therapeutic relationships re-defined. *Occupational Therapy in Mental Health, 19,* 33–56. http://dx.doi.org/10.1300/J004v19n02_03

Cole, M. B. (2005). *Group dynamics in occupational therapy: The theoretical basis and practice application of group intervention* (4th ed.). Thorofare, NJ: Slack.

Collins, M. (1998). Occupational therapy and spirituality: Reflecting on quality of experience in therapeutic interventions. *British Journal of Occupational Therapy, 61,* 280–285. http://dx.doi.org/10.1177/030802269806100614

Collins, M. (2007). Spirituality and the shadow: Reflection and the therapeutic use of self. *British Journal of Occupational Therapy, 70,* 88–90. http://dx.doi.org/10.1177/030802260707000208

Donohue, M. V. (2003). Being there. In P. Precin (Ed.), *Surviving 9/11: Impact and experiences of occupational therapy practitioners* (pp. 43–50). New York: Haworth.

Duff, C. T., & Bedi, R. P. (2010). Counsellor behaviors that predict therapeutic alliance: From the client's perspective. *Counselling Psychology Quarterly, 23*(1). http://dx.doi.org/10.1080/09515071003688165

Farah, J., & McColl, M. A. (2008). Exploring prayer as a spiritual modality. *Canadian Journal of Occupational Therapy, 75,* 5–13. http://dx.doi.org/10.1177/000841740807500103

Farah, J., & McColl, M. A. (2011). In M. A. McColl (Ed.), *Spirituality and occupational therapy* (2nd ed., pp. 193–200). Ottawa, ON: CAOT Publications.

Fine, S. B. (1991). Resilience and human adaptability: Who rises above adversity? *American Journal of Occupational Therapy, 45,* 493–503. http://dx.doi.org/10.5014/ajot.45.6.493

Forster, D., Fardella, J., & McColl, M. A. (2011). Transformation and maturity. In M. A. McColl (Ed.), *Spirituality and occupational therapy* (2nd ed., pp. 131–140). Ottawa, ON: CAOT Publications.

Frank, J. D. (1958). The therapeutic use of self. *American Journal of Occupational Therapy, 13,* 215–225. http://www.ncbi.nlm.nih.gov/pubmed/13559345?report=abstract

Gee, J., & Loewenthal, D. (2013). Working with despair: A phenomenological investigation. *Psychology and Psychotherapy: Theory, Research and Practice, 86,* 229–243. http://dx.doi.org/10.1111/j.2044-8341.2011.02053.x

Gockel, A. (2011). Client perspectives on spirituality in the therapeutic relationship. The *Humanistic Psychologist, 39,* 154–168. http://dx.doi.org/10.1080/08873267.2011.564959

Green, C. A., Polen, M. R., Janoff, S. L., Castleton, D. K., Wisdom, J. P., Vuckovic, N., & Oken, S. L. (2008). Understanding how clinician–patient relationships and relational continuity of care affect recovery from serious mental illness: STARS study results. *Psychiatric Rehabilitation Journal, 32*(1), 9–22. http://dx.doi.org/10.2975/32.1.2008.9.22

Greenberg, N. S. (2003). Spiritual spontaneity. *Occupational Therapy in Mental Health, 19,* 153–189. http://dx.doi.org/10.1300/J004v19n03_15

Grepmair, L., Mitterlehner, F., Loew, T., & Nickel, M. (2007). Promotion of mindfulness in psychotherapists in training: Preliminary study. *European Psychiatry, 22,* 485–489. http://dx.doi.org/10.1016/j.eurpsy.2007.02.004

Hasselkus, B. R. (2002). *The meaning of everyday occupation.* Thorofare, NJ: Slack.

Hayward, C., & Taylor, J. (2011). Eudaimonic well-being: Its importance and relevance to occupational therapy for humanity. *Occupational Therapy International, 18,* 133–141. http://dx.doi.org/10.1002/oti.316

Hooper, B. (1997). The relationship between pretheoretical assumptions and clinical reasoning. *American Journal of Occupational Therapy, 51,* 328–338. http://dx.doi.org/10.5014/ajot.51.5.328

Hopkins, H. L., & Tiffany, E. G. (1988). Occupational therapy—A problem-solving process. In H. H. Hopkins & H. D. Smith (Eds.), *Willard and Spackman's occupational therapy* (7th ed., pp. 102–111). Philadelphia: J. B. Lippincott.

Howard, B. S., & Howard, J. R. (1997). Occupation as spiritual activity. *American Journal of Occupational Therapy, 51,* 181–185. http://dx.doi.org/10.5014/ajot.51.3.181

Kang, C. (2003). A psychospirtiual integration frame of reference for occupational therapy. Part 1: Conceptual foundations. *Australian Occupational Therapy Journal, 50,* 92–103. http://dx.doi.org/10.1046/j.1440-1630.2003.00358.x

Kirsh, B. (1996). A narrative approach to addressing spirituality in occupational therapy: Exploring personal meaning and purpose. *Canadian Journal of Occupational Therapy, 63,* 55–61. http://dx.doi.org/10.1177/000841749606300107

Kirsh, B. (2011). Narrative: What makes narratives spiritual and how can we use them in OT? In M. A. McColl (Ed.), *Spirituality and occupational therapy* (2nd ed., pp. 201–208). Ottawa, ON: CAOT Publications.

Kroeker, P. T. (1997). Spirituality and occupational therapy in a secular culture. *Canadian Journal of Occupational*

Therapy, 64, 122–126. http://dx.doi.org/10.1177/000841 749706400308

Low, J. F. (1997). Religious orientation and pain management. *American Journal of Occupational Therapy, 51,* 215–219. http://dx.doi.org/10.5014/ajot.51.3.215

Luboshitzky, D. (2008). Exploring the spiritual meaning of suffering: A strategy of self-help, recovery, and hope. *Occupational Therapy in Health Care, 22,* 21–38. http://dx.doi.org/10.1080/J003v22n01_03

Mattingly, C., & Fleming, M. (1994). *Clinical reasoning: Forms of inquiry in a therapeutic practice.* Philadelphia: F. A. Davis.

Muñoz, J. (2007). Culturally responsive caring in occupational therapy. *Occupational Therapy International, 14,* 256–280. http://dx.doi.org/10.1002/oti.238

Palmadottir, G. (2003). Client perspectives on occupational therapy in rehabilitation services. *Scandinavian Journal of Occupational Therapy, 10,* 157–166. http://dx.doi.org/10.1080/11038120310017318

Peloquin, S. M. (2003). The therapeutic relationship: Manifestations and challenges in occupational therapy. In E. B. Crepeau, E. S. Cohn, & B. A. Boyt Schell (Eds.), *Willard and Spackman's occupational therapy* (10th ed., pp. 157–170). Philadelphia: Lippincott Williams & Wilkins.

Pentland, W., & McColl, M. A. (2008). Occupational integrity: Another perspective on "life balance." *Canadian Journal of Occupational Therapy, 74,* 135–138. http://dx.doi.org/10.1177/000841740807500304

Pizzi, M. A., & Briggs, R. (2004). Occupational and physical therapy in hospice: The facilitation of meaning, quality of life, and well-being. *Topics in Geriatric Rehabilitation, 20,* 120–130. http://journals.lww.com/topicsingeriatricrehabilitation/Abstract/2004/04000/Occupational_and_Physical_Therapy_in_Hospice__The.7.aspx

Pollard, N. (2006). Is dying an occupation? *Journal of Occupational Science, 13,* 149–152. http://dx.doi.org/10.1080/144 27591.2006.9726508

Price, P. (2009). The therapeutic relationship. In E. B. Crepeau, E. S. Cohn, and B. A. Boyt Schell (Eds.), *Willard & Spackman's occupational therapy* (11th ed., pp. 328–358). Philadlephia: Lippincott Williams & Wilkins.

Provencher, H. L., & Keyes, C. L. M. (2011). Complete mental health recovery: Bridging mental illness with positive mental health. *Journal of Public Mental Health, 10,* 57–69. http://dx.doi.org/10.1108/17465721111134556

Richards, P. S., & Bergin, A. E. (2005). *A spiritual strategy for counseling and psychotherapy* (2nd ed.). Washington, DC: American Psychological Association.

Romanoff, B. D., & Thompson, B. E. (2006). Meaning construction in palliative care: The use of narrative, ritual, and the expressive arts. *American Journal of Hospice and*

Palliative Care, 23, 309–316. http://dx.doi.org/10.1177/1049909106290246

Schulz, E. K. (2004). Spirituality and disability: An analysis of select themes. *Occupational Therapy in Health Care, 18,* 57–83. http://dx.doi.org/10.1080/J003v18n04_05

Schwartzberg, S. L. (1988). Generic tools. In H. H. Hopkins & H. D. Smith (Eds.), *Willard and Spackman's occupational therapy* (7th ed., pp. 385–389). Philadelphia: Lippincott Williams & Wilkins.

Schwartzberg, S. L. (1993). Tools of practice. In H. L. Hopkins and H. D. Smith (Eds.), *Willard and Spackman's occupational therapy* (8th ed., pp. 269–274). Philadelphia: Lippincott Williams & Wilkins.

Shattell, M. M., Starr, S. S., & Thomas, S. P. (2007). "Take my hand, help me out": Mental health service recipients' experience of the therapeutic relationship. *International Journal of Mental Health Nursing, 16,* 274-284. http://dx.doi.org/10.1111/j.1447-0349.2007.00477.x

Simó-Algado, S., & Burgman, I. (2005). Occupational therapy intervention with children survivors of war. In In F. Kronenberg, S. A. Algado, & N. F. Pollard (Eds.), *Occupational therapy without borders: Learning from the spirit of survivors* (pp. 313– 325). New York: Elsevier/Churchill Livingstone.

Smith, C., & Taylor, R. (2010). Using the Intentional Relationship Model in the treatment of medically complicated depression. *Journal of Psychiatric Intensive Care, 7,* 41–43. http://dx.doi.org/10.1017/S1742646410000154

Smith, S. (2008). Toward a flexible framework for understanding spirituality. *Occupational Therapy in Health Care, 22,* 39–54. http://dx.doi.org/10.1080/J003v22n01_04

Spector, M. (1996). Developing therapeutic use of self through spirituality. *Journal of Occupational Therapy Students, 22,* 21–36.

Steffen, E. (2013). Both "being with" and "doing to": Borderline personality disorder and the integration of humanistic values in contemporary therapy practice. *Counseling Psychology Review, 28(1),* 64-71. http://bit.ly/1Q64vAy https://www.researchgate.net/profile/Edith_Steffen2/publication/260228766_Both_being_with_and_doing_to_Borderline_personality_disorder_and_the_integration_of_humanistic_values_in_contemporary_therapy_practice/links/0a85e5303ca393f80e000000.pdf

Taylor, R. R. (2008). *The intentional relationship: Occupational therapy and the use of self.* Philadelphia: F. A. Davis.

Taylor, R. R. (2013). Therapeutic relationship and client collaboration: Applying the Intentional Relationship Model. In B. A. Boyt Schell, G. Gillen, & M. E. Scaffa (Eds.), *Willard and Spackman's occupational therapy* (12th ed., pp. 425–236). Philadelphia: Lippincott Williams & Wilkins.

Taylor, R. R., & Van Puymbroeck, L. (2013). Therapeutic use of self: Applying the Intentional Relationship Model in group therapy. In J. C. O'Brien & J. W. Solomon (Eds.), *Occupational analysis and group process* (pp. 36–52). St. Louis: Elsevier.

Thibeault, R. (1997). A funeral for my father's mind: A therapist's attempt at grieving. *Canadian Journal of Occupational Therapy, 64,* 107–114. http://dx.doi.org/10.1177/000841749 706400306

Thibeault, R. (2011). Resilience and maturity. In M. A. McColl (Ed.), *Spirituality and occupational therapy* (2nd ed., 121–130). Ottawa, ON: CAOT Publications.

Townsend, E. (2003). Reflections on power and justice in enabling occupations. *Canadian Journal of Occupational Therapy, 70,* 74–87. http://dx.doi.org/10.1177/000841740307000203

Tse, S., Lloyd, C., Petchkovsky, L., & Manaia, W. (2005). Exploration of Australian and New Zealand indigenous people's spirituality and mental health. *Australian Occupational Therapy Journal, 52,* 181–187. http://dx.doi.org/10.1111/j.1440-1630.2005.00507.x

Unruh, A. (2011). Appreciation of nature: Restorative occupations. In M. A. McColl (Ed.), *Spirituality and occupational therapy* (2nd ed., pp. 249–256). Ottawa, ON: CAOT Publications.

Unruh, A. M., Versnel, J. & Kerr, N. (2002). Spirituality unplugged: A review of commonalties and contentions, and a resolution. *Canadian Journal of Occupational Therapy, 69,* 5–20. http://dx.doi.org/10.1177/000841740206900101

Unruh, A. M., Versnel, J., & Kerr, N. (2004). Spirituality in the context of occupation: A theory to practice application. In M. Molineux (Ed.), *Occupation for occupational therapists* (pp. 32–45). Malden, MA: Blackwell.

Walker, A. D. (1971). Occupational therapy in geriatrics. In H. S. Willard & C. S. Spackman (Eds.), *Occupational therapy* (4th ed., pp. 507–539). Philadelphia: Lippincott.

Ward, M. R., Linville, D. C., & Rosen, K. H. (2007). Clients' perceptions of the therapeutic process: A common factors approach. *Journal of Couple and Relational Therapy, 63,* 25–43. http://dx.doi.org/10.1300/J398v06n03_02

Williams, B. J. (2008). An exploratory study of older adults' perspectives of spirituality. *Occupational Therapy in Health Care, 22,* 3–19. http://dx.org/10.1080/J003v22n01_02

Wilson, L. (2010). Spirituality, occupation and occupational therapy revisited: Ongoing consideration of the issues for occupational therapists. *British Journal of Occupational Therapy, 73,* 437–444. http://dx.doi.org/10.4276/0308022 10X12839367526219

Wilson, L. (2011). Occupational analysis and spirituality. In L. Mackenzie & G. O'Toole (Eds.), *Occupational analysis in practice* (pp. 53–65). Oxford, UK: Wiley-Blackwell.

Young, B. (2010). Using the Tidal Model of Mental Health Recovery to plan primary health care for women in residential substance abuse recovery. *Issues in Mental Health Nursing, 31,* 569–575. http://dx.doi.org/10.3109/01612840.2010. 487969

Part III.

FURTHER CONSIDERATIONS AND CHALLENGES

CHAPTER 9.

CLIENT-CENTERED CARE AND SPIRITUALITY

Mary Ann McColl, PhD, MTS

Chapter Highlights

✦ Canadian Model of Occupational Performance
✦ Defining *client-centered practice*
✦ Defining *spirituality*
✦ Similarities between spirituality and client-centered practice
✦ Barriers to spirituality and client-centered practice
✦ Approaching with humility.

Key Terms and Concepts

✦ Canadian Model of Occupational Performance
✦ Client-centered practice
✦ Ego
✦ Environment
✦ Fixing

✦ Helping
✦ Occupation
✦ Occupational performance
✦ Person
✦ Serving
✦ Spirituality

In Chapter 1, "Addressing Spirituality in Occupational Therapy," and Chapter 2, "Contemporary History of Spirituality and Occupational Therapy," Humbert observed that two important terms emerged in occupational therapy in the early 1980s: (1) spirituality and (2) client-centered practice. She attributes both, at least in part, to the ***Canadian Model of Occupational Performance (CMOP;*** Department of National Health and Welfare [DNHW]/Canadian Association of Occupational Therapists [CAOT], 1983). The model

features occupation as an interaction between the person (including his or her spirituality) and the environment. Client-centered practice is endorsed as the best model for the relationship between occupational therapists and their clients (DNHW/CAOT, 1983; Polatajko, Townsend, & Craik, 2007).

Is it a coincidence that these two ideas—client-centered practice and spirituality—arose in occupational therapy in tandem? Or did some underlying commonality bring them both to attention contemporaneously? I am aware of no systematic exploration to date of the relationship between the two concepts. In this chapter, I explore the definitions of *spirituality* and *client-centered practice,* the similarities between them, and the challenges of practicing according to these two worthy ideals.

Canadian Model of Occupational Performance

The CMOP arose out of collaboration between the Government of Canada's DNHW and CAOT (1983). Together they formed a task force to create a standard of practice for occupational therapy in Canada—a benchmark against which the profession could be judged and resource allocation decisions could be made. In its deliberations, the task force quickly realized that the practice of occupational therapy could not be easily reduced to a simple checklist. The complexity of occupational therapy was better served by a conceptualization that worked across settings, across clients, and across age groups.

Thus was born the original CMOP, with its three concentric circles representing the **person** at the center; the **environment** around the outside; and, between them, **occupational performance**—the medium through which individuals and environments interact. Simple, elegant, evocative. The model established the primacy of occupation as the basis for occupational therapy in Canada and reinforced the definition of **occupation** as a balance of self-care, productivity, and leisure (McColl, Law, & Stewart, 2014).

The CMOP also introduced two other new and important concepts to occupational therapy, spirituality and client-centered practice. In elaborating the person, the model referred to physical, mental, emotional, and spiritual components. The first three were familiar—they built on the popular biopsychosocial model prevalent in the 1970s. The fourth component, spirituality, was, however, new and surprising. It hearkened back to the early 20th-century motto of occupational therapy, which featured body, mind, and spirit (Friedland, 2011). It challenged occupational therapists to think about what it meant to engage not only the body and mind of a client but also the spirit. Subsequent versions of the CMOP (and CMOP–E; Canadian Association of Occupational Therapists, 1997, 2002; Townsend & Polatajko, 2007) reinforced the importance of spirituality by moving spirituality to a more central position—at the very core of the client.

The other new idea introduced by the CMOP was client-centered practice, as reflected in the title of that original publication: *Guidelines for the Client-Centred Practice of Occupational Therapy* (DNHW/CAOT, 1983). Client-centered practice was taken as a core assumption underlying the practice of occupational therapy in Canada. It was understood that Canadian occupational therapists use their professional expertise not to control and dominate their clients but to serve them. They place their professional knowledge and experience at the disposal of their clients to help them realize their goals and aspirations.

Defining *Client-Centered Practice*

Client-centered practice was first defined by Carl Rogers (1946, 1965) as an approach to therapy characterized by three essential elements: (1) empathic understanding, (2) unconditional positive regard, and (3) therapeutic genuineness.

For therapy to be successful, Rogers (2013) claimed, six conditions needed to be present:

1. Warm and trusting rapport
2. Freedom to express feelings without judgment
3. Recognition and acceptance by the client of his or her spontaneous self
4. Responsibility for choices
5. Development of insight
6. Supported growth toward maturity and independence.

Since the early 1980s, client-centered practice has become the default assumption of how occupational therapists relate to their clients and the implicit best practice in occupational therapy. Occupational therapists have calibrated the classic definition of *client-centered practice* to speak to the context of occupational therapy. Sumsion and Law (2006) identified five core elements of client-centered practice in occupational therapy:

1. A shift in the balance of power in favor of clients
2. A joint partnership between therapist and client in decision making
3. Active listening as a validation of the importance of the client's voice
4. Client choice in the goals and processes of therapy
5. Hope, an emotional investment in the future.

Defining *Spirituality*

Much of this book is devoted to defining *spirituality,* so I defer to those more detailed discussions to raise the many issues inherent in spirituality. For the purpose of this chapter, I define *spirituality* as I have in the past, as the desire for and sensitivity to the presence of spirit (McColl, 2011). This definition attempts to be clear and precise about what spirituality is. It is easy to become overwhelmed by the complexity and abstraction of the concept of spirituality. Many definitions talk about what spirituality is like or what it is related to rather than what it is. This definition resists the urge to do that. At the same time, it acknowledges the limitations of language to capture the essence of spirituality and to embrace the mystery of spirit.

The spiritual aspect of clients refers to how clients relate to themselves, to others, to the world, and to a higher power (if they believe that one exists). Some examples of spiritual questions are

- What does it mean to be human, and how is my humanity affected by having a disability?
- To whom does my life belong?
- Who or what is responsible for things being the way they are?
- What is my responsibility or duty to others, and theirs to me?
- What are my sources of strength in difficult situations?
- What do I believe in and not believe in?
- What spiritual practices are meaningful to me, and how have these practices developed over the course of my life?
- How have my early experiences, adult experiences, growing older, and acquiring a disability affected who I am and what I believe?
- What do I hope for—for myself, for others, for the world?

Similarities Between Spirituality and Client-Centered Practice

The most obvious similarity between spirituality and client-centered practice is that both are abstract concepts. They are complex and multidimensional and not easily captured in words. Despite that (or perhaps because of it), both concepts are unanimously endorsed and virtually universally upheld in contemporary occupational therapy. It would be counter to the culture of the profession to admit that you were opposed to either client-centered practice or spirituality, or that you simply did not take them into account in practice.

Perhaps the main similarity between spirituality and client-centered practice is that both seek to reinforce the client's humanity. Both seek to understand who the client is and what is meaningful to him or her. This understanding depends on a therapeutic relationship that has some depth. It depends on a relationship that engages the full humanity of both the therapist and the client.

Several key elements of people's humanity are their free will, their autonomy, and their inalienable right to be—to live, to choose, and to be respected. Both spirituality and client-centered practice honor people's free will, respect their autonomy, and accept their beliefs. Regardless of disability, age, or culture, client-centered practice accepts people's right to choose who they want to be and what changes they want to make in therapy. Spirituality acknowledges the deep meaning of people's existence.

Barriers to Spirituality and Client-Centered Practice

Both client-centered practice and spirituality are notoriously difficult to put into practice. With regard to client-centered practice, Richard and Knis-Matthews (2010) found that only 35% of therapists agreed with the goals set by their clients. Bright, Boland, Rutherford, Kayes, and McPherson (2012) were surprised to discover that therapists were governed by system and profession priorities rather than client priorities. Kjellberg, Kahlin, Haglund, and Taylor (2012) found that only 12%–14% of therapists allowed their clients to identify problems and set goals autonomously. Instead, therapists made decisions, either unilaterally (20%–22%) or in consultation with clients (66%).

With regard to spirituality, numerous surveys of occupational therapists have shown that although therapists readily acknowledge the importance of spirituality, they do not address it in practice (Bruce, 2009; Farrar, 2001; Hoyland & Mayers, 2005; O'Connor et al., 2010; Schwarz & Fleming Cottrell, 2007; Wilding, 2002). Occupational therapists consistently recognize spirituality as an important aspect of occupational therapy (Baptiste, 1997; Canadian Association of Occupational Therapists, 1997; Enquist, Short-DeGraff, Gliner, & Oltjenbruns, 1997; Rose, 1999), but in practice the topic of spirituality evokes guilt, embarrassment, and ambivalence (McColl, 2001).

In previous work, I have explored barriers to both spirituality (McColl, 2011, 2016) and client-centered practice (McColl & Pollock, 2015) in occupational therapy. In this chapter, I explore the extent to which those barriers are the same and seek to discover the underlying difficulties with both of these admittedly valuable approaches.

Lack of Consensus

The first barrier to a practice that incorporates both spirituality and client-centered practice is the lack of consensus on definitions of the two terms. This lack of agreement on definitions can be both a benefit and a difficulty. On the one hand, it means that individuals are free to define these terms in their own way. On the other hand, it means a person can never be sure when talking to someone else about these terms that they are talking about the same thing. The lack of agreement about what these terms mean provides an easy excuse for failing to address these difficult topics in practice. After all, if the experts cannot even agree about what they are, how is the therapist supposed to know what to do?

Time

The second, and perhaps most common, barrier to addressing both spirituality and client-centered practice is that they take too much time. It does take more time to become involved with clients to the extent that you know what is important to them, that you understand the context of their lives, and that you immerse yourself in their belief systems and values. It is, in fact, much more efficient to simply tell the client what you think they should work on and to keep those goals concrete and achievable.

Gupta and Taff (2015) suggested that client-centered practice is incompatible with contemporary practice, which they characterized as reimbursement driven, impairment focused, and institutionally constrained. Bright and colleagues (2012) noted that they felt the pressure of time in their therapeutic relationships. They attributed the sense of urgency to organizational goals, such as early discharge, efficient use of resources, and funder restrictions. As a result, they set small goals in an attempt to be realistic rather than engage deeply with clients. They acknowledged that they had been co-opted by the system in which they worked at the expense of their clients.

The therapist-dominated approach has the added efficiency of restricting goals to issues that the therapist feels comfortable addressing and has the required expertise to confront with a minimum of effort or new learning. It is much more demanding to actually get to know the client in a deep and multidimensional way, to hear his or her hopes and dreams, and to figure out how to marshal resources to help. Only by embarking on that deeper relationship, however, is it possible to enact the principles of client-centered practice or engage with the client on a spiritual level.

Assumptions About Client Insight and Ability

Another often-cited impediment to both spirituality and client-centered practice is the perception that some clients lack the insight or ability to participate in these more demanding or abstract aspects of the therapeutic process (Kjellberg et al., 2012). In particular, this concern is often expressed in relation to clients with mental illness or cognitive impairment. In these instances, therapists perceive that they are acting in the best interests of their clients by taking charge of the therapeutic agenda and avoiding difficult or abstract discussions. They maintain that they need to be free to exercise their judgment about safety and risk even if it runs contrary to clients' goals and desires (Durocher, Kinsella, Ells, & Hunt, 2015). Colquhoun, Letts, Law, MacDermid, and Edwards (2010) showed that 100% of their clients with cognitive impairments could identify occupational performance problems, and 94% could score those problems on importance, performance, and satisfaction.

Previous research with people with acquired brain injuries showed that although they might not be capable of managing a bank account, they were coherent and expressive when talking about what had happened to them, what it meant, and how their spirit was affected by the onset of their disability

(McColl et al., 2000a, 2000b). People who had experienced a spinal cord injury or traumatic brain injury in the preceding 2 years were asked what had happened to their spirit when their body or their brain became disabled. Interviewees were remarkably thoughtful and consistent in their responses. They identified five themes in their relationships with a supreme being, with the world, or with all of humanity (transpersonal):

1. Awareness of their place in the world
2. Connection to others, to a supreme power, or both
3. Trust in the beneficence of others and of the world
4. Sense of their finite humanity and their mortality
5. Feeling of meaning and purpose in life (McColl et al., 2000a, 2000b).

Power and Professionalism

A fourth barrier to both spirituality and client-centered practice has to do with power and professionalism. Professions are established to assert power and control over a domain of knowledge and practice. According to Whalley Hammell (2015), power derives from social inequalities between professionals and clients in education, social location, privilege, and institutional affiliation.

As Brodley (2011) put it, client-centered practice runs counter to the conventional forces in professions. In discussions of client-centered practice, professionals often endorse the idea of "giving power" to clients. Despite the benevolent intent of this statement, it betrays an underlying assumption that power lies with the professional and that he or she may choose to bestow some of it on the client under certain circumstances. Client-centered practice asks professionals to acknowledge the structural and systemic forces that create power in the health and social services—forces such as referral networks, institutional policies and practices, technical terminology, and social and educational advantages.

McCorquodale and Kinsella (2015) named four factors that uphold the power differential between professionals and their clients:

1. Dichotomous thinking (e.g., good–bad, easy–difficult)
2. Objectification of clients as the other
3. Time and other economic imperatives
4. Formal ways of knowing.

To be client centered, professionals must recognize the power they have and acknowledge the inequities created by the system in which they work. Moreover, they must be willing to set aside that power in favor of the rights of clients to control their own destiny (Whalley Hammell, 2013). The client-centered relationship restores the balance of power and, in fact, permits the balance to tip in favor of the client. Brodley (2011) further suggested that client-centered practice is an "expression of the therapist's character, values and attitudes" (p. 10) and inferred that not all therapists will be up to the task.

Crocker and Johnson (2006) distinguished among fixing, helping, and serving. *Fixing* involves doing something to another person; *helping* involves doing something with another person. In both instances, the other is assumed to be incapable, or at least less capable. *Serving,* however, means offering what is needed to allow the other to do. Serving focuses on the served rather than the server. It assumes the served person's capability, provided the necessary support. The client-centered therapist serves—a therapeutic stance that requires setting aside the ego.

A key impediment to both spirituality and client-centered practice is the *ego.* It strives to be all powerful and to control the conditions of life; the ego says that humans are capable of understanding all that there is. Layered on the human ego is the professional ego, cultivated through higher education, exclusive knowledge, and hierarchical institutions. The ego seeks to control, whereas spirituality and client centeredness require therapists to let go—to be sensitive, to embrace mystery, to accept that they do not control the agenda. Client-centered practice instead acknowledges that therapists serve the goals and desires of another—the client. Spirituality requires therapists to serve spirit, whatever that may be or however they conceptualize that mysterious force that governs and animates the universe.

Approaching With Humility

Several authors have advocated approaching spirituality humbly, with awareness of the inability to fully understand it—listening without knowing, accepting what one has to learn from clients, creating safe or sacred space, and acknowledging reciprocity in the therapeutic relationship (Davis & Hook, 2014; Hook & Davis, 2014; McColl, 2011; Thibeault, 2011). These are all ways in which therapists may begin to adopt a therapeutic approach that minimizes the impact of ego and allows spirituality to thrive. Of course, this stance is also entirely compatible with client-centered practice.

One way to think about the therapeutic role in a client-centered or spiritually focused practice may lie in an old chestnut of an idea—one that continues to be a mystery and a source of personal growth and development: the therapeutic use of self. This idea acknowledges that in each therapist lies some quality or characteristic that permits the other to make changes, to meet challenges, and to endure difficulties. Each therapist has something unique that is essentially therapeutic and that propels others to name and claim their goals, to summon courage to face difficult times, and to hope and trust in the future. Therapists spend their whole professional lives attempting to understand the essence of that quality. What they perhaps forget is that they can only be of service when they are able to set aside their own ego and enter into the personal and spiritual space of the client.

Practicing from a client-centered or spiritually focused perspective requires therapists to reconsider the client–therapist boundary. Although professional boundaries need to be observed to prevent confusion about the nature of the therapeutic relationship, perhaps these boundaries have become overly rigid and impermeable. In the strictest sense, the personal–professional boundary is a one-way membrane, allowing therapeutic goods to flow from therapist to client but not allowing any traffic in the other direction. Such a rigid boundary may be necessary in very extreme cases of boundary confusion, but in most instances there is much to be gained from adopting a willingness to learn from the experience of patients and an acceptance of one's own limited understanding.

Summary

This chapter has built on Humbert's observation about the contemporaneous development of two important ideas in occupational therapy: spirituality and client-centered practice. After defining both,

I have explored similarities between the two concepts. The main similarity is that both approaches reinforce the full humanity of the client. Both are dependent on a view of the client that is not limited to the individual encountered for a few hours in the clinical situation. Instead, both approaches have, at their core, an understanding of the client as a complex, multidimensional individual who is worth taking the time to get to know.

If you acknowledge the full humanity of the client, it is difficult to sustain an approach that either denies the spiritual dimension or denies the client's agency and autonomy. Such an approach would disregard who the client is in his or her deepest self. When you encounter clients as spiritual beings, you can no longer simply tell them what to do. To be client centered means to reinforce the agency, autonomy, and full humanity of the client.

The barriers to client-centered practice and to spiritual care have previously been explored in the literature, as well as in my own work. The barriers to practicing according to each are remarkably similar. They consist primarily of issues related to the therapeutic relationship, to power, and to ego. To overcome these barriers, I suggest that we

- Be clear about what is meant by both client-centered practice and spirituality;
- Be prepared to take time to move beyond superficial relationships with clients;
- Acknowledge that spirituality and autonomy are present in all clients, not just those who are emotionally or intellectually intact;
- Let go of the need to be in charge and acknowledge that the process is at least 50% owned by the client;
- Embrace a service approach rather than a helping approach or a fixing approach; and
- Acknowledge the reciprocity in the therapeutic relationship and the rich opportunity to continue to learn from clients throughout one's entire career.

References

Baptiste, S. (1997). Spiritually speaking. *Canadian Journal of Occupational Therapy, 64,* 104–105. http://dx.doi.org/10.1177/000841749706400303

Bright, F. A., Boland, P., Rutherford, S. J., Kayes, N. M., & McPherson, K. M. (2012). Implementing a client-centered approach in rehabilitation: An autoethnography. *Disability and Rehabilitation, 34,* 997–1004. http://dx.doi.org/10.3109/09638288.2011.629712

Brodley, B. T. (2011). *Practicing client-centred therapy.* Ross-on-Wye, England: PCCS Books.

Bruce, A. (2009). Opening conversations: Dilemmas and possibilities of spirituality and spiritual care. In M. McIntyre & C. McDonald (Eds.), *Realities of Canadian nursing: Professional, practice, and power issues* (3rd ed., pp. 455–469). Philadelphia: Lippincott Williams & Wilkins.

Canadian Association of Occupational Therapists. (1997). *Enabling occupation: An occupational therapy perspective.* Ottawa, ON: CAOT Publications.

Canadian Association of Occupational Therapists, (2002). *Enabling occupation: An occupational therapy perspective* (rev.ed). Ottawa, ON: CAOT Publications.

Colquhoun, H., Letts, L., Law, M., MacDermid, J., & Edwards, M. (2010). Feasibility of the Canadian Occupational Performance Measure for routine use. *British Journal of Occupational Therapy, 73,* 48–54. http://dx.doi.org/10.4276/030802210X12658062793726

Crocker, L., & Johnson, B. (2006). *Privileged presence: Personal stories of connections in health care.* Boulder, CO: Bull.

Davis, D., & Hook, J. (2014). Humility, religion, and spirituality: An endpiece. *Journal of Psychology and Theology, 42,* 111–117.

Department of National Health and Welfare and Canadian Association of Occupational Therapists. (1983). *Guidelines for the client-centred practice of occupational therapy* (No. H39-33/1983E). Ottawa, ON: Author.

Durocher, E., Kinsella, E. A., Ells, A., & Hunt, M. (2015). Contradictions in client-centred discharge planning: Through the lens of relational autonomy. *Scandinavian Journal of Occupational Therapy, 22,* 293–301. http://dx.doi.org/10.3109/11038128.2015.1017531

Enquist, D. E., Short-DeGraff, M., Gliner, J., & Oltjenbruns, K. (1997). Occupational therapists' beliefs and practices with respect to spirituality and therapy. *American Journal of Occupational Therapy, 51,* 173–180. http://dx.doi.org/10.5014/ajot.51.3.173

Farrar, J. E. (2001). Addressing spirituality and religious life in occupational therapy practice. *Physical and Occupational Therapy in Geriatrics, 18,* 65–85. http://dx.doi.org/10.1080/J148v18n04_06

Friedland, J. (2011). *Restoring the spirit: The beginnings of occupational therapy in Canada, 1890–1930.* Montreal: McGill Queen's University Press.

Gupta, J., & Taff, S. (2015). The illusion of client-centred practice. *Scandinavian Journal of Occupational Therapy, 22,* 244–251. http://dx.doi.org/10.3109/11038128.2015.1020866

Hook, J., & Davis, D. (2014). Humility, religion, and spirituality: Introduction to the special issue. *Journal of Psychology and Theology, 42,* 3–6.

Hoyland, M., & Mayers, C. (2005). Is meeting spiritual need within the occupational therapy domain? *British Journal of Occupational Therapy, 68,* 177–180. http://dx.doi.org/10.1177/030802260506800406

Kjellberg, A., Kahlin, I., Haglund, L., & Taylor, R. (2012). The myth of participation in occupational therapy: Reconceptualizing a client-centred approach. *Scandinavian Journal of Occupational Therapy, 19,* 421–427. http://dx.doi.org/10.3109/11038128.2011.627378

McColl, M. A. (2001). Spirit, occupation and disability. In *Muriel Driver Memorial Lecture: Anthology* (pp. 1–13). Ottawa, ON: CAOT Publications.

McColl, M. A. (2011). *Spirituality and occupational therapy* (2nd ed.). Ottawa, ON: CAOT Publications.

McColl, M. A. (2016). Spirituality. In B. Bonder & V. Dal Bellow-Haas (Eds.), *Functional performance in older adults* (4th ed.). Philadelphia: F. A. Davis.

McColl, M. A., Bickenbach, J., Johnston, J., Nishihama, S., Schumaker, M., Smith, K., & Yealland, B. (2000a). Changes in spiritual beliefs after traumatic disability. *Archives of Physical Medicine and Rehabilitation, 81,* 817–823. http://dx.doi.org/10.1016/S0003-9993(00)90117-5

McColl, M. A., Bickenbach, J., Johnston, J., Nishihama, S., Schumaker, M., Smith, K., & Yealland, B. (2000b). Spiritual issues associated with traumatic-onset disability. *Disability and Rehabilitation, 22,* 555–564. http://dx.doi.org/10.1080/096382800416805

McColl, M. A., Law, M. C., & Stewart, D. (2014). *The theoretical basis of occupational therapy* (3rd ed.). Thorofare, NJ: Slack.

McColl, M. A., & Pollock, N. (in press). Measuring occupational performance using a client-centered perspective. In M. Law, C. Baum, & W. Dunn (Eds.), *Measuring occupational performance* (3rd ed.). Thorofare, NJ: Slack.

McCorquodale, L., & Kinsella, E. A. (2015). Critical reflexivity in client-centred therapeutic relationships. *Scandinavian Journal of Occupational Therapy, 22,* 311–317. http://dx.doi.org/10.3109/11038128.2015.1018319

O'Connor, T., Chow, M., Payne, G., Young, J., Rivera, M., Meakes, E., & Howitt, J. (2010). In the beginning: A Canadian ethnographic study on sources and definitions of spiritual reflection used by health care professionals who are not chaplains. *Journal of Pastoral Care and Counseling, 64,* 1–14. http://dx.doi.org/10.1177/154230501006400102

Polatajko, H. J., Townsend, E. A., & Craik, J. (2007). Canadian Model of Occupational Performance and Engagement (CMOP–E). In E. A. Townsend & H. J. Polatajko (Eds.), *Enabling occupation II: Advancing an occupational therapy vision for health, well-being and justice through occupation* (3rd ed., p. 23). Ottawa, ON: CAOT Publications.

Richard, L. F., & Knis-Matthews, L. (2010). Are we really client-centered? Using the Canadian Occupational Performance Measure to see how the client's goals connect with the goals of the occupational therapist. *Occupational Therapy in Mental Health, 26,* 51–66. http://dx.doi.org/10.1080/01642120903515292

Rogers, C. (1946). Significant aspects of client-centered therapy. *American Psychologist, 1,* 415–422. Retrieved from http://psychclassics.yorku.ca/Rogers/therapy.htm

Rogers, C. (1965). *Client-centered therapy: Its current practice, implications and theory.* Boston: Houghton-Mifflin.

Rogers, C. (2013). *Significant aspects of client-centered therapy by Carl Rogers.* Retrieved from http://www.all-about-psychology.com/client-centered-therapy.html

Rose, A. (1999). Spirituality and palliative care: The attitudes of occupational therapists. *British Journal of Occupational Therapy, 62,* 307–312. http://dx.doi.org/10.1177/030802269906200707

Schwarz, L., & Fleming Cottrell, R. P. (2007). The value of spirituality as perceived by elders in long-term care. *Physical and Occupational Therapy in Geriatrics, 26,* 43–62. http://dx.doi.org/10.1080/J148v26n01_04

Sumsion, T., & Law, M. (2006). A review of evidence on the conceptual elements informing client-centred practice. *Canadian Journal of Occupational Therapy, 73,* 153–162. http://dx.doi.org/10.1177/000841740607300303

Thibeault, R. (2011). Ritual: Ceremonies of life. In M. A. McColl (Ed.), *Spirituality and occupational therapy* (2nd ed., pp. 233–240). Ottawa, ON: CAOT Publications.

Townsend, E.A., & Polatajko, H.J. (2007). *Enabling occupation II: Advancing an occupational therapy vision for health, well-being, and justice through Occupation.* Ottawa, ON: CAOT Publications.

Whalley Hammell, K. R. (2013). Client-centered practice in occupational therapy: Critical reflections. *Scandinavian Journal of Occupational Therapy, 20,* 174–181. http://dx.doi.org/10.3109/11038128.2012.752032

Whalley Hammell, K. R. (2015). Client-centered occupational therapy: The importance of critical perspectives. *Scandinavian Journal of Occupational Therapy, 22,* 237–243. http://dx.doi.org/10.3109/11038128.2015.1004103

Wilding, C. (2002). Where angels fear to tread: Is spirituality relevant to OT practice? *Australian Occupational Therapy Journal, 49,* 44–47. http://dx.doi.org/10.1046/j.0045-0766.2002.00292.x

CHAPTER 10.

CONNECTING WITH CLIENTS TO FACILITATE OCCUPATION AND WELL-BEING

Mary Egan, PhD, OT(C); Suzette Brémault-Philips, PhD, OT(C); and Joëlle Richard, MScS, OT(C)

Chapter Highlights

✦ Contexts and environments
✦ Creating and maintaining safe spaces
✦ Considering motivation.

Key Terms and Concepts

✦ Amotivation
✦ Constructivist perspective
✦ Contexts
✦ Countertransference
✦ Deficit needs
✦ Extrinsic motivation
✦ First-order therapy

✦ Holistic thinking
✦ Intrinsic motivation
✦ Mindfulness
✦ Motivation
✦ Second-order therapy
✦ Transformative dialogue

Throughout this text, theory and research have been shown to consider spirituality as a way to engage with people in an effort to facilitate therapeutic encounters that support reaching one's maximum potential. Occupational engagement and health are best promoted through relationships that support personal awareness and growth, and such relationships require understanding and trust.

To engage in such a relationship, we need to consider the systems in which both therapists and clients are embedded. This chapter provides an overview of issues related to connecting at a deep level and establishing therapeutic partnerships to promote occupational engagement and health. This work comprises three related and iterative elements: (1) appreciation of context, (2) creation of safe spaces, and (3) consideration of motivation.

Exemplary occupational therapy requires both an excellent grasp of biomedical knowledge as it relates to daily function and an appreciation of and thirst for continuing education related to how people connect with themselves, one another, nature, and the transcendent. Such practice requires that practitioners understand historical and current contexts and intentionally work to establish and maintain trust. This chapter aims begin to provide a framework for readers to organize personal reading and reflection in these key areas.

Contexts and Environments

The Canadian Model of Occupational Performance and Engagement (CMOP–E; Townsend & Polatajko, 2007) and the *Occupational Therapy Practice Framework: Domain and Process* (American Occupational Therapy Association, 2014) provide guidance for occupational therapists regarding how to consider *contexts* and environments as facilitators of or barriers to occupational engagement and health. Within these models, the occupational therapist is directed to consider multiple interconnected contexts, including the physical and social environments and the cultural, institutional, personal, temporal, and virtual contexts.

Unlike biomedical frameworks that view people as the sum of their parts, *holistic thinking* seeks to appreciate that people are embedded within and cannot be separated from these multiple interconnected contexts (Newman, 1999). As members of a profession based on this belief in holism, occupational therapists are challenged daily to recognize and shed patterns of thinking that rely on disconnected assessments of component parts of people and their contexts (McColl, 1994). Instead, practitioners must adopt the difficult practice of conceptualizing people as not only embedded within a certain context but actually inextricably linked to this context.

For example, a person is embedded in one or more cultures, socioeconomic strata, families, and communities. His or her values, ideas, and goals related to health and occupation arise from a unique mix of the values, ideas, and goals of these contexts, as well as the person's unique life experience to this point in time. In addition, both people and their contexts are in constant flux, being shaped by both their personal history and the histories of their ancestors.

To make matters even more interesting and complex, people remain largely unaware of the influence of their own contexts. It might be helpful to think of our contexts figuratively as unique pools in which we each swim, often with little awareness of them or of the ways in which they differ from the pools in which others are immersed. A first step in becoming a context-aware practitioner is to initiate an ongoing examination of your personal context. Three ongoing practices are recommended to help occupational therapists become and remain at least partially aware of their personal interconnected contexts:

1. Becoming aware of one's own cultural history
2. Reflecting on the cultures of others
3. Seeking varied cultural experiences.

Becoming Aware of One's Cultural History

The first step is to become more aware of one's cultural history. This awareness is accomplished first through an examination of the cultural history of one's own groups and can be carried out through an examination of history, art, literature, and other records of these groups' collective stories.

Next, personal reflection on the influence of one's culture on spirituality contributes to greater awareness. Martsolf (1997) developed a series of questions that may be helpful here (Table 10.1). Being more aware of one's unique and personal contextual pool is the first step to being open to and aware of clients' different contexts.

Reflection on Others' Cultures

Becoming a context-aware practitioner involves ongoing study of and reflection on the cultures and cultural histories of other groups, particularly those common to the clients with whom you tend to work. Again, through an examination of history, art, literature, and other records of groups' collective stories, the therapist begins to gain an understanding of the different values, ideas, and goals related to health and occupation that a client who is embedded in a different context may hold. The word *may* is important here because, depending upon other factors (e.g., personal history, family, economic and educational conditions), the individual's context may be very different from the

Table 10.1. Self-Reflection on Culture

Cultural Aspects	Self-Reflection Questions
Cultural affiliation	With what groups am I most closely affiliated now?
	Has any change occurred in my group affiliation throughout my life?
Life meaning in cultural context	What do I believe is the meaning and purpose of life?
	How did I obtain this belief?
	What persons in my life would readily understand my beliefs about the meaning of life? Least understand?
	What words do I use to communicate these beliefs?
	How does my sense of meaning in life affect the rules that I live by? The roles I enact? What I do each day?
Values in cultural context	What do I value most?
	How did I obtain these values?
	What persons in my life would readily understand my values?
	How do my values affect the rules I live by? The roles I enact? What I do each day?
Transcendence in cultural context	What is my experience of a dimension beyond myself?
	What persons in my life would readily these experiences? least understand?
	What words do I use to communicate these experiences?
	How do these experiences affect the rules I live by? The roles I enact? What I do each day?
Connection in cultural context	What are the characteristics of my relationship with myself? Others? God or a higher power? Nature?
	What persons in my life would readily understand my relationships? Least understand?
	What words do I use to communicate these relationships?
	How do these relationships affect the rules I live by? The roles I enact? What I do each day?
A sense of becoming in cultural context	What is my life story?
	How have I grown and developed as a person?
	Where am I headed in life?
	Is my life story, my development as a person and my direction in life similar to that of any particular group of people?

Source. Reprinted from "Cultural Aspects of Spirituality in Cancer Care," by D. S. Martsolf, 1997, *Seminars in Oncology Nursing, 13,* p. 234. Copyright © 1997 by Elsevier. Used with permission.

ideas, values, and goals typically associated with a particular culture (Bonder & Martin, 2013).

Exposure to Varied Cultural Practices

The third step in becoming a context-aware practitioner is to regularly expose oneself to varied cultural practices. Take opportunities to meet people from other cultures and participate in typical cultural activities. Again, the idea is to further appreciate ideas, values, and goals regarding health and occupation that vary in different cultural contexts while becoming more comfortable with cross-cultural conversations. Such comfort is indispensable to the second element—creation of safe spaces—that both supports establishing therapeutic partnerships and connecting at a deeper level and promotes occupational engagement and health.

Creating and Maintaining Safe Spaces

In our own lives, we have all had experiences of feeling relatively safe or unsafe in professional encounters. Three considerations may help occupational therapists create and maintain safe spaces within which the therapeutic relationship can develop and valued occupations can be enabled:

1. Attention to power differentials
2. Support of transformative dialogue from a position of safe uncertainty
3. Deeply listening.

Difference in Power

Appreciating the power differential in professional relationships is a critical first step in the creation and maintenance of safe spaces. Teachers, professors, and health care professionals have power as a result of their knowledge and position to judge and define people both formally (e.g., "a student with an A average") and informally (e.g., "hopeless in math" or "unmotivated in therapy"). They often control access to services and other professionals. For example, a poor recommendation from a teacher might limit one's access to specific university or college programs.

Occupational therapy practitioners hold variable degrees of power in the health care system. An occupational therapist's recommendation is often required to access payment for adaptive equipment or continuing workers' compensation benefits. As health professionals, occupational therapists generally have a duty to report suspected child abuse or neglect, and clients may feel quite vulnerable to therapists' judgments regarding their parenting abilities or ability to make independent decisions regarding their personal or financial matters. People raised in an era when the doctor's word was unquestioned and people could be sent to institutional care facilities without their consent may fear that occupational therapists could recommend that they be sent to long-term care. These are just a few examples of power that occupational therapists might be perceived to or actually wield.

To create and maintain a safe space for therapy, therapists must remain aware of this power differential. Explicitly discussing with clients that your concern is with enabling valued occupation rather than sending them to a nursing home, challenging their ability to make independent decisions, recommending their children be taken into care, or withholding services (depending upon context) may help reassure them that it is safe to engage with you. When this is not the case, as, for example, when your report may contribute to loss of disability support payments, it needs to be clearly discussed, and your role and process needs to be made understandable at the outset of any assessment or intervention.

Transformative Dialogue

Transformative dialogue is conversation that invites examination of the participants to construct a shared and growth-promoting narrative of a difficult problem (Botella & Herrero, 2000). This work is well illustrated in the family therapy concepts of first-order and second-order therapy (Hoffman, 1985).

In *first-order therapy,* therapists apply their expertise to examine and define the problem and identify and prescribe the solution. Therapists may be certain that they can identify and fix the problem. Because families are complex, developing entities, this way of working tends to lead to a simplistic understanding of the situation and less-than-ideal solutions. Moreover, the therapist's certainty in his or her understanding of the situation makes it hazardous for clients to disagree. At best, this approach leads to a shallow understanding of the issues and ineffective treatment plans. At worst, it can lead to solutions that cause more harm than benefit (Hoffman, 1985).

Further complicating the first-order therapy approach, clients may come to therapy firmly convinced of ideas that are counterproductive to growth (e.g., "I'm a failure and will never hold a job" or "I can't do anything with my arm this way"). Clients may feel certain that they do not have the information or the ability to move forward. Such attitudes act against the hope and creativity required to move forward. In this way, the therapist's and the client's beliefs represent unsafe certainty, that is, certainty that does not promote growth (Mason, 1993).

In *second-order therapy,* therapists use their expertise to help clients explore the situation, its meanings to everyone involved, and the value of potential solutions. This approach leads to a condition of safe uncertainty. This position of safe uncertainty encourages multiple perceptions and assessments of the situation. It appreciates that people's ideas are subject to perceptions formed within their unique contexts. This approach also acknowledges that solutions are, at best, evolving steps in getting to a better situation. Safe uncertainty is not a fixed position but one that

> is always in a state of flow, and is consistent with the notion of a respectful, collaborative, evolving narrative, one which allows a context to emerge whereby new explanations can be placed alongside rather than instead of, in competition with, the explanations that clients and therapists bring. (Mason, 1993, p. 194)

In a place of safe uncertainty, a transformative dialogue can occur (Gergen, McNamee, & Barrett, 2001).

This **constructivist perspective** (i.e., that reality is constructed through action and perception) of therapy (Leitner & Epting, 2001) is well recognized within occupational therapy. Methods such as narrative (Clark, 1993; Kirsh, 1996; Smith, 2006) and ethnographic interviewing (Gitlin, Corcoran, & Leinmiller-Eckhardt, 1995) help occupational therapy practitioners create safe spaces from which clients in difficulty can comfortably explore options and opportunities and move forward. These approaches rely on the occupational therapist's expertise with the methods of facilitating growth and supporting occupational engagement and health. They also highlight the importance of appreciating the client's expertise.

Constructivist therapy underlines the importance of the awareness of context (both the therapist's and the client's) in the experience of daily life. Again, continual sensitivity and lifelong learning about other cultures, worldviews, and histories are essential.

Deeply Listening

A profound openness to other ways of perceiving and experiencing life is also an important aspect of the third step, listening deeply. Key aspects here include mindfulness and awareness of countertransference.

Mindfulness practices for occupational therapists include preparing oneself for the therapeutic encounter (Reid, 2009). Such preparation might include a practitioner working to become aware of the current state of his or her mind and body

and calming the mind to prepare for listening. An important element of this presence while listening to the client is remaining aware of one's own inner dialogue. We must be cognizant of the experience of **countertransference,** or the feelings stirred in us by our clients' strong emotions:

> The therapist, being with the patient in a real and authentic manner, may come into contact with feelings that are disturbing and frightening. In order to protect themselves from those feelings, the therapist may unconsciously avoid any further contact with the patient, or make a remark that prevents a patient from saying anything further. (Nicholls, 2013, p. 24)

One disturbing emotion that commonly arises during clinical encounters is that of feeling incompetent (Thériault & Gazzola, 2006). Fear that we do not have adequate skills to help the client can shut down our ability to listen or cause us to flee from the client. Sessions may be concluded prematurely, and clients may even be discharged when such feelings become overwhelming. This feeling keeps us from providing what is perhaps the most important element of promoting growth and wholeness—the caring presence of another human being who is listening deeply.

Practitioners who are listening deeply engage with clients in an intentional way. Rather than anticipating what a client will say, the therapist greets the encounter with a sense of wonder: "I wonder what this person may say?" He or she then reflects on personal sensations, emotions, and inner dialogue, bringing the same sense of wonder and openness to his or her own reactions. "How am I feeling? What words or ideas I am reacting to?" The approach is "Isn't this interesting?" rather than "I shouldn't be feeling or thinking this." Practitioners' recognizing and accepting their concerns and fears allows them to first validate fears and concerns and then momentarily place them aside to better hear the client's concerns, fears, and hopes.

Appreciating that one may be scared or saddened by what one is hearing may allow therapists to avoid making unreflective exhortations, such as suggesting that clients who are distressed look on the bright side. Such responses may be more a way to protect oneself from clients' fear and sadness. When clients' underlying feelings resonate in a particular manner with the therapist's less conscious concerns, the therapist might reflect back to a client at only a superficial level, making it clear that he or she does not understand, feel safe with, or honor the client's deeper concerns (Nicholls, 2013). Rather than trying to brush one's personal experience aside, acceptance of and remaining in touch with these feelings of sadness and helplessness may be more helpful for both the client and the therapist alike.

Considering Motivation

When clients do not make the progress practitioners think they are capable of, and when they do not seem impressed by practitioners' suggestions or grateful for their help, practitioners usually begin to feel disappointed (Gabbard, 2000). This feeling can lead practitioners through conscious or unconscious feelings of incompetence or powerlessness, followed by conscious or unconscious anger, and on to a certain level of exasperation with the client whom we ultimately might label unmotivated. Here, we would like to share with you how a deeper understanding of motivation has led us to listen more deeply to clients' concerns in support of their return to valued occupations.

Through a synthesis of research on the psychology of motivation and the ongoing development and testing of theoretical models, Ryan and Deci (2000) presented an excellent framework for understanding motivation that resonates well with the work of promoting occupational engagement. For them, *motivation* is an attitude toward a particular activity. Motivation regarding any activity is divided into two categories: (1) intrinsic and (2) extrinsic. Activities for which one has *intrinsic motivation* form a special group. These activities are those people engage in simply for the pleasure of doing them; engaging in them is a reward in itself. These activities are unique to each individual, and given autonomy and the necessary supports, people simply just do them.

All other activities, which people do for reasons other than the pleasure of doing them, occur from *extrinsic motivation.* Depending upon the degree to which one has internalized activities—that is, the extent to which the activities reflect who one wants to be and what one values—people will be more or less drawn to them. Alternatively, activities that

people feel compelled to do and that have no value to them are sources of *amotivation.* This is an extreme situation, but it may occur when clients have no interest in or control over therapeutic activities.

Creating space for clients to talk to the therapist about their intrinsically motivated or highly internalized, extrinsically motivated activities can lead to the identification of therapeutic goals that harness their attention and energy. Asking about the occupations that have special importance to them gives clients permission to dream (Fearing, 2001; Smith, 2006) and helps them feel safe in envisioning that dream.

Client-Centered Goals

There is evidence that even the discussion of client-centered goals can have therapeutic benefit (Brock et al., 2009). This may occur for several reasons. Naming goals can energize and orient a person toward action (Rosewilliam, Roskell, & Pandyan, 2011). Goal setting may also give clients permission to dream, which may be particularly important among clients who have been counseled to restrict their aspirations (Kessler, 2015).

Many occupational therapy clients have been advised against taking up or continuing certain occupations. They may worry that such activities may worsen their condition, or they may not be aware that restrictions initially recommended after an acute episode no longer need to be followed. As well, people are often told in therapy that certain occupations are too risky or unrealistic, and considerable time can be spent talking people out of their goals instead of supporting them (Russell, Fitzgerald, Williamson, Manor, & Whybrow, 2002). Trying occupations may be a necessary step in problem solving and adaptation. Supporting identification of goals may help initiate the process of reengagement in valued activities (Kubina, Dubouloz, Davis, Kessler, & Egan, 2013).

Unmet Needs

People require motivation to fulfill their goals. Identifying or moving toward valued goals may signify the presence of unmet needs. Maslow (1943) reasoned that for a person to grow and contribute (an occupational therapist might say, "to engage in occupation"), certain conditions had to be in place.

These conditions make up his famous pyramid of needs, starting from the bottom up: physiological, safety, love and belongingness, self-esteem, and self-actualization. What is essential to understand is that Maslow felt that these needs comprised two separate sets of needs: (1) basic (i.e., physiological, safety) and (2) higher (i.e., all the others). He called the basic needs *deficit needs* because a person has to feel that they have been met before he or she can move on to meeting higher level needs.

Maslow (1943) believed that people naturally want to do things that allow them to grow into their unique selves and contribute to life around them, but he observed that to do this, they had to be acting from a place of safety. One of the most important things to know about this place of safety is that it is subjective. The person must feel that his or her basic needs for food, shelter, human contact, and security are met, but what one person needs to feel that these needs have been met may be very different from what another person needs. In addition, some people may need to have a sense of hope before they can even be open to receiving these basic needs.

Motivating From a Space of Safety: Karine's Story

Feeling safe and having a sense of possibility allows people to take risks in the service of occupational engagement, according to Maslow (1943). How an occupational therapist can help a client move from feeling unsafe to safe is beautifully illustrated in the work of Karine, an occupational therapy student.

During her final clinical placement, Karine encountered a client who was generally considered unmotivated for therapy. David, a man in his 60s, had a car accident that resulted in T2 paraplegia. After 2 weeks at a rehabilitation center, he was doing very little for himself and was using a tilt-recline power wheelchair. The team believed he could become more functionally independent, and their goal was to help him to do this. However, David seemed very passive in therapy and was extremely hesitant to move out of his wheelchair.

When Karine listened to David, she was struck by how anxious he was about returning home. He really could not envision how he could live in his house again. In David's mind, he had lost his home—he was homeless. Karine understood this. She scheduled a home visit with David for the following week (rather than waiting until just before discharge, as was usually done on this unit). The visit centered on the renovations that could be carried out. After the visit, David and his wife met with a contractor. David began to see that it might be possible for him to return to his home. He began to understand how mobility at home would be easier with a manual chair. Encouraged by Karine, all of the therapists made wheelchair mobility their primary goal, and David began to really engage in his therapy for the first time.

This intervention sounds simple, but it would not have been possible without the safe space that Karine created for her work with David or the hope that was instilled and could take root as a result of her deep listening. She was sensitive to the power differential between them. Although she was a student, she still appreciated the authority that she had over him. She could have used this authority to threaten him with potential discharge to a nursing home if he did not start working harder in therapy. Instead, she acted from a position of safe uncertainty, appreciating that there was more to the situation than she knew. She did not know what he would tell her, but she demonstrated that she was open to his concerns and would calmly consider them.

As David spoke to her, she listened to her inner voice, which told her she was rather anxious. This was a senior placement, and she was not sure what to do. "Hearing" her own anxiety, she was able to set it aside long enough to hear the anxiety behind David's words. She used her understanding of motivation to carefully put together a hypothesis about what she was seeing, and she revised her plan according to David's concerns.

Application to Practice

When we find ourselves thinking about a client as unmotivated, two strategies may allow us to really hear what the client may be trying to communicate or need. The first is to reflect on Ryan and Deci's (2000) framework for examining motivation.

- What is the client intrinsically motivated to do?
- What are his or her internalized motivations?

Listening for these motivations provides a safe space to pursue wholeness while helping to identify meaningful therapy goals.

The second strategy is to reflect on Maslow's (1943) deficiency needs as experienced by the client. Appreciating these needs and working toward their resolution produces highly effective occupational therapy. Listening for and addressing unmet needs in occupational therapy seems to fulfill Peloquin's (2002) vision of occupational therapy as "reaching for heart as well as hands" (p. 517). It cultivates hope and creates possibility.

Summary

Although there have been many different conceptualizations of the place of spirituality in occupational therapy, most promote the importance of something else beyond the technical competence and conscientiousness important in any field of health care. We assert that this something else relates to a deeper engagement with people with the goal of facilitating wholeness and growth. We have presented three interrelated elements critical for this work: (1) appreciation of context, (2) creation of safe spaces, and (3) consideration of motivation.

References

American Occupational Therapy Association. (2014). Occupational therapy practice framework: Domain and process (3rd ed.). *American Journal of Occupational Therapy, 68*(Suppl. 1), S1–S48. http://dx.doi.org/10.5014/ajot.2014.682006

Bonder, B., & Martin, L. (2013). *Culture in clinical care* (2nd ed.). Thorofare, NJ: Slack.

Botella, L., & Herrero, O. (2000). A relational constructivist approach to narrative therapy. *European Journal of Psychotherapy, Counselling and Health, 3*, 407–418. http://dx.doi.org/10.1080/13642530010012048

Brock, K., Black, S., Cotton, S., Kennedy, G., Wilson, S., & Sutton, E. (2009). Goal achievement in the six months after inpatient rehabilitation for stroke. *Disability and Rehabilitation, 31*, 880–886. http://dx.doi.org/10.1080/09638280802356179

Clark, F. (1993). Occupation embedded in a real life: Interweaving occupational science and occupational therapy. *American Journal of Occupational Therapy, 47*, 1067–1078. http://dx.doi.org/10.5014/ajot.47.12.1067

Fearing, V. G. (2001). Change: Creating our own reality. *Canadian Journal of Occupational Therapy, 68*, 208. http://dx.doi.org/10.1177/000841740106800403

Gabbard, G. O. (2000). On gratitude and gratification. *Journal of the American Psychoanalytic Association, 48*, 697–716. http://www.ncbi.nlm.nih.gov/pubmed/11059393

Gergen, K. J., McNamee, S., & Barrett, F. J. (2001). Toward transformative dialogue. *International Journal of Public Administration, 24*, 679–707. http://dx.doi.org/10.1081/PAD-100104770

Gitlin, L. N., Corcoran, M., & Leinmiller-Eckhardt, S. (1995). Understanding the family perspective: An ethnographic framework for providing occupational therapy in the home. *American Journal of Occupational Therapy, 49*, 802–809. http://dx.doi.org/10.5014/ajot.49.8.802

Hoffman, L. (1985). Beyond power and control: Toward a "second order" family systems therapy. *Family Systems Medicine, 3*, 381–396. http://dx.doi.org/10.1037/h0089674

Kessler, D. (2015). *Occupational performance coaching for stroke survivors (OPC–Stroke): A novel patient-centered intervention to improve participation in valued activities* (Doctoral dissertation). Ottawa, ON: University of Ottawa.

Kirsh, B. (1996). A narrative approach to addressing spirituality in occupational therapy: Exploring personal meaning and purpose. *Canadian Journal of Occupational Therapy, 63*, 55–61. http://dx.doi.org/10.1177/000841749606300107

Kubina, L. A., Dubouloz, C. J., Davis, C. G., Kessler, D., & Egan, M. Y. (2013). The process of re-engagement in personally valued activities during the two years following stroke. *Disability and Rehabilitation, 35*, 236–243. http://dx.doi.org/10.3109/09638288.2012.691936

Leitner, L. M., & Epting, F. R. (2001). Constructivist approaches to therapy. In K. J. Schneider, J. F. T. Bugental, & J. F. Pierson (Eds.), *Handbook of humanistic psychology* (pp. 421–431). Thousand Oaks, CA: Sage.

Martsolf, D. S. (1997). Cultural aspects of spirituality in cancer care. *Seminars in Oncology Nursing, 13*, 231–236. http://dx.doi.org/10.1016/S0749-2081(97)80016-2

Maslow, A. H. (1943). A theory of human motivation. *Psychological Review, 50*, 370–396. http://dx.doi.org/10.1037/h0054346

Mason, B. (1993). Towards positions of safe uncertainty. *Human Systems, 4*, 189–200.

McColl, M. A. (1994). Holistic occupational therapy: Historical meaning and contemporary implications. *Canadian Journal of Occupational Therapy, 61*, 72–77. http://dx.doi.org/10.1177/000841749406100202

Newman, M. A. (1999). The rhythm of relating in a paradigm of wholeness. *Image: The Journal of Nursing Scholarship, 31*, 227–230. http://dx.doi.org/10.1111/j.1547-5069.1999.tb00485.x

Nicholls, L. (2013). The "therapeutic use of self" in occupational therapy. In L. Nicholls, J. C. Piergrossi, C. de Sena Gibertoni, & M. A. Daniel (Eds.), *Psychoanalytic thinking in occupational therapy* (pp. 15–31). Chichester, UK: Wiley.

Peloquin, S. M. (2002). Reclaiming the vision of reaching for heart as well as hands. *American Journal of Occupational Therapy, 56,* 517–526. http://dx.doi.org/10.5014/ajot.56.5.517

Reid, D. (2009). Capturing presence moments: The art of mindful practice in occupational therapy. *Canadian Journal of Occupational Therapy, 76,* 180–188. http://dx.doi.org/10.1177/000841740907600307

Rosewilliam, S., Roskell, C. A., & Pandyan, A. (2011). A systematic review and synthesis of the quantitative and qualitative evidence behind patient-centred goal setting in stroke rehabilitation. *Clinical Rehabilitation, 25,* 501–514. http://dx.doi.org/10.1177/0269215510394467

Russell, C., Fitzgerald, M. H., Williamson, P., Manor, D., & Whybrow, S. (2002). Independence as a practice issue in occupational therapy: The safety clause. *American Journal of Occupational Therapy, 56,* 369–379. http://dx.doi.org/10.5014/ajot.56.4.369

Ryan, R. M., & Deci, E. L. (2000). Self-determination theory and the facilitation of intrinsic motivation, social development, and well-being. *American Psychologist, 55,* 68–78. http://dx.doi.org/10.1037/0003-066X.55.1.68

Smith, G. (2006). The Casson Memorial Lecture 2006: Telling tales—How stories and narratives co-create change. *British Journal of Occupational Therapy, 69,* 304–311. http://dx.doi.org/10.1177/030802260606900702

Thériault, A., & Gazzola, N. (2006). What are the sources of feelings of incompetence in experienced therapists? *Counselling Psychology Quarterly, 19,* 313–330. http://dx.doi.org/10.1080/09515070601090113

Townsend, E. A., & Polatajko, H. J. (2007). *Advancing an occupational therapy vision for health, well-being, and justice through occupation.* Ottawa, ON: CAOT Publications.

CHAPTER 11.

SPIRITUALITY IN MULTIDISCIPLINARY AND INTERDISCIPLINARY HEALTH CARE

Tamera Keiter Humbert, MA, DEd, OTR/L

Chapter Highlights

✧ Other disciplines' approaches to spirituality
✧ Interdisciplinary approach to spirituality
✧ Spirituality and major life events and transitions: systematic literature review
✧ Where do we go from here? Considerations for future research.

Key Terms and Concepts

✧ Acceptance and positivity
✧ Chaplains
✧ Connectedness
✧ Coping mechanisms and activities
✧ Counselors
✧ Developing resilience
✧ Embracing acceptance
✧ Emotional suffering
✧ Fear
✧ Fight
✧ Guilt
✧ HealthCare Chaplaincy Model
✧ Holistic perspective
✧ Hope
✧ Interdisciplinary approach
✧ Major life event

✧ Moving forward or away
✧ Multidisciplinary approach
✧ Nurses
✧ Physical suffering
✧ Physical therapists
✧ Physicians
✧ Psychologists
✧ Purpose and life meaning
✧ Relationships
✧ Religious affiliations
✧ Social workers
✧ Spiritual competency
✧ Time fillers
✧ Transition
✧ Trust in God or a higher power

Issues of how to engage spirituality in practice, how to promote significant or definable professional roles within spirituality, and how spirituality is understood and communicated are consistently articulated in the literature of various disciplines, such as nursing, psychology, social work, physical therapy, chaplaincy, and medicine (Elkonin, Brown, & Naicker, 2014; Hunt, 2014; Lavinder, Patel, Campo, & Lichtman, 2013; Senreich, 2013; Winter, 2014). This chapter provides perspectives on multidisciplinary and interdisciplinary approaches to understanding spirituality and using it in practice.

In a *multidisciplinary approach,* each discipline carves out a unique role and select responsibilities in addressing assessment and intervention with a client and, when applicable, with significant others and families (BusinessDictionary.com, 2016b). This chapter first highlights other disciplines' viewpoints on spirituality in the contemporary health care literature. It then provides examples of interdisciplinary approaches that emphasize a collaborative response to the concerns and questions about spirituality, that is, multiple disciplines working together to contribute to a larger conversation about spirituality. Interdisciplinary teams work collaboratively to address specific questions and concerns (BusinessDictionary.com, 2016a).

Next, the chapter provides an overview of a comprehensive systematic literature review addressing the spiritual needs of people going through a major life event or transition. The last portion of the chapter highlights future considerations for ongoing research within this aspect of care.

Other Disciplines' Approaches to Spirituality

A review of the literature provides a snapshot of the approaches used by different health care disciplines when considering spirituality in practice and their concerns regarding incorporating spirituality into daily routines and professional roles. The disciplines include counseling and psychology, nursing, medicine, social work, physical therapy, and chaplaincy.

Counselors and Psychologists

Counselors and *psychologists* provide individual, family, and group therapy supporting personal growth and adjustment to life events, focusing heavily on emotional and mental health and wellness. They have recognized the value and importance of attending to clients' spirituality and have identified professional standards for doing so (American Counseling Association, 2005; American Psychological Association, 2000, 2003). The literature related to spirituality and these professional roles points to the confluence between spirituality and personal growth and transformation (Corry, Mallett, Lewis, & Abdel-Khalek, 2013; Drobin, 2014; Wessels & Müller, 2013) and spirituality and the psyche (Helminiak, 2008). The professions of psychology and counseling have also been called on to further develop interdisciplinary theories in understanding spirituality (McIntosh & Newton, 2013) and integrate spirituality and religious constructs into education and training (Schafer, Handa, Brawer, & Ubinger, 2011).

Potential conflicts

Aspects of spirituality that may become problematic for some clients when dealing with a major life event or transition, and that may also ultimately affect health and well-being, include the underlying motivation for change (Giordano & Cashwell, 2014), conflicts between personal beliefs and actions (Ybañez-Llorente & Smelser, 2014), and conflicts between personal beliefs and larger social, cultural, or community beliefs (Werdel, Dy-Liacco, Ciarrocchi, Wicks, & Breslford, 2014; Ybañez-Llorente & Smelser, 2014). In particular, psychologists and counselors assist individuals, couples, families, and others to recognize the need to make changes in their life, identify the reasons for making or not making those changes, and confront the sometimes complex dilemmas in making changes that challenge personal beliefs and perspectives.

Focus of spirituality in therapy

The focus of spirituality in therapy may include bringing to light the conflicts that exist between spiritual and religious beliefs and wellness (Werdel et al., 2014; Wessels & Müller, 2013); reframing or co-creating new images and ideas around religious ideas or spirituality (Drobin, 2014; Giordano & Cashwell, 2014; Ybañez-Llorente & Smelser, 2014); implementing spiritual wellness practices

(Garlick, Wall, Corwin, & Koopman, 2011); and promoting and using established spiritual and religious practices for strength, coping, and resilience (Elkonin et al., 2014; Helminiak, 2008; Ybañez-Llorente & Smelser, 2014).

Spiritual development and coping

The counseling and psychology literature on spirituality emphasizes personal development and coping as they relate to religion or spirituality, theories related to understanding spirituality, and training therapists to incorporate spirituality into practice. Psychologists and counselors have articulated a greater need to better understand the implications of faith-based spirituality on health and wellness, including faith development and maturity (Anderson & Grice, 2014; Drobin, 2014); personal integration of beliefs and experiences, especially when conflict occurs (Elkonin et al., 2014); cultivation of religious or spiritual attributes such as humility (Hook & Davis, 2014); and understanding spirituality as it is created and enhanced within relationships (Wessels & Müller, 2013).

In the counseling and psychology disciplines, spirituality is considered to be dynamic and changeable (Elkonin et al., 2014; Helminiak, 2008), affected by religious beliefs and practices (Anderson & Grice, 2014; Drobin, 2014; Werdel et al., 2014), and developmental (Drobin, 2014) or related to faith or religious maturity (Anderson & Grice, 2014; Werdel et al., 2014).

Nurses

Nurses provide direct care to patients and significant others, addressing their physical health and resulting emotional and spiritual needs. The nursing literature frequently attributes the start of the profession, and recognition of spirituality, with Florence Nightingale (Meehan, 2012; Pesut, 2013; Timmins & McSherry, 2012). Contemporary nursing includes a *holistic perspective* (i.e., biopsychosocial–spiritual; Carpenter, Girvin, Kitner, & Ruth-Sahd, 2008; McSherry & Smith, 2007; Meehan, 2012) in which nurses are called upon to appreciate patients' religious and spiritual beliefs and culture as they relate to health and wellness, healing, and end of life care (Meehan, 2012; Murphy, Begley, Timmins, Neill, & Sheaf, 2015; Yilmaz & Gurler, 2014).

Additionally, in nursing, spirituality encompasses all aspects of patient care, including administrative decisions and policies and the health care environment (Reimer-Kirkham, Pesut, Sawatzky, Cochrane, & Redmond, 2012).

Empathy

Nurses are encouraged to cultivate an attitude of empathetic and compassionate care while they journey with patients and significant others through decision making and delivery of medical care (Carpenter et al., 2008; McSherry & Jamieson, 2013; Meehan, 2012; Prentis, Rogers, Wattis, Jones, & Stephenson, 2014; Rogers & Wattis, 2015; Tiew, Kwee, Creedy, & Chan, 2013). This attitude is accomplished by showing respect for patients and their life circumstance (Meehan, 2012; Timmins & McSherry, 2012), including their cultural perspectives that influence spirituality (Reimer-Kirkham et al., 2012; Timmins & McSherry, 2012).

As a result of the nursing role; time spent with clients and significant others; and the profession's holistic focus on mind, body, and spirit, nurses may be in a unique position to recognize when a patient is in spiritual distress or emotional and spiritual pain and suffering, especially during periods of crisis and trauma (Blanchard, Dunlap, & Fitchett, 2012; Carpenter et al., 2008). Therefore, nurses typically complete a spiritual assessment within the first 24 hours of hospital admission to gain perspective about clients' spiritual challenges, resources, and needs.

Critiques of nursing and spirituality

Nurses have been encouraged to help patients or significant others deal with pain and suffering by listening to them and engaging them in discourse related to life meaning (Rogers & Wattis, 2015; Tiew et al., 2013). However, this role has engendered several critiques. In particular, the exact role of nurses in spiritual assessment and intervention beyond a general respect for patients' beliefs has been questioned (Çetinkaya, Azak, & Dündar, 2013; McSherry & Jamieson, 2013; Pesut, 2013). Additionally, debates have arisen about whether their training, personal comfort, and expertise are adequate to assess patients' spirituality, spiritual distress, or religious beliefs that support or hinder health (Blanchard et al., 2012; Clarke, 2009; Draper & McSherry, 2013; Yilmaz & Gurler, 2014).

Another critique within the nursing literature about the role of spirituality and medical care centers on recognizing both the importance of spirituality as it pertains to seeking the transcendent and the importance of religious beliefs and practices (Clarke, 2009; Pesut, 2008; Reinert & Koenig, 2013). In other words, it is not necessarily a good idea to conceptually separate spirituality and religious beliefs and practices. It is important for nurses to understand that either may be important when addressing a patient's health, wellness, and end-of-life care. Additionally, if the definitions and constructs of *spirituality* used in practice are phrased in only universal ways related to meaning, purpose, or coping, as is frequently done, then nurses (and all health care practitioners) potentially lose some fundamental understanding of how a patient's religious and spiritual beliefs contribute to or interfere with health (Clarke, 2009; Reinert & Koenig, 2013). Although this critique is applied to all of health care, the nursing literature explicitly articulates this concern. Further research is recommended to better understand religious beliefs and their impact on health and well-being and to further explore comprehensive constructs of spirituality (Clarke, 2009; Pesut, 2008, 2013).

Physicians

Many *physicians,* who attend to the medical care and oversight of patients, also recognize the integration of spirituality and health and wellness (Meldrum, 2012; Nicastri, 2014). Areas of medicine in which spirituality and religious and faith perspectives particularly come into focus include mental health and psychiatry (Curlin et al., 2007; Singh & Ajinkya, 2012), oncology (Balboni, 2014; King, Dimmers, Langer, & Murphy, 2013), gerontology (Singh & Ajinkya, 2012), hospice and palliative care (Balboni, 2014; Best, Butow, & Olver, 2014; Singh & Ajinkya, 2012), pediatrics (King et al., 2013), gerontology and dementia care (De Sousa, 2011; Jolley et al., 2010), and trauma care (Chapple, Swift, & Ziebland, 2011). Note that spirituality affects not only the patient but the medical professional (De Sousa, 2011; Jolley et al., 2010).

Physicians who have graduated from medical educational programs that offer didactic and experiential components toward an understanding and use of spirituality in practice, along with physicians who have incorporated spirituality into their lives, tend to provide care that attends to spirituality (Ellis, Campbell, Detwiler-Breidenbach, & Hebrand, 2002; King et al., 2013; LoboPrabhu & Lomax, 2010; Meldrum, 2012). However, although there is general support that spiritual and religious practices and beliefs are helpful in recovery, healing, and well-being, there is also some recognition that religious and spiritual beliefs may have a negative effect on a patient's recovery, ability to cope with long-term illness, and ability to deal with death (Anandarajah, 2014; Curlin et al., 2007; Huguelet & Koenig, 2009). Additionally, although the medical community generally supports spirituality as an integral part of health care, many physicians are still apprehensive about how best to address spiritual challenges and distress articulated by patients (Anandarajah & Roseman, 2014; Best, Butow, & Olver, 2015; Ledford et al., 2015; King et al., 2013).

Social Workers

Social workers provide individual, couple, group, and family therapy to people who are dealing with a major life event or transition, focusing on individual and social supports to address challenges. Social workers have traditionally focused their work on completing client assessments that note the social and cultural environments in which the client and significant others live and engage. Spirituality and religious beliefs are now part of those assessments, recognizing their effect on clients' performance, health, and well-being (Hodge, 2006, 2013; Hunt, 2014; Husain & Sherr, 2015; Seitz, 2014) and end-of-life care (Callahan, 2015).

Some social work educational programs include developing sensitivity in asking about spiritual aspects of the client's life and cultivating self-awareness of one's own spiritual or religious background as it influences perspectives and client relationships (Barker & Floersch, 2010; Hunt, 2014; Lun, 2015; Seitz, 2014). Professionals should also be aware of their own personal understanding of spirituality and religious beliefs and be nondiscriminatory when providing services. This self-awareness further promotes *spiritual competency,* or the ability to effectively use spirituality within the therapeutic process (Callahan, 2015; Mulder, 2015).

Intervention recommendations and conflicts

Some literature recommends the following interventions regarding spirituality: determining with clients whether there is conflict between the client's spiritual and religious beliefs and physical and emotional needs, eliciting the client's spiritual perspective about the focus of the therapeutic process, and validating the spiritual experiences of the client (Callahan, 2015; Hodge, 2013; Mulder, 2015; Senreich, 2013). Social workers may also provide spiritual activities, such as meditation and prayer, to promote self-care and healing (Callahan, 2015; Dombo & Gray, 2013).

However, some literature is not clear about how or whether social workers should integrate spirituality into practice. Some challenge the notion that spirituality can or should be assessed (Oxhandler & Pargament, 2014). Some question whether the determination of a client's spirituality is in the purview of the social worker (Senreich, 2013). Tension also exists regarding social workers understanding clients' religious and cultural beliefs and practices without making judgments about their value or validity (Husain & Sherr, 2015; Mulder, 2015; Senreich, 2013).

Limited research

The social work literature has expressed concern about the limited research on understanding how people make sense of the world and use personal beliefs for ethical decision making (Seitz, 2014). Studies have been conducted on spiritual activities used in practice and their perceived effectiveness and on social workers' comfort level with spirituality; the overall results are limited and inconclusive (Oxhandler & Pargament, 2014).

The social work literature has proposed furthering dialogue about defining spirituality: Should spirituality be inclusive (Hodge, 2013; Senreich, 2013), or should the profession recognize and uphold values and ethics of specific religious and faith-based groups (Seitz, 2014)? The literature has also proposed further investigating how social workers make evidenced-based decisions about when to address and how to use spirituality in practice (Husain & Sherr, 2015; Oxhandler & Pargament, 2014) and how social workers can become more culturally and spiritually competent practitioners (Callahan, 2015; Mulder, 2015).

Physical Therapists

Physical therapists work with people with injuries, illnesses, or long-standing disabilities, focusing on the restoration of the body. Physical therapists have asserted the connection between faith, spirituality, and hope and health promotion and the motivation needed to deal with life-threatening illnesses and disabilities and long-term disabilities (Coyne, 2005; Svalina & Webb, 2012). It is important for therapists to be sensitive to and respectful of their clients' diverse spiritual and faith perspectives and practices (Lavinder et al., 2013). For example, respect may be demonstrated by not scheduling therapy visits on holy days or honoring clients' requests to engage in worship services or rest instead of engaging in therapy (Coyne, 2005). Additionally, physical therapy students, practitioners, and educators consider spirituality important and a valid topic for study and research (Lavinder et al., 2013; Oakley, Katz, Sauer, Dent, & Millar, 2010; Pitts, 2008; Tapley, Fell, & Pitts, 2012), even though there has been limited inclusion of the topic within physical therapy curricula (Lavinder et al., 2013).

In one study regarding spirituality and physical therapy, Svalina and Webb (2012) identified the spiritual construct of forgiveness and associated forgiveness of self with better health behaviors that resulted in greater health and physical status and less physical pain. The implications for practice are an increased awareness of and sensitivity to the interplay between psychological and spiritual factors and healing and health and an appreciation for providing applicable recommendations and referrals in addressing underlying concerns.

Chaplains

Chaplains have a unique role within the health care system because they intentionally address the spiritual and religious concerns of not only patients but also families, significant others, health care team members, and the community at large (Balboni, 2014; Emanuel et al., 2015; Taylor et al., 2015). The primary role of chaplains is to attend to the spiritual care of the people they encounter (see Chapter 4, "Spirituality Through the Lens of Health Care Chaplaincy"). Contemporary literature has described two main challenges for chaplains: (1) developing and using spiritual assessments and (2) clarifying their role.

Spiritual assessments

As health care has moved to become more evidence based, cost-effective, and efficient, chaplains have been expected to validate their work (Cheng, Purcell, Dimitriou, & Grossoehme, 2015; Powell et al., 2015). One response to this expectation has been to create and implement spiritual assessments. However, questions have arisen about what type of assessments should be used, what their purpose is, and who should implement them. Additionally, debate about spiritual assessments has included whether they can really assess spiritual domains (Bishop & Trancik, 2013), whether they can truly address spirituality or psychological adaptation (Trancik, 2013), whether and how a patient's culture affects their completion (Schultz, Lulav-Grinwald, & Bar-Sela, 2014), and whether an opportunity is lost when a patient's particular theological assumptions are not assessed (Rumbold, 2013; Trancik, 2013).

Moreover, if spiritual assessments are used to identify people in spiritual distress or crisis who might benefit from chaplain services, what constitutes spiritual distress or crisis must be established (Blanchard et al., 2012). For example, is spiritual distress or crisis a matter of a patient's personal perspective only or can chaplains or health care workers make that determination? For example, in Blanchard et al., (2012), chaplains provided education on a spiritual assessment to nurses working in an oncology department. The screening tool included three questions for the patient:

1. Do you have beliefs, spiritual or otherwise, that are helpful to you?
2. Are those beliefs currently helping you?
3. Were the beliefs helpful in the past?

Nurses and patients did not discuss specific beliefs or state any judgment about whether patients' beliefs were applicable or healthy. Therefore, on the basis of their perceived spiritual struggle, patients were able to request spiritual help or not.

Generally, limited numbers of chaplains are on staff to effectively provide screening, assessment, and intervention for all patients. As a result, the health care team is integral in first identifying and referring patients, families, or staff for services, but education and awareness is still needed to increase levels of comfort in recognizing and addressing spiritual concerns and making applicable referrals (Ellman et al., 2012; King et al., 2013; Parameshwaran, 2015).

Role of chaplain

The unique role of chaplains must be clearly articulated within an interdisciplinary or multidisciplinary approach, and credible research must support that role as efficacious (Powell et al., 2015). Chaplains' tasks and roles have been documented for palliative care (Massey et al., 2015), traumatic death (Chapple et al., 2011), pediatric care (Nash, Darby, & Nash, 2012), and psychiatric care (Hirschmann, 2011). One unique role of chaplains in a multidisciplinary approach is to use sacred and religious texts and images in conversations about spirituality, when applicable, whether with clients or within their own reflective practice (Hirschmann, 2011; Kestenbaum et al., 2015; O'Connor et al., 2012).

Recommendations have been made in the literature to develop practice models for further role clarification and research purposes (Kestenbaum et al., 2015). Emanuel and colleagues (2015) described the practice model the *HealthCare Chaplaincy Model,* which proposes a complex, multidimensional, and ever-changing process of spirituality when a person is confronted with injury, illness, or sudden loss. The chaplain's role in this model is described as providing interventions "to care for the human spirit" (Emanuel et al., 2015, p. 10).

What is not articulated well in the reviewed literature on chaplaincy are approaches and role distinctions for health care team members in collaboratively caring for the human spirit. Moreover, the role of any team member in addressing perceived spiritual distress or attending to spiritual matters in general continues to be ambiguous.

Interdisciplinary Approach to Spirituality

An *interdisciplinary approach* brings together diverse perspectives in an attempt to add clarity, depth, or more comprehensive understanding to an area of practice. For example, research focusing on interdisciplinary perspectives has been carried out to address real-world spiritual issues and to expand understanding of spiritual concepts and ideals. This section describes three such studies.

Challenging Personal and Professional Biases Related to Spirituality

Omu, Al-Obaidi, and Reynolds (2014) conducted a study in Kuwait with 40 women who suffered a stroke and were engaged in rehabilitation. The authors completed surveys with the women that focused on religious faith, self-efficacy, and life satisfaction. The quantitative results were that religious life did not relate to life satisfaction or self-efficacy.

These results were then shared with 12 professionals from diverse cultural backgrounds, including physical therapists, occupational therapists, speech and language therapists, and nurses. These professionals were from Canada, the United States, Kuwait, and Malaysia. Each of the professionals provided his or her own interpretation of the meaning of the quantitative data results and gave personal examples of therapeutic encounters that supported their interpretations.

The cultural (personal and professional) lens that each professional used provided a different interpretation of the clients' behaviors in relation to the study results. Omu et al. (2014) noted that the contrast in professional views demonstrates the need to better understand the perspectives that each client brings to the rehabilitation process and to better comprehend clients' unique religious practices, beliefs, and assumptions as they relate to the recovery process.

National Health System Trust

Harlow (2010) provided a case study about the process of setting up a National Health System Trust in Britain to address spirituality and spiritual needs of people seeking mental health and social services care. An interdisciplinary team consisting of nurses, occupational therapists, administrators, social workers, chaplains, service users, and advocates met to begin deliberating how to address spirituality within care.

Ten high-impact changes were identified, and strategies to address these changes were ultimately implemented. The case described not only the group members' diverse perspectives but also their challenges and struggles to find common ground in defining spirituality and addressing the need for spiritual care. As a result, a spiritual advocate role and job description were developed to ensure that someone was designated to attend to spiritual needs within units and service areas. The advocate could be of any professional discipline that had an interest in and desire to support spirituality.

After the program was implemented, activities associated with spirituality (e.g., yoga, meditation, Reiki) were provided for clients who desired them, chaplain visits increased, and conversations began or continued with community religious groups. Harlow (2010) stated that the spiritual care provided and the suggestions to address spirituality can be profound within an interdisciplinary team approach. In addition, such care and suggestions need not come from an administrator or chaplain but from staff and workers with a deep desire to see spirituality promoted and integrated into services.

Systems Model Approach

Rousseau (2014) provided a systems model approach in understanding spirituality and health care by providing a philosophical perspective to the current literature. While recognizing the contributions and insights from the health care community, primarily from physicians and nursing, regarding spirituality, he added an ontological exploration of how spirituality could be considered and assessed. He stated, "I propose the development of a 'philosophy of spirituality' that can clarify the conceptual terrain, identify important research directions, and facilitate a comprehensive and interdisciplinary investigation into the nature, validity, and implications of spirituality's conceptual and practical entailments" (p. 476). Rousseau's contribution to the health care community is to bring consensus to the discussion of spirituality; offer a model to consider spirituality within health care; and to further examine personal spiritual behaviors, competencies, agency, beliefs, growth, and larger philosophical constructs of the nature of people, the world, and reality.

Spirituality and Major Life Events and Transitions: Systematic Literature Review

Nicole Pagana, Christa Velenger, Christine Maley (former graduate students at Elizabethtown College, Elizabethtown, PA), and I were interested in exploring how people dealing with a major life event or life transition used spirituality. Because the empirical literature within occupational therapy, including studies that highlighted the intersection of meaning, engagement in occupations, and use of spirituality during life challenges (see Chapter 6, "The Meaning of Meaning: Thinking About Phenomenology and Meaning," and Chapter 7, "Spirituality and Occupational Therapy: A Conceptual Model for Practice"), was limited, we thought it would be beneficial to examine the literature outside of occupational therapy.

Review Background

The systematic literature review began by identifying key terms, selecting databases to be used, and choosing criteria for the studies (Humbert, Maley, Pagana, & Velenger, in press). In particular, we were interested in understanding how people made sense of their own spirituality and life event or transition and to see whether there was any consideration for the use of occupations during these experiences. As a result, the literature review focused on research that used personal perspectives within narrative analysis and phenomenological research methodologies.

A *transition* was determined as any situation or circumstance that altered a person's life in a substantial way, implying some level of role change or adaptation (i.e., beginning college, becoming a parent, moving out of poverty, recovering from substance abuse, adjusting to the aftermath of a stroke, dealing with an illness such as cancer) and implied an ongoing adjustment (Orentlicher & Gibson, 2015). A *major life event* entailed a sudden and dramatic change.

We began the search with the term *spirituality*, the type of methodology that was sought (phenomenology or narrative analysis), and a specific term regarding major life change or transition, including *life change, disability, illness, death, crisis, conflict, rehabilitation, stress, trauma, substance abuse, abuse, mental health, marriage,* and *children.* Sixty articles were found. We randomly chose 15 articles to review, performing an initial analysis to establish a coding sheet to use with all 60 articles. For the final review and analysis, a total of 59 articles were used that spanned health care disciplines and academic departments, countries, and type of research (Table 11.1). The articles also ranged in participants' major life event or transition reported (Table 11.2), country or area of residence, religious affiliation, and age and gender (Tables 11.1 and 11.2). We used a constructivist and positivist or optimistic

lens for this study, believing that we could find some common themes in such diverse studies, disciplines, and demographics (Savin-Baden & Howell Major, 2013). About half of the articles (31) focused primarily on the life event or transition, such as having a heart attack, with spirituality being a secondary theme. The remaining 28 articles focused on spirituality and its use during a major life event or transition, such as using spirituality when dealing with a divorce (Table 11.3). Moreover, three main categories of spirituality were identified:

1. Avenues to and through spirituality
2. Experience of spirituality
3. Meaning of spirituality (Humbert et al., in press).

Avenues to and Through Spirituality

Participants in the studies articulated various avenues in which spirituality was sought, experienced, or enhanced. Although study participants, and most of the authors, did not use the term *occupation* or *occupations,* we believe that this category best represents how occupational therapy practitioners understand occupations. The primary avenues in which spirituality was experienced included

- Religious affiliations,
- Coping mechanisms and activities, and
- Relationships.

Religious affiliations

Study participants identified avenues that had explicit *religious affiliations* or orientations, including, but not limited to, reading or reciting sacred texts, praying, fasting, engaging in structured services, taking sacrament, speaking with religious authorities, and sharing stories of God or a higher being. Participants attributed a strong faith in God as a result of or precursor to engaging in these occupations. This faith was associated with a general belief of trusting in God regardless of the hardship or situation. Use of these religious affiliation avenues were most noted in people from religions such as Islam, Judaism, and Christianity (Aghamohammadi-Kalkhoran, Valizadeh, Mohammadi, Ebrahimi, & Karimollahi, 2012; Carron & Cumbie, 2011; Hong & Welch, 2013; Koslander, Lindstrom, & Barbosa da Silva, 2012; Mitchell, Silver, & Ross, 2012; Price, Kinghorn, Patrick, & Cardell, 2012; Williamson & Hood, 2013).

Table 11.1. Articles in the Systematic Literature Review and Related Demographics

Author/Link	Religious Affiliation	Participant			Type of Research	Authors' Background/ Country
		Country/ Area	Gender (n)	Age, yr		
Aghamohammadi-Kalkhoran, Valizadeh, Mohammadi, Ebrahimi, & Karimollahi (2012) http://bit.ly/1Qh0uta	Muslim	Iran	Women (19)	35–59	Phenomenological	Nursing, midwifery Iran
Allen & Brooks (2012) http://bit.ly/1QugbAX	Christian, Hindu, Jewish, Muslim	USA	Women (67) Men (28)	18–22	Narrative analysis	MD USA
Asgeirsdottir et al. (2013) http://bit.ly/1LI8lhm	Christian, none	Iceland	Women (5) Men (5)	42–83	Phenomenological	Religious studies, nursing, social services Iceland, UK
Baum, Weidberg, Osher, & Kohelet (2012) http://bit.ly/1XP4Yfw	Christian, Muslim	Israel	Women (30)	21–41	Phenomenological	Social work Israel
Bong (2011a) http://bit.ly/1QAqPlk	Buddhist	Malaysia	Women (1)	NR	Narrative analysis	Malaysia
Bong (2011b) http://bit.ly/21umTdI	Buddhist, Christian, Hindu, Muslim, none, spiritualist	Malaysia, Singapore	Women (16) Men (14)	21+	Phenomenological	Malaysia, Singapore
Bornsheuer, Henriksen, & Irby (2012) http://bit.ly/1p96vBr	Christian	USA	Women (7) Men (7)	28–70	Phenomenological	Counseling USA
Bruun, Pedersen, Osther, & Wagner (2011) http://1.usa.gov/1TVVFu3	NR	Denmark	Women (5)	54–73	Phenomenological hermeneutic	Nursing, MD Denmark
Bsiri-Moghaddam, Basiri-Moghaddam, Sadeghmoghaddam, & Ahmadi (2011) http://1.usa.gov/1XP5dHy	NR	Iran	Women (7) Men (5) Parents (8)	7–11 24–47	Phenomenological husserl eidetic	Nursing, paramedic Iran

(Continued)

Table 11.1. Articles in the Systematic Literature Review and Related Demographics (*Cont.*)

Author/Link	Religious Affiliation	Participant			Type of Research	Authors' Background/ Country
		Country/ Area	Gender (*n*)	Age, yr		
Carron & Cumbie (2011) http://bit.ly/1VTphHt	Christian	USA	Women (11) Men (4)	28–84	Phenomenological	USA
Cheney et al. (2013) http://bit.ly/21jZhfj	Christian	USA	Women (14) Men (14)	20–61	Narrative analysis	Psychiatry USA
Civish (2013) http://bit.ly/1Qo8lav	Christian	USA	Women (10) Men (4)	30–63	Narrative analysis	Theology USA
Collin (2012) http://bit.ly/1T9ZHQV	None	Scotland	Women (2) Men (4)	47–73	Phenomenological	Nursing Scotland
de Castella & Simmonds (2012) http://bit.ly/1Rshj4j	Christian	Australia	Women (10)	29–51	Phenomenological	Psychology Australia
de Guzman et al. (2011) http://bit.ly/21k04gb	Christian	Philippines	Men (4)	60+	Phenomenological	Nursing, education Philippines
Denney, Aten, & Leavell (2011) http://bit.ly/1QArL94	Christian Latter Day	USA	Women (10) (Men) 3	44–73	Phenomenological	Psychology USA
Dittman (2012)	NR	USA	Men (9)	NR	Phenomenological	Nursing
Fallah, Keshmir, Kashani, Azargashb, & Akbari (2012) http://bit.ly/1SlVTe6	Muslim	Iran	Women (23)	34–61	Phenomenological	MD Iran
Fernando & Ferarri (2011) http://bit.ly/1Rshs80	Buddhist, Christian	Sri Lanka	Women (21) Men (12)	5–18, 25–80	Narrative interviews	Canada
Gall, Malette, & Guirguis-Younger (2011) http://bit.ly/1njU58n	Christian, Jewish, Muslim, other, none	Canada, Europe, USA, other	Women (142) Men (94)	M 39.5	Grounded theory/ axial coding	Canada
Gottheil & Groth-Marnat (2011) http://bit.ly/1TTkmbP	Amma, Benedictine, Buddhist, Christian, Jewish, none, pagan, Vedanta	European–American	Women (14) Men (11)	20–82	Narrative analysis/ grounded theory	USA

(Continued)

Table 11.1. Articles in the Systematic Literature Review and Related Demographics (*Cont.*)

Author/Link	Religious Affiliation	Participant Country/Area	Gender (*n*)	Age, yr	Type of Research	Authors' Background/Country
Hattie & Beagan (2013) http://bit.ly/1P02B3Q	Buddhist, Christian, Jewish	Canada	Women (19)	23–62	Phenomenological	Occupational therapy, social work, women's studies Canada
Heriot-Maitland, Knight, & Peters (2012) http://bit.ly/1S477Un	NR	England	Women (6) Men (6)	20–63	Phenomenological	Psychiatry UK
Hertz, Addad, & Ronel (2012) http://1.usa.gov/1TbZWe2	Jewish	Israel	Women (20)	26–62	Phenomenological	Social work Israel
Hong & Welch (2013) http://bit.ly/1p9beTN	Christian, Buddhist	Taiwan	Women (13)	18+	Phenomenological	Nursing Taiwan, Australia
Humbert, Bess, & Mowery (2013) http://bit.ly/1Lg8kXg	Christian, Muslim	USA	Women (6)	24–59	Phenomenological	Occupational therapy USA
Hutchinson, Hersch, Davidson, Chu, & Mastel-Smith (2011) http://bit.ly/24rGlub	NR	USA	Women (11) Men (12)	60–80	Phenomenological	Nursing USA
Kim & Pak (2013) http://bit.ly/1oKxLWY	Christian	Korea*	Women (5)	49–62	Narrative analysis	Psychology USA
Koslander, Lindstrom, & Barbosa da Silva (2012) http://bit.ly/1mZW0i5	NR	NR	NR	NR	Narrative analysis/ hermeneutic	Social Science, Nursing Sweden, Finland, Norway
Kwilecki (2011) http://bit.ly/1Lg8Jce	Christian, spiritualist	USA	NR	NR	Narrative analysis	Religious studies, philosophy USA
Lee & Smith (2012) http://bit.ly/1Ta25XK	Christian, Confucianism	USA	Women (8)	M 60	Phenomenological/ case study	Social work USA

(Continued)

Table 11.1. Articles in the Systematic Literature Review and Related Demographics (*Cont.*)

Author/Link	Religious Affiliation	Participant Country/Area	Participant Gender (*n*)	Participant Age, yr	Type of Research	Authors' Background/Country
Leung et al. (2011) http://bit.ly/1QAuCPw	NR	Canada	Women (18) Men (1)	24–64	Phenomenological	Nursing, MD Canada
Lietz & Hodge (2011) http://bit.ly/1Qog48A	NR	USA	Women (13) Men (6)	NR	Narrative analysis	Social work USA
Mihalache (2012) http://bit.ly/1SXSQcV	Buddhist Christian, Jewish Muslim, Native American, Taoist, Vedanta	NR	Women (9) Men (4)	38–75	Heuristic Qualitative	Psychology USA
Miller & Chavier (2013) http://bit.ly/1XP8rL8	Buddhist, Christian, Hindu, Jewish, Latter Day, Muslim	USA	Women (11) Men (6)	NR	Phenomenological	Psychology USA
Minaye (2012) http://bit.ly/1p9cYMU	NR	Ethiopia	Women (8)	20–30	Phenomenological	Social work Ethiopia
Mitchell, Silver, & Ross (2012) http://bit.ly/24rH8eB	Christian	Honduras	Women (23)	11–19	Qualitative	Social work USA
Morden (2012)	Christian	NR	Men (1)	NR	Narrative analysis	Theology USA
Nabolsi & Carson (2011) http://bit.ly/1R4IZMq	Muslim	Jordan	Men (19)	42–59	Phenomenological	Nursing Jordan, UK
Park, Chesla, Rehm, & Chun (2011) http://bit.ly/1Lg9T7k	NR	USA	NR	NR	Phenomenological	Psychiatry, nursing, medical ethics USA
Price, Kinghorn, Patrick, & Cardell (2012) http://bit.ly/1KOdZUr	Christian	USA	Men (1)	70	Narrative analysis	Occupational therapy USA

(*Continued*)

Table 11.1. Articles in the Systematic Literature Review and Related Demographics (*Cont.*)

Author/Link	Religious Affiliation	Participant Country/Area	Gender (*n*)	Age, yr	Type of Research	Authors' Background/Country
Rehnsfeldt & Arman (2012) http://bit.ly/1TBlz63	NR	Sweden	Women (13) Men (6)	24–69	Interpretive hermeneutic	Nursing Norway, Sweden
Renz, Mao, Bueche, Cerny, & Strasser (2012) http://bit.ly/1XP9iLL	NR	Switzerland	NR	NR	Phenomenological	Psychology
Saeteren, Lindström, & Naden (2011) http://bit.ly/1R4JR3C	NR	Norway	Women (6) Men (9)	46–76	Hermeneutic	Nursing Norway, Finland
Schapmire, Head, & Faul (2012) http://bit.ly/1OxUo5G	NR	USA	Women (8) Men (2)	M 44	Phenomenological	Social work USA
Schick Makaroff, Sheilds, & Molzahn (2013) http://bit.ly/1RqBYZ3	Christian	North America	Women (4) Men (10)	M 66	Narrative inquiry	Nursing Canada
Sharpe, Joe, & Taylor (2013) http://bit.ly/1mZXetW	NR	USA	Women (3) Men (9)	NR	Phenomenological	Social work USA
Smith & Suto (2012) http://bit.ly/1JIBoWW	Christian, Jewish, spiritual order	Canada	Women (6) Men (5)	19+	Phenomenological	Occupational therapy Canada
Tan, Wilson, Olver, & Barton (2011) http://bit.ly/1p9fzXb	Christian, none	Australia	Women (7) Men (5)	21–81	Phenomenological	Nursing, midwifery Australia
Tate, Swift, & Bayomi (2013) http://bit.ly/1SXUX0c	NR	Canada	Men	M 78	Survey with narrative descriptions	NR Canada
Teti et al. (2012) http://bit.ly/1oSWiZw	NR	USA	Men (30)	18–44	Phenomenological	Public health USA

(*Continued*)

Table 11.1. Articles in the Systematic Literature Review and Related Demographics (*Cont.*)

Author/Link	Religious Affiliation	Participant Country/Area	Gender (*n*)	Age, yr	Type of Research	Authors' Background/Country
Thornton & Pratt Hopp (2011) http://bit.ly/1LXnoUx	NR	USA	Women (7)	40–52	Phenomenological	Social work USA
Unruh & Hutchinson (2011) http://bit.ly/1Qha6nM	NR	Canada	Women (27) Men (15)	32–80	Phenomenological	Occupational therapy Canada
Van Lith (2014) http://bit.ly/1oD6iWA	NR	Australia	Women (7) Men (5)	Early 20s–late 50s	Phenomenological/ case study	Art therapy Australia
Wade (2013) http://bit.ly/1VHre9K	Christian	USA	Women (6) Men (6)	25+	Phenomenological	Psychology USA
Welton-Mitchell, McIntosh & DePrince (2013) http://bit.ly/1p9gXJ6	NR	USA	Women (48) Men (23)	M 32.28	Narrative analysis	Psychology USA
Williamson & Hood (2013) http://bit.ly/1TBmJhX	Christian, none	USA	Men (10)	24–50	Phenomenological	USA
Wu, Guo, Xia, Lu, & Xi (2011) http://bit.ly/1nk1Kn6	Christian, Buddhist	China	Women (14) Men (10)	18+	Phenomenological	Nursing, ophthalmology China
Yarhouse & Carrs (2012) http://bit.ly/1TcbKNI	Christian	NR	Men to women transgender (32)	40–67	Phenomenological	Psychology, counseling USA

Note. * = originally from Korea but may not be currently living there; *M* = mean; MD = medicine; NR = not reported; yr = years.

Table 11.2. Research Focus and Participant Demographics in the Reviewed Literature

Major Life Event or Transition, n[a]

Focus	Disability/Aging	Caregiving	Cancer/Palliative Care	Violence	Poverty	Cultural/Social Conflict	Sexuality/Gender Identity	General Health Care	Mental Health/Substance Abuse	Other	Undetermined
Life event	3	2	5	4	2	3	0	7	3	2	1
Spirituality	0	1	4	3	0	5	4	4	6	1	5

Religious Affiliation, n[a]

	Buddhist	Christian	Hindu	Jewish	Muslim	Native American	Spiritualist	None	Other	Undetermined
Life event	4	9	1	3	6	1	1	17	3	
Spirituality	5	23	3	5	3	0	3	6	5	

Residence, n[a]

	United Kingdom	Asia/Pacific	Scandinavia	Africa	Middle East	USA/Canada	Central America	Undetermined
Life event	1	4	4	1	5	14	0	2
Spirituality	3	2	1	0	0	12	1	9

Age (yr) and Gender, n[a]

	Age 0–17	Age 18–60	Age ≥61	Age Undetermined	Transgender
Life event[b]	1	15	9	10	0
Spirituality[c]	2	18	12	9	1

Note. [a]n = number of articles. [b]Total women = 277; total men = 155. [c]Total women = 282; total men = 146. yr = years.

Table 11.3. Overview of Themes and Subthemes in the Literature Review

Theme	Subtheme	Description	Examples
Avenues to and through spirituality	Religiously affiliations • Faith in God • Speaking with religious officials • Prayer • Religious rituals and actions*	Activities and beliefs that people engage in when relating to a higher being or religious principles as they handle their current situation	*Engaging in worship, reading scripture, fasting, telling sacred stories about God, taking sacrament, obeying the Ten Commandments, reciting the Qur'an.
	Coping mechanisms and activities • Expressive activities* • Bold actions[†] • Ignoring problems and time fillers[‡]	Actions and behaviors that people use as a means to deal with their current situation and stressors	*Meditation, creative writing and journaling, gardening, yoga, crying, exercising, caring for and responding affectionately to others. [†]Converting from Buddhism to Christianity after going through divorce, placing amulets in incubators of very-low-weight babies, inflicting self-harm. [‡]Smoking or using alcohol and other drugs, reading, watching television, working, listening to music.
	Relationships • Connecting with others • Engaging in a structured organization* • Attending church	Connections and associations that people experience with others	*Support groups, group and individual therapy, Alcoholics Anonymous.
Experience of spirituality	Embracing acceptance	Validation and acknowledgment of the person or life situation	Coming to terms with a diagnosis or illness, realizing that death is imminent, acknowledging trauma, admitting substance abuse or dependency, recognizing errors made, realizing self-worth.
	Developing resilience	A personal quality influenced or heightened through spirituality that enables the person to work through the life event/transition	Overcoming the long-term effects of dealing with the aftermath of war, dealing with long-term and progressive illnesses, challenging social and cultural stigmas.
	Dealing with suffering, fear, and guilt	People frequently need to deal with physical and emotional suffering, fear, or guilt	Attending to and dealing with depression and suicidal ideation, rejection from families, loss of employment, physical pain, relationship breakup or betrayal, death of a loved one, violence.

(Continued)

Table 11.3. Overview of Themes and Subthemes in the Literature Review (*Cont.*)

Theme	Subtheme	Description	Examples
	Finding hope and fight	Hope is an expectation and strong feeling or want for something to happen; fight refers to the action a person takes to achieve a goal	Realizing others are counting on you as a father or mother, finding the energy to live one more day to accomplish an immediate goal, embracing a new role (e.g., caregiver, partner), spending time and energy to leave a legacy.
	Moving forward or away	A positive change in a physical, personal, or spiritual sense results in a plan of action for change or continued growth	Finding alternative housing, making plans to leave an abusive relationship, setting new life goals.
Meaning of spirituality	Purpose and life meaning	People finding a reason behind what is happening in their lives	A reason for existence, a responsibility to give back to others, a message or life lesson.
	Trust in God or a higher power	A previous or ongoing reliance on God or a higher power	Reliance within the ultimate plan, a sense of complete dependency on God or a higher power, a greater sense of trust with a higher being.
	Acceptance and positivity	An altruistic or aesthetic response to challenges	Finding or recognizing opportunities despite incredible challenges, identifying blessings within or despite pain and suffering.
	Connectedness	Having a significant and reciprocal connection with a higher power or other people	Guidance from others who have the ability to offer strength and resources.
	Questioning God	Questioning current circumstances, especially hardships	Why is this happening to me? Did I do something wrong? Did God inflict this illness on me? Why is God not helping me?
	Critical thoughts and questions	Experiencing anger, questioning, wrestling with challenges	The reason for existence, the nature of good and evil, who is in control of our lives, who deserves forgiveness.

Coping mechanisms and activities

Another avenue, **coping mechanisms and activities,** or the things people think about and do to deal with the stress of life events and transitions, was identified and associated with spirituality or an increasing ability to cope with major life stressors. Although not all coping mechanisms and activities are directly related to spirituality, participants in the reviewed studies shared that engaging in coping activities or actions fostered a sense of emotional or physical release, or increased self-identity and awareness, which ultimately influenced their overall spiritual well-being. It was not clear from the studies how this improvement actually occurred, but various types of occupations influenced or were influenced by spirituality. Some of these occupations included meditation (Miller & Chavier, 2013), creative writing and journaling (Smith & Suto, 2012), gardening (Unruh & Hutchinson, 2011), yoga (Mihalache, 2012), and expressive activities (crying, showing affection) that primarily promoted physical or emotional release (Rehnsfeldt & Arman, 2012).

The literature noted examples in which people attributed bold actions or withdrawal from the stressful situation as a means not only to cope with the situation but also to initiate or heighten their spiritual journey. Examples of bold actions included converting from Buddhism to Christianity after going through divorce (Hong & Welch, 2013), placing amulets in the incubators of very-low-weight babies (Baum, Weidberg, Osher, & Kohelet, 2012), and inflicting self-harm (Lee & Smith, 2012; Sharpe, Joe, & Taylor, 2013).

Ignoring problems or using withdrawing activities, sometimes considered **time fillers** by study participants, included smoking (Hutchinson, Hersch, Davidson, Chu, & Mastel-Smith, 2011), using alcohol and other drugs (Sharpe et al., 2013), reading (Gottheil & Groth-Marnat, 2011), watching television (Hutchinson et al., 2011), working (Teti et al., 2012), and listening to music (Renz, Mao, Bueche, Cerny, & Strasser, 2012) and brought relief from boredom and anxiety associated with the life challenge. All of these coping mechanisms and activities brought temporary relief to participants, contributing to an associated sense of spiritual well-being or allowing the participant to better engage in spiritual activities. Note that although only some of these coping mechanisms may be considered traditional or

healthy, participants expressed that all of them were significant in some way to their spiritual journey.

Relationships

The third avenue to and through spirituality was **relationships,** or the connections and associations that people experience with others. In the reviewed studies, relationships included both personal connections with families and friends that provided a beneficial support system (Tan, Wilson, Olver, & Barton, 2011) and deep and transformative connections to others going through the same life event or transition or to the professionals who provided care (Saeteren, Lindström, & Naden, 2011). Relationships were also developed and nurtured through support groups, group and individual therapy, Alcoholics Anonymous, and church involvement. Frequently, a reciprocal relationship existed between receiving support and fulfilling a spiritual need or quest (Humbert, Bess, & Mowery, 2013; Lee & Smith, 2012; Wade, 2013).

Summary

Overall, multiple acts of spiritual doing, such as speaking with religious leaders and engaging in prayer, religious rituals, and actions, were emphasized in the avenues identified in the literature. In addition, doing, being, becoming, centeredness, and connectedness (Kang, 2003) were reflected in both relationships and coping mechanisms and strategies. Moreover, the reviewed studies indicate that physical or emotional release, relief from pain and anxiety, or an increased sense of self-identity and awareness may be associated with engaging in spirituality or possibly may be precursors to experiencing spirituality.

The interplay among these avenues of occupational engagement is dynamic; therefore, each client's chosen avenues are complex and personal. In addition, because implications of spirituality are highly social, cultural, and political, the avenues that are highlighted in the literature review should not be considered the only ones.

Experience of Spirituality

The experience of spirituality highlights the expressed and observable outcomes or results of engaging in

Figure 11.1. The experience of spirituality.

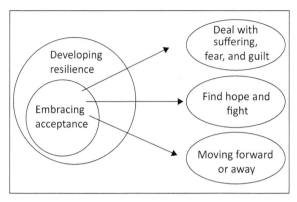

spirituality, that is, what happens when a person engages in spirituality. The experience of spirituality is represented by

- Embracing acceptance and
- Developing resilience.

These experiences allow people to deal with suffering, fear, and guilt; find hope and fight; and move forward or away (Figure 11.1).

Embracing acceptance

Embracing acceptance, the validation of the person in crisis as someone with worth and dignity or acknowledgment of the life circumstance as complex and challenging, appears to be central or preliminary to the experience of spirituality and may be foundational to developing resilience. Sometimes acceptance comes from an internal, renewed, or redefined self-identity (Allen & Brooks, 2012; Bong, 2011a, 2011b; Wade, 2013). Alternatively, acceptance comes through others or a higher being or power (de Guzman et al., 2011; Dittman, 2012) and reflects people's beliefs that God or a higher power is merciful, forgiving, noncondemning, and loving regardless of the situation (Cheney et al., 2013; Dittman, 2012; Wade, 2013) or has the authority or ability to heal, help, and guide.

Acceptance, whether internally or externally generated, results in not feeling alone (Tan et al., 2011), finding purpose and meaning (Tan et al., 2011; Williamson & Hood, 2013), having greater pride in oneself or in one's beliefs (Bong, 2011a, 2011b), being able to endure the challenge (de Guzman et al., 2011), or accepting unconditional care (Hertz, Addad, & Ronel, 2012).

Developing resilience

Developing resilience has been depicted as an important quality for a person to have or acquire to enhance his or her abilities, overcome illness, and accept change. There is some suggestion that resilience as a personal quality is influenced or heightened by a person's ongoing engagement in spirituality, embracing acceptance, and working through challenging life events (Fallah, Keshmir, Kashani, Azargashb, & Akbari, 2012; Price et al., 2012; Teti et al., 2012).

Deal with suffering

As part of the spiritual experience, participants in the reviewed studies frequently needed to deal with suffering, fear, or guilt specifically related to the life transition or event. These feelings were diminished or resolved through spirituality or spirituality provided them with the strength to endure or face these challenges.

Emotional suffering was often experienced before, during, or after an illness, diagnosis, traumatic experience, or loss of a loved one (Mihalache, 2012) and was described as emotional pain, sadness, loneliness, powerlessness, failing hope, being wounded, defeated, tired, in despair, numb, loss of purpose, loss of comfort, grief, angst, being devastated, exhausted, disturbed, having anxiety, being trapped, isolated, overwhelmed, and hurt. The ability for people to tolerate emotional suffering varied, and sometimes this suffering was described as unbearable.

Physical suffering was described as pain, irritation, and bodily aversion, often as the result of an insult to the body. One participant in Cheney et al. (2013) described his physical suffering from drug use as "a burning that never quits" (p. 8). People either sought out deliverance from God to alleviate this suffering (Cheney et al., 2013) or came to understand the suffering as being a blessing or a motivator in their life (de Castella & Simmonds, 2012; Gottheil & Groth-Marnat, 2011; Kwilecki, 2011). Physical suffering, at times, was also viewed as a physical test of a person's tolerance that could be overcome or endured through avenues of spirituality (Fallah et al., 2012).

Fear may be related to the here and now or to anticipation of the future, centering on experienced or expected hardship, or possible death, or continued or increased pain or suffering. Fear often encompasses both physical and emotional suffering. For example, a participant in Asgeirsdottir et al. (2013) shared, "I went through a phase as many of us do. That is to be angry, hurt and bitter and in the end I was dealing with the fear of dying" (p. 1450). The experience of spirituality was found to assist in overcoming fear (Collin, 2012; Denney, Aten, & Leavell, 2011).

Guilt is feeling shame (Bong, 2011b), blame, or remorse. Sometimes guilt arises in a person from feelings of responsibility for a situation that is out of his or her control (Rehnsfeldt & Arman, 2012; Sharpe et al., 2013). A tsunami survivor stated, "I would have been together more with my children than I have been" (Rendsfeldt & Arman, 2012, p. 542). Frequently, when guilt is imposed or projected on a person by others, that person faces a great personal challenge to deal with the conflict, reject the projected guilt, or accept responsibility. This situation often grounds people's spirituality and frequently reinforces their own belief system (Allen & Brooks, 2012; Wade, 2013).

Find hope and fight

Hope and *fight* were common terms mentioned in the reviewed articles, and they are related because a person fights because of hope. *Hope* was often described as a spiritual belief that enabled people to believe that "things are going to work out somehow" (Wade, 2013, p. 1143). This sentiment was expressed many times in reference to a better future, as a way to live, as recognition of God's support, and as a mantra to overcome hardship (de Guzman et al., 2011; Hong & Welch, 2013; Minaye, 2012). Finding hope enables people to take on a challenge, or *fight,* and then take action to deal with the difficult life circumstance (Hong & Welch, 2013).

Finding hope and fight also implies making meaning of the changing life event or transition by considering future possibilities and engaging in actions (or occupations) to realize those possibilities (Revheim, Greenberg, & Citrome, 2010). However, it is important to note that these actions include a variety of occupations such as finding housing and employment and being able to navigate social and physical environments (Beagan, Etowa, & Bernard, 2012; Glover-Graf, Marini, Baker, & Buck, 2007), not just actions commonly associated with spiritual and religious activities.

Move forward or away

Moving forward or away has been depicted as a positive change in a physical, personal, or spiritual sense that involves engaging in a plan of action for change or growth to occur. Multiple authors have described people's experiences of personal growth as they moved forward in dealing with a major life event (de Castella & Simmonds, 2012; Fallah et al., 2012; Hong & Welch, 2013; Price et al., 2012). Other authors have described people moving away from failure and suffering toward a more positive future after finding hope and growing through a difficult experience (Humbert et al., 2013).

Participants in several reviewed studies attributed spirituality to their ability to constantly move and rise to the challenge no matter how bad their circumstance or feelings of suffering (Lietz & Hodge, 2011; Rehnsfeldt & Arman, 2012; Teti et al., 2012). In addition, some connection seems to exist between engagement (doing) and the internal aspect of growing and moving or experience of spirituality (Ivtzan, Chan, Gardner, & Prashar, 2013). The idea of moving forward or away may be indicative of both engagement in action and growing associated with the experience of spirituality (de Castella & Simmonds, 2012; Fallah et al., 2012; Hong & Welch, 2013; Price et al., 2012). In other words, when a person is attending to a life event or transition, he or she experiences an element of doing along with a sense of being or belonging. This reciprocal relationship, while unclear how it is actually accomplished, signifies the importance of both occupational engagement and the spiritual experience.

Meaning of Spirituality

As depicted in this literature review, the meaning of spirituality represents how people make sense of what has happened to them or family members within the larger context of life. Meaning provides a framework for understanding the reasons or purpose for the life challenges, enabling people to respond to the life event or transition.

Purpose and life meaning

Purpose and life meaning is described as people finding a reason behind what has happened in their lives. For some of the participants in the reviewed studies, this reason was frequently associated with some concept of God or a higher being or power. For example, Nabolsi and Carson (2011) interviewed Jordanian Muslim men with coronary artery disease and found that many of them relied on the "will of God" (p. 719) to control their destiny and believed that becoming sick was their purpose or fate. In addition, in de Castella and Simmonds (2012), one participant regarded her suffering as God's way of "cleansing" (p. 544) her from the past.

Throughout the reviewed literature, purpose and life meaning encompassed coming to terms with a sense of a distinct purpose. In a study by Denney et al. (2011), cancer survivors suggested that God used their experience with their diagnosis and treatment for a spiritual or divine purpose. Terms frequently used to describe life purpose and meaning also referenced a religious connotation or belief, including *God's calling, God's plan, life call, God's will, destiny, life mission,* and *divine purpose,* with the idea that experiencing a challenging life event was part of a larger scheme, often outside of the person's control. Purpose and life meaning in this context may or may not have been fully understood by the person but was still acknowledged as being part of or important in providing something better to others, to communities, or to themselves.

Outside of explicit religious beliefs, some of the participants in the reviewed articles described purpose and life meaning as a reason for existence (Teti et al., 2012), a responsibility to give back to others (Unruh & Hutchinson, 2011), or a message or life lesson (Baum et al., 2012). These ideas represent an understanding of a larger, grander design, even though it was not attributed to a higher being or power. The person experiencing the challenging circumstances was engaged in or part of this design, and the challenge was a means for some betterment to others or for personal growth.

Trust in God or a higher power

Participants consistently mentioned a sense of ***trust in God or a higher power,*** often implying that God or a higher power was in control of the situation. This theme corresponds with purpose and life meaning but goes further to describe a previous or ongoing reliance on God or a higher power within an ultimate plan or a sense of complete dependency on God or a higher power. This acknowledgment

often included descriptions of God or a higher power such as goodness, strength, grace, mercy, and unconditional love.

In one example of trust in God, a woman living in a short-term shelter and crisis center stated, "Allah is the God of my people.... He's got me here, He's gotten me through a lot, and He will get me through this too" (Humbert et al., 2013, p. 258). In another example, Schapmire, Head, and Faul (2012) interviewed a man with an advanced cancer who stated, "I never really worried about it. I knew it was going to be taken care of. I'm a firm believer that if they [health care providers] can't take care of it, God can" (p. 45). The implication for this theme is that the challenging life experience facilitated or enhanced a greater sense of trust in a higher being who held the person's best interest in mind.

Acceptance and positivity

Acceptance and positivity is an altruistic or aesthetic response to challenges. It recognizes the incredible suffering a person has experienced or is experiencing while still finding some sense of beauty or gift within that experience or within daily life (Price et al., 2012). Fernando and Ferrari (2011) discussed the resilience of children living in a war orphanage. The children were provided with a secure environment, with an emphasis on emotional, social, and religious support from a board of professional women. Most of the children (all but one) did well in school, had plans for the future, and created vocational goals while working with teachers and other leaders. The spiritual meaning of acceptance and positivity is that despite difficult life circumstances and pain suffered, people can find new life goals, develop personal strength, and have the ability to see life's beauty.

Connectedness

Connectedness is the idea of having a significant bond with a higher power or other people that ultimately brings strength or resources to the challenging event and can also provide a means for a reciprocal relationship. Participants in Bornsheuer, Henriksen, and Irby's (2012) study believed that their relationships with church leaders helped guide them in the right direction or directly helped them to deal with problems. *Connectedness* references recognition of the intricate web of relations that are encountered and the interconnectedness and significance of those relationships to all of life, including others, places, or experiences (Tan et al., 2011). In the studies reviewed that were associated with connectedness, challenging life events enabled participants to be more aware and appreciative of connections or value relationships in deeper ways (Asgeirsdottir et al., 2013; Denney et al., 2011).

Questioning God

Throughout the reviewed literature, participants had moments when they questioned God, a higher power, or reality about their current circumstances, and especially their hardships. Their life challenges were the impetus to pose questions and further their understanding about God or a higher power. They asked questions such as

- "Why me?" and "What did I do wrong?" (de Guzman et al., 2011, p. 277),
- "Did God inflict this stroke on me?" (Price et al., 2012, p. 114),
- "Why is this happening?" (Collin, 2012, p. 386), and
- "Why is [God] not helping me?" (Hattie & Beagan, 2013, p. 253).

de Guzman et al. (2011) discussed how clients often experienced an initial denial of their circumstances and then, after some awareness, would pose questions. One participant spoke of the anger that he felt toward God. "I felt angry with God because something like this happened.... What did I do wrong? I'm not that sinful" (p. 277). Questioning frequently led people to seek something beyond themselves (Gottheil & Groth-Marnat, 2011) to gain answers, insights, and clarity about their situation. Therefore, their questioning provided increased self-awareness or perspectives that they had not considered previously, enlightenment that provided reassurance or hope (Mitchell et al., 2012), or new images of God (Kim & Pak, 2013).

Critical thoughts and questions

Some participants in the studies reviewed had moments of anger and questioning and wrestled with their challenges. These critical thoughts and

questions were directed at others, God or a higher power, or no one in particular. A woman who had lost two children in a tsunami made a statement that life would never be good again, emphasizing the impact that natural disasters have on survivors and implying questioning of why these events happen (Rehnsfeldt & Arman, 2012).

In another study, Van Lith (2014) addressed people with mental illness and the influence of art making during psychosocial rehabilitation. Participants saw direct connections between their art and their spirituality, which led to critical thoughts and questions. For example, participants asked, "What is life?" and used phrases such as "finding my spirit" when discussing the role of art making in their recovery (Van Lith, 2014, p. 26). Their questions included concepts about the reason for existence (Van Lith, 2014), the nature of good and evil (Cheney et al., 2013), who is in control of our lives (Saeteren et al., 2011), and who deserves forgiveness (Mihalache, 2012). In addition, participants recognized that some questions are unanswerable, acknowledging the mysteries of life (Allen & Brooks, 2012; Wade, 2013).

Making sense of challenging life events frequently evokes critical thoughts and questions that do not have tangible answers. Nevertheless, by virtue of contemplating these critical thoughts and questions, people may gain insight into life's mysteries, which can provide meaning to life.

Implications for Occupational Therapy

The *Occupational Therapy Practice Framework: Domain and Process* (AOTA, 2014) identifies spirituality as a client factor and notes its relationship to instrumental activities of daily living (i.e., religious and spiritual occupations) and rituals. However, the results of this literature review suggest that people engage in spirituality in diverse and complex ways and that spirituality is subsumed within many daily occupations. In addition, the review highlighted the interconnection among occupations, client factors, contexts, and rituals.

Social participation as a spiritual occupation

Social relationships are recognized as avenues to or through spirituality in this review, and the complexity and connectedness of social relationships can be significant and may have specific spiritual meaning. Thus, occupations of social participation may affect client factors related to spirituality and beliefs. For example, two people might meet at a support group meeting and share their struggles with caring for a loved one dealing with Alzheimer disease. One person describes the importance of still recognizing and honoring the essence of the loved one, seeing the unique qualities of that person despite the cognitive changes and confusion witnessed. He or she shares his or her belief that caring for someone provides opportunities to connect in new ways to the loved one and that care offers moments of beauty.

Understanding social participation and spirituality can be complex. For example, social participation as it relates to spirituality may or may not be contextualized within a sacred or spiritual place or routine. Social relationships may exist within the context of traditional religious actions and activities; however, they may be created or developed as part of a therapy or support group or with another person experiencing the same life event. In addition, the context may be intentional and sought out by the person or not overtly attended to. The relationship may be a onetime encounter or part of a regular routine as a person engages in his or her life.

Spirituality and angst

Spirituality is frequently portrayed in the literature as an avenue for developing resilience and the ability to cope, suggesting mediation of pain and suffering. The experience of spirituality in occupational therapy can be closely connected with the acceptance of events and oneself. However, the reviewed articles have highlighted the deep and painful challenges experienced when significant others do not accept lifestyles, life events, or personal qualities and life choices (Bong, 2011a, 2011b). Authors and participants spoke about the significant turning point when acceptance was finally achieved, even if only partially.

Valuing others, including their perceived acceptance, may support or enhance a person's experience of spirituality. This factor might be understood within the current descriptions of spirituality as a way of seeking meaning and purpose and connectedness to others, but the current descriptions of spirituality in the *Framework* (AOTA, 2014) do not give credence to the difficulty and potential angst

associated with seeking acceptance from others or a higher being. However, the *Framework* somewhat acknowledges the importance of accepting oneself or a major life event as central to the spiritual experience as a person tries to make meaning of the challenge and may reflect the connection between occupational engagement and the construction and reconstruction of self-identity (Boswell, Hamer, Glacoff, & McChesney, 2007; Boswell, Knight, & Hamer, 2001).

Occupational engagement, adaptation, and spirituality

The interconnection among occupational engagement, adaptation, and the experience of spirituality (i.e., acceptance) suggests a complex and individualistic path in which spirituality may affect the life event or transition or the life event or transition becomes the impetus to the spiritual experience. There is evidence that occupations do help people adapt to major life events and transitions that parallels the results of this systematic review. Occupations assist people in dealing with grief (Chaffey & Fossey, 2004; Johansson & Johansson, 2009), accepting the life event (Parson & Stanley, 2008; Smith, Ludwig, Anderson, & Copolillo, 2009), finding hope (Muñoz, Dix, & Reichenbach, 2006; Smith et al., 2009), engaging in meaningful religious rituals (Chapman & Nelson, 2014), developing coping strategies (Dubouloz, Vallerand, Laporte, Ashe, & Hall (2008), and relying on relationships and social support (Chaffey & Fossey, 2004; Isaksson, Josephsson, Lexell, & Skär, 2008).

The results of the literature review emphasized that spirituality heightened, substantiated, or sustained the engagement in occupations in addition to adaptation to the life event. However, how the process of occupational engagement, spirituality, and adaptation actually unfolds is unknown. It is important to note that the process for each person may be complex.

Implications for Occupational Therapy Intervention

Because the three aspects of spirituality (avenues to and through spirituality, experience of spirituality, and meaning of spirituality) are relevant to people dealing with a major life event or transition, it is

Figure 11.2. Interconnections of avenues to and through spirituality (occupational engagement), the experience of spirituality, and the meaning of spirituality.

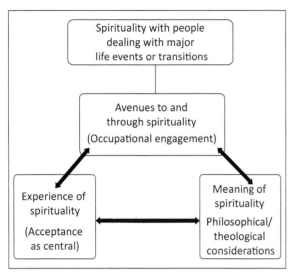

important to consider how they might play out in occupational therapy intervention. For example, if avenues to and through spirituality are engaged, whether traditionally religious or spiritual in nature or not, those avenues may affect a person's experience of spirituality and the meaning of spirituality (Figure 11.2). As a result, acceptance of the life circumstance might be realized, resilience strengthened, hope renewed, fight engaged, growth realized, or movement made. In addition, clients may find new purpose and meaning, connectedness, and acceptance.

If the desire of the client is to engage in select and meaningful occupations or avenues to spirituality that will bring reassurance or support in clarifying life meaning or bring relief from pain and suffering, should the focus of occupational therapy then be on these occupations?

When spirituality is addressed in occupational therapy, the focus of the intervention becomes the use of specific occupations. Occupational therapy practitioners should take note of the significance or value that the client holds for those occupations and how the experience of spirituality is realized for that person to further promote recovery (Burns, 2007; Smith & Suto, 2012; Unruh & Hutchinson, 2011). Practitioners may take notice of the client's experience of spirituality and the meaning of spirituality, especially if the relationship has been

well-established over time (Beagan et al., 2012; Nesbit, 2006; Ramugondo, 2005).

What if this life experience and subsequent spirituality were experienced in a different manner and the results affected the therapeutic process? For example, if the person going through a major life event or transition is primarily dealing with the meaning of spirituality and that becomes the central focus of his or her life, it may or may not lead to meaningful occupational engagement or the experience of spirituality. Struggling with the questions of "Why?" "Why me?" or "What does this mean for my life?" may leave little ability for the client to actively engage in therapy tasks. In addition, occupational therapy practitioners may not be ready to attend to these questions or be overwhelmed by them, not knowing how best to respond (Meredith, 2010; Morris, 2013).

It may be a reasonable argument that addressing philosophical and theological questions alone may be beyond the purview of the occupational therapy practitioner and cause inherent conflict within managed care and cost-driven health care (see Chapter 1, "Addressing Spirituality in Occupational Therapy"). However, a multidisciplinary or interdisciplinary focus on attending to the meaning of spirituality for clients is reasonable (Harlow, 2010; Morgan, 2010). Considering alternative ways to address spirituality within a cost-driven health care system is a valid point of conversation and valued by some in the occupational therapy profession and in other professions (Blanchard et al., 2012; Harlow, 2010).

Where Do We Go From Here? Considerations for Future Research

Multiple considerations must be discussed as the conversation about spirituality in occupational therapy continues. First, the recognition that spirituality is a complex construct that incorporates multiple contexts has been highlighted in this chapter and throughout the text. Further research is needed to understand the dynamics of culture, relationships, religious beliefs, interpersonal growth and development, engagement in occupations, and spirituality in affecting health and wellness and providing support and guidance through challenging life events and transitions. Second, although some work has been completed on establishing conceptual models related to spirituality, additional research is needed to substantiate and elaborate on these models of practice.

Third, conversation and research have been limited regarding an interdisciplinary approach in addressing spirituality within the context of client-centered care. The question remains, How can occupational therapy practitioners best work collaboratively when attending to the spiritual needs of clients, families, communities, and organizations? Providing opportunities to engage in robust conversations about such care, and developing the willingness to further explore this dynamic and fluid aspect of health care, has been suggested in the literature and will continue to be promoted in the future.

Summary

Spirituality has been deemed an important aspect of health care as articulated by the various members of the health care team. Whether the focus of spirituality is addressed through the specific roles and responsibilities of each team member, as in a multidisciplinary approach, or addressed collectively within an interdisciplinary approach, the value of attending to clients' spiritual needs is noted in the literature. The ways in which people use spirituality when dealing with a major life event or transition is complex, entailing the engagement of occupations (avenues to and through spirituality), the process of spirituality (experience of spirituality), and meaning making (meaning of spirituality). Occupational therapy practitioners have a role within the health care team to understand how clients use spirituality to deal with major life events and transitions and how best to support them through the use of meaningful occupations.

References

Aghamohammadi-Kalkhoran, M., Valizadeh, S., Mohammadi, E., Ebrahimi, H., & Karimollahi, M. (2012). Health according to the experiences of Iranian women with diabetes: A phenomenological study. *Nursing and Health Sciences, 14,* 285–291. http://dx.doi.org/10.1111/j.1442-2018.2011.00672.x

Allen, K. R., & Brooks, J. E. (2012). At the intersection of sexuality, spirituality, and gender: Young adults' perceptions of religious beliefs in the context of sexuality education. *American Journal of Sexuality Education, 7,* 285–308. http://dx.doi.org/10.1080/15546128.2012.740859

American Counseling Association. (2005). *ACA code of ethics.* Retrieved from http://www.counseling.org/Resources/aca-code-of-ethics.pdf

American Occupational Therapy Association. (2014). *Occupational therapy practice framework: Domain and process.* (3rd ed.). *American Journal of Occupational Therapy, 68*(Suppl. 1), S1–S48. http://dx.doi.org/10.5014/ajot.2014.682006

American Psychological Association. (2000). Guidelines and principles for accreditation of programs in professional psychology. Washington, DC: Author.

American Psychological Association. (2003). Guidelines on multicultural education, training, research, practice, and organizational change for psychologists. *American Psychologist, 58,* 377–402. Retrieved from http://www.apa.org/pi/oema/resources/policy/multicultural-guidelines.aspx

Anandarajah, G. (2014). Introduction to spirituality and medical practice. *Rhode Island Medical Journal, 97,* 16. Retrieved from https://www.rimed.org/rimedicaljournal/2014/03/2014-03-16-spirituality-anandarajah.pdf

Anandarajah, G., & Roseman, J. L. (2014). A qualitative study of physicians' views on compassionate patient care and spirituality: Medicine as a spiritual practice? *Rhode Island Medical Journal, 97,* 17–22.

Anderson, J. A., & Grice, J. W. (2014). Toward an integrated model of spirituality. *Journal of Psychology and Christianity, 33,* 3–21.

Asgeirsdottir, G., Sigurbjörnsson, E., Traustadottir, R., Sigurdardottir, V., Gunnarsdottir, S., & Kelly, E. (2013). "To cherish each day as it comes": A qualitative study of spirituality among persons receiving palliative care. *Support Cancer Care, 21,* 1145–1451. http://dx.doi.org/10.1007/s00520-012-1690-6

Balboni, T. (2014). Spirituality plays key role in patients' cancer care. *HemOnc Today, 15*(11), 20. Retrieved from http://www.healio.com/hematology-oncology/palliative-care/news/print/hemonc-today/%7B2eb957ac-cbc2-4736-806e-43bfdc48bd60%7D/spirituality-plays-key-role-in-patients-cancer-care

Barker, S. L., & Floersch, J. E. (2010). Practitioners' understandings of spirituality: Implications for social work education. *Journal of Social Work Education, 46,* 357–370.

Baum, N., Weidberg, Z., Osher, Y., & Kohelet, D. (2012). No longer pregnant, not yet a mother: Giving birth prematurely to a very-low-birth-weight baby. *Qualitative Health Research, 22,* 595–606. http://dx.doi.org/10.1177/1049732311422899

Beagan, B. L., Etowa, J., & Bernard, W. T. (2012). "With God in our lives he gives us the strength to carry on": African Nova Scotian women, spirituality, and racism-related stress. *Mental Health, Religion and Culture, 15,* 103–120. http://dx.doi.org/10.1080/13674676.2011.560145

Best, M., Butow, P., & Olver, I. (2014). The doctor's role in helping dying patients with cancer achieve peace: A qualitative study. *Palliative Medicine, 28,* 1139–1145. http://dx.doi.org/10.1177/0269216314536455

Best, M., Butow, P., & Olver, I. (2015). Doctors discussing religion and spirituality: A systematic literature review. *Palliative Medicine,* Advance online publication. http://dx.doi.org/10.1177/0269216315600912

Bishop, J. P., & Trancik, E. K. (2013). Assessing the spirit? *Christian Bioethics, 19,* 247–250. http://dx.doi.org/10.1093/cb/cbt026

Blanchard, J. H., Dunlap, D. A., & Fitchett, G. (2012). Screening for spiritual distress in the oncology inpatient: A quality improvement pilot project between nurses and chaplains. *Journal of Nursing Management, 20,* 1076–1084. http://dx.doi.org/10.1111/jonm.12035

Bong, S. A. (2011a). Beyond queer: An epistemology of bi choice. *Journal of Bisexuality, 11,* 39–63. http://dx.doi.org/10.1080/15299716.2011.545304

Bong, S. A. (2011b). Negotiating resistance/resilience through the nexus of spirituality–sexuality of same-sex partnerships in Malaysia and Singapore. *Marriage and Family Review, 47,* 648–665. http://dx.doi.org/10.1080/01494929.2011.619305

Bornsheuer, J. N., Henriksen, R. C., Jr., & Irby, B. J. (2012). Psychological care provided by the church: Perceptions of Christian church members. *Counseling and Values, 57,* 199–213. http://dx.doi.org/10.1002/j.2161-007X.2012.00017.x

Boswell, B. B., Knight, S., & Hamer, M. (2001). Disability and spirituality: Reciprocal relationships with the implications for the rehabilitation process. *Journal of Rehabilitation, 67*(4), 20–25.

Boswell, B., Hamer, M., Knight, S., Glacoff, M., & McChesney, J. (2007). Dance of disability and spirituality. *Journal of Rehabilitation, 73*(4), 33–40.

Bruun, P., Pedersen, B. D., Osther, P. J., & Wagner, L. (2011). The lonely female partner: A central aspect of prostate cancer. *Urologic Nursing, 31,* 294–299. http://www.ncbi.nlm.nih.gov/pubmed/22073900 (PubMed link)

Bsiri-Moghaddam, K., Basiri-Moghaddam, M., Sadeghmoghaddam, L., & Ahmadi, F. (2011). The concept of hospitalization of children from the view point of parents and children. *Iranian Journal of Pediatrics, 21,* 201–208. Retrieved from http://www.ncbi.nlm.nih.gov/pmc/articles/PMC3446164/

Burns, J. (2007). OT leads the way: A child's triumph in war-torn Iraq. *OT Practice, 12*(1), 7–9. Retrieved from https://majorburns.wordpress.com/2011/07/17/ot-leads-the-way-a-childs-triumph-in-war-torn-iraq/

BusinessDictionary.com (2016a). Interdisciplinary team. Retrieved from http://www.businessdictionary.com/definition/interdisciplinary-team.html

BusinessDictionary.com. (2016b). Multidisciplinary team. Retrieved from http://www.businessdictionary.com/definition/multidisciplinary-team.html

Callahan, A. M. (2015). Key concepts in spiritual care for hospice social workers: How an interdisciplinary perspective can inform spiritual competence. *Social Work and Christianity, 42,* 43–62.

Carpenter, K., Girvin, L., Kitner, W., & Ruth-Sahd, L. (2008). Spirituality: A dimension of critical care nursing. *Dimensions of Critical Care Nursing, 27,* 16–20. http://dx.doi.org/10.1097/01.DCC.0000304668.99121.b2

Carron, R., & Cumbie, S. A. (2011). Development of a conceptual nursing model for the implementation of spiritual care in adult primary healthcare settings by nurse practitioners. *Journal of the American Academy of Nurse Practitioners, 23,* 552–560. http://dx.doi.org/10.1111/j.1745-7599.2011.00633.x

Çetinkaya, B., Azak, A., & Dündar, S. A. (2013). Nurses' perceptions of spirituality and spiritual care. *Australian Journal of Advanced Nursing, 31,* 1–10. Retrieved from http://www.ajan.com.au/Vol31/Issue1/1Azak.pdf

Chaffey, L., & Fossey, E. (2004). Caring and daily life: Occupational experiences of women living with sons diagnosed with schizophrenia. *Australian Occupational Therapy Journal, 51,* 199–207. http://dx.doi.org/10.1111/j.1440-1630.2004.00460.x

Chapman, L., & Nelson, D. (2014). Person-centered, community-based occupational therapy for a man with Parkinson's disease: A case study. *Activities, Adaptation, and Aging, 38,* 94–112. http://dx.doi.org/10.1080/01924788.2014.901045

Chapple, A., Swift, C., & Ziebland, S. (2011). The role of spirituality and religion for those bereaved due to a traumatic death. *Mortality, 16,* 1–18. http://dx.doi.org/10.1080/13576275.2011.535998

Cheney, A. M., Curran, G. M., Booth, B. M., Sullivan, S. D., Stewart, K. E., & Borders, T. F. (2013). The religious and spiritual dimensions of cutting down and stopping cocaine use: A qualitative exploration among African Americans in the south. *Journal of Drug Issues, 20*(10), 1–20. http://dx.doi.org/10.1177/0022042613491108

Cheng, J., Purcell, H. N., Dimitriou, S. M., & Grossoehme, D. H. (2015). Testing the feasibility and acceptability of a chaplaincy intervention to improving treatment: Attitudes and self-efficacy of adolescents with cystic fibrosis: A pilot study. *Journal of Health Care Chaplaincy, 21,* 76–90. http://dx.doi.org/10.1080/08854726.2015.1015365

Civish, G. (2013). The calling: A study of personal spiritual experiences of seminary students. *Journal of Spirituality in Mental Health, 15,* 186–214. http://dx.doi.org/10.1080/19349637.2013.776446

Clarke, J. (2009). A critical view of how nursing has defined spirituality. *Journal of Clinical Nursing, 18,* 1666–1673. http://dx.doi.org/10.1111/j.1365-2702.2008.02707.x

Collin, M. (2012). The search for a higher power among terminally ill people with no previous religion or belief. *International Journal of Palliative Nursing, 18,* 384–389. http://dx.doi.org/10.12968/ijpn.2012.18.8.384

Corry, D. A. S., Mallett, J., Lewis, C. A., & Abdel-Khalek, A. M. (2013). The creativity–spirituality construct and its role in transformative coping. *Mental Health, Religion and Culture, 16,* 979–990. http://dx.doi.org/10.1080/13674676.2013.834492

Coyne, C. (2005, July). Addressing spirituality: Issues in patient interventions. *PT Magazine, 13*(7), 38–44.

Curlin, F. A., Lawrence, R. E., Odell, S., Chin, M. H., Lantos, J. D., Koenig, H. G., & Meador, K. G. (2007). Religion, spirituality, and medicine: Psychiatrists' and other physicians' differing observations, interpretations, and clinical approaches. *American Journal of Psychiatry, 164,* 1825–1831. http://dx.doi.org/10.1176/appi.ajp.2007.06122088

de Castella, R., & Simmonds, J. G. (2012). "There's a deeper level of meaning as to what suffering's all about": Experiences of religious and spiritual growth following trauma. *Mental Health, Religion and Culture, 16,* 536–556. http://dx.doi.org/10.1080/13674676.2012.702738

de Guzman, A. B., Shim, H., Sia, C. M., Sizaon, W. S., Sibal, M. P., Siglos, J. C., & Simeon, F. C. (2011). Ego integrity of older people with physical disability and therapeutic recreation. *Educational Gerontology, 37,* 265–291. http://dx.doi.org/10.1080/03601270903534945

De Sousa, A. (2011). Spirituality and geriatric psychiatry: A review. *Indian Journal of Gerontology, 25,* 345–354.

Denney, R. M., Aten, J. D., & Leavell, K. (2011). Posttraumatic spiritual growth: A phenomenological study of cancer survivors. *Mental Health, Religion and Culture, 14,* 371–391. http://dx.doi.org/10.1080/13674671003758667

Dittman, P. W. (2012). Mountains to climb: Male nurses and their perspective on professional impairment. *International Journal for Human Caring, 16,* 34–41.

Dombo, E. A., & Gray, C. (2013). Engaging spirituality in addressing vicarious trauma in clinical social workers: A self-care model. *Social Work and Christianity, 40,* 89–104.

Draper & McSherry, P. (2013). Making windows into men's souls: Ethical perspectives on spiritual assessment in nursing.

Christian Bioethics, 19, 270–281. http://dx.doi.org/10.1093/cb/cbt025

Drobin, P. (2014). Recovery, spirituality and psychotherapy. *Journal of Religion and Health, 53,* 789–795. http://dx.doi.org/10.1007/s10943-013-9800-4

Dubouloz, C., Vallerand, J., Laporte, D., Ashe, B., & Hall, B. (2008). Occupational performance modification and personal change among clients receiving rehabilitation services for rheumatoid arthritis. *Australian Occupational Therapy Journal, 55,* 30–38. http://dx.doi.org/10.1111/j.1440-1630.2006.00639.x

Elkonin, D., Brown, B., & Naicker, S. (2014). Religion, spirituality and therapy: Implications for training. *Journal of Religion and Health, 53,* 119–134. http://dx.doi.org/10.1007/s10943-012-9607-8

Ellis, M. R., Campbell, J. D., Detwiler-Breidenbach, A., & Hebrand, D. K. (2002). What do family physicians think about spirituality in clinical practice? *Journal of Family Practice, 51,* 249–254.

Ellman, M. S., Schulman-Green, D., Blatt, L., Asher, S., Viveiros, D., Clark, J., & Bia, M. (2012). Using online learning and interactive simulation to teach spiritual and cultural aspects of palliative care to interprofessional students. *Journal of Palliative Medicine, 15,* 1240–1247. http://dx.doi.org/10.1089/jpm.2012.0038

Emanuel, L., Handzo, G., Grant, G., Massey, K., Zollfrank, A., Wilke, D.,... Pargament, K. (2015). Workings of the human spirit in palliative care situations: A consensus model from the Chaplaincy Research Consortium. *BMC Palliative Care, 14*(29), 1–13. http://dx.doi.org/10.1186/s12904-015-0005-3

Fallah, R., Keshmir, F., Kashani, F. L., Azargashb, E., & Akbari, M. E. (2012). Post-traumatic growth in breast cancer patients: A qualitative phenomenological study. *Middle East Journal of Cancer, 3*(2/3), 35–44. http://mejc.sums.ac.ir/index.php/mejc/article/view/40

Fernando, C., & Ferarri, M. (2011). Spirituality and resilience in children of war in Sri Lanka. *Journal of Spirituality in Mental Health, 13*(1), 52–77. http://dx.doi.org/10.1080/19349637.2011.547138

Gall, T. L., Malette, J., & Guirguis-Younger, M. (2011). Spirituality and religiousness: A diversity of definitions. *Journal of Spirituality and Mental Health, 13,* 158–181. http://dx.doi.org/10.1080/19349637.2011.593404

Garlick, M., Wall, K., Corwin, D., & Koopman, C. (2011). Psycho-spiritual integrative therapy for women with primary breast cancer. *Journal of Clinical Psychology in Medical Settings, 18,* 78–90. http://dx.doi.org/10.1007/s10880-011-9224-9

Giordano, A. L., & Cashwell, C. S. (2014). Entering the sacred: Using motivational interviewing to address spirituality in counseling. *Counseling and Values, 59,* 65–79. http://dx. doi.org/10.1002/j.2161-007X.2014.00042.x

Glover-Graf, N. M., Marini, I., Baker, J., & Buck, T. (2007). Religious and spiritual beliefs and practices of persons with chronic pain. *Rehabilitation Counseling Bulletin 51*(1), 21–33. http://dx.doi.org/10.1177/00343552070510010501

Gottheil, E. A., & Groth-Marnat, G. (2011). A grounded theory study of spirituality: Using personal narratives suggested by spiritual images. *Journal of Religion and Health, 50,* 452–463. http://dx.doi.org/10.1007/s10943-010-9366-3

Harlow, R. (2010). Developing a spirituality strategy—why, how, and so what? *Mental Health, Religion and Culture, 13,* 615–624. http://dx.doi.org/10.1080/13674676.2010.488426

Hattie, B., & Beagan, B. L., (2013). Reconfiguring spirituality and sexual/gender identity: "It's a feeling of connection to something bigger, it's part of a wholeness." *Journal of Religion and Spirituality in Social Work: Social Thought, 32,* 244–268. http://dx.doi.org/10.1080/15426432.2013.801733

Helminiak, D. A. (2008). Confounding the divine and the spiritual: Challenges to a psychology of spirituality. *Pastoral Psychology, 57,* 161–182. http://dx.doi.org/10.1007/s11089-008-0163-9

Heriot-Maitland, C., Knight, M., & Peters, E. (2012). A qualitative comparison of psychotic-like phenomena in clinical and non-clinical populations. *British Journal of Clinical Psychology, 51,* 37–53. http://dx.doi.org/10.1111/j.2044-8260.2011.02011.x

Hertz, P., Addad, M., & Ronel, N. (2012). Attachment styles and changes among women members of Overeaters Anonymous who have recovered from binge-eating disorder. *Health and Social Work, 37,* 110–122.

Hirschmann, J. (2011). Psychological and theological dynamics in an inpatient psychiatric chaplaincy group. *Journal of Religion and Health, 50,* 964–974. http://dx.doi.org/10.1007/s10943-011-9500-x

Hodge, D. R. (2006). A template for spiritual assessment: A review of the JCAHO requirements and guidelines for implementation. *Social Work, 51,* 317–326. http://dx.doi.org/10.1093/sw/51.4.317

Hodge, D. R. (2013). Implicit spiritual assessment: An alternative approach for assessing client spirituality. *Social Work, 58,* 223–230. http://dx.doi.org/10.1093/sw/swt019

Hong, R., & Welch, A. (2013). The lived experiences of single Taiwanese mothers being resilient after divorce. *Journal of Transcultural Nursing, 24,* 51–59. http://dx.doi.org/10.1177/1043659612452007

Hook, J. N., & Davis, D. E. (2014). Humility, religion and spirituality: Introduction to the special issue. *Journal of Psychology and Theology, 42,* 3–6.

Huguelet, P., & Koenig, H. G. (Eds.). (2009). *Religion and spirituality in psychiatry.* New York: Cambridge University Press.

Humbert, T. K., Bess, J. L., & Mowery, A. M. (2013). Exploring women's perspectives of overcoming intimate partner violence: A phenomenological study. *Occupational Therapy in Mental Health, 29,* 246–265. http://dx.doi.org/10.1080/0164212X.2013.819465

Humbert, T. K., Maley, C. M., Pagana, N. K., & Velenger, C. A. (in press). Individuals dealing with major life events and transitions: A systematic literature review and occupational analysis on the topic of spirituality. *American Journal of Occupational Therapy.*

Hunt, J. (2014). Bio-psycho-social-spiritual assessment? Teaching the skill of spiritual assessment. *Social Work and Christianity, 41,* 373–384.

Husain, A., & Sherr, M. E. (2015). Introduction: Religion and spirituality in competency-based social work practice. *Social Work and Christianity, 42,* 3–6.

Hutchinson, S., Hersch, G., Davidson, H. A., Chu, A. Y., & Mastel-Smith, B. (2011). Voices of elders: Culture and person factors of residents admitted to long-term care facilities. *Journal of Transcultural Nursing, 22,* 397–404. http://dx.doi.org/10.1177/1043659611414138

Isaksson, G., Josephsson, S., Lexell, J., & Skär, L. (2008). Men's experiences of giving and taking social support after their wife's spinal cord injury. *Scandinavian Journal of Occupational Therapy, 15,* 236–246. http://dx.doi.org/10.1080/11038120802194265

Ivtzan, I., Chan, C., Gardner, H., & Prashar, K. (2013). Linking religion and spirituality with psychological well-being: Examining self-actualisation, meaning in life, and personal growth initiative. *Journal of Religion and Health 52,* 915–929. http://dx.doi.org/10.1007/s10943-011-9540-2

Johansson, A. M., & Johansson, U. (2009). Relatives' experiences of family members' eating difficulties. *Scandinavian Journal of Occupational Therapy, 16,* 25–32. http://dx.doi.org/10.1080/11038120802257195

Jolley, D., Benbow, S. M., Grizzell, M., Willmott, S., Bawn, S., & Kingston, P. (2010). Spirituality and faith in dementia. *Dementia, 9,* 311–325. http://dx.doi.org/10.1177/1471301210370645

Kang, C. (2003). A psychospiritual integration frame of reference for occupational therapy, part 1: Conceptual foundations. *Australian Occupational Therapy Journal, 50,* 92–103. http://dx.doi.org/10.1046/j.1440-1630.2003.00358.x

Kestenbaum, A., James, J., Morgan, S., Shields, M., Hocker, W., Rabow, M., & Dunn, L. B. (2015). "Taking your place at the table": An autoethnographic study of chaplains' participation on an interdisciplinary research team. *BMC Palliative Care, 14*(20), 1–10. http://dx.doi.org/10.1186/s12904-015-0006-2

Kim, H., & Pak, J. (2013). Journeys toward spiritual maturity among Korean immigrant women in midlife. *Journal of Psychology and Christianity, 32,* 3–19.

King, S. D., Dimmers, M. A., Langer, S., & Murphy, P. E. (2013). Doctors' attentiveness to the spirituality/religion of their patients in pediatric and oncology settings in the Northwest USA. *Journal of Health Care Chaplaincy, 19,* 140–164. http://dx.doi.org/10.1080/08854726.2013.829692

Koslander, T., Lindstrom, U. A., & Barbosa da Silva, A. (2012). The human being's spiritual experiences in a mental healthcare context; their positive and negative meaning and impact on health—a hermeneutic approach. *Scandinavian Journal of Caring Sciences, 27,* 560–568. http://dx.doi.org/10.1111/j.1471-6712.2012.01067.x

Kwilecki, S. (2011). Ghosts, meaning, and faith: After-death communications in bereavement narratives. *Death Studies, 35,* 219–243. http://dx.doi.org/10.1080/07481187.2010.511424

Lavinder, G., Patel, U., Campo, M., & Lichtman, S. W. (2013). The perceived role of spirituality in physical therapy education. *International Journal of Health, Wellness and Society, 2,* 133–154. Available from http://ijw.cgpublisher.com/product/pub.198/prod.111

Ledford, C. J. W., Canzona, M. R., Seehusen, D. A., Cafferty, L. A., Schmidt, M. E., . . . Villagran, M. M. (2015). Differences in physician communication when patients ask versus tell about religion/spirituality: A pilot study. *Family Medicine, 47,* 138–142.

Lee, Y., & Smith, L. (2012). Qualitative research on Korean American dementia caregivers' perception of caregiving: Heterogeneity between spouse caregivers and child caregivers. *Journal of Human Behavior in the Social Environment, 22,* 115–129. http://dx.doi.org/10.1080/10911359.2012.646840

Leung, D., Esplen, M. J., Peter, E., Howell, D., Rodin, G., & Fitch, M. (2011). How haematological cancer nurses experience the threat of patients' mortality. *Journal of Advanced Nursing, 68*(10), 2175–2184. http://dx.doi.org/10.1111/j.1365-2648.2011.05902.x

Lietz, C. A., & Hodge, D. R. (2011). Spirituality and child welfare reunification: A narrative analysis of successful outcomes. *Child and Family Social Work, 16,* 380–390. http://dx.doi.org/10.1111/j.1365-2206.2010.00752.x

LoboPrabhu, S., & Lomax, J. (2010). The role of spirituality in medical school and psychiatry residency education. *International Journal of Applied Psychoanalytic Studies, 7,* 180–192. http://dx.doi.org/10.1002/aps.241

Lun, M. W. A. (2015). A qualitative study of students' perceptions of spirituality and religion. *Social Work and Christianity, 42,* 178–192.

Massey, K., Barnes, M. J. D., Villines, D., Goldstein, J. D., Hisey Pierson, A. L., Scherer, C., . . . Summerfelt, W. T. (2015). What do I do? Developing a taxonomy of chaplaincy activities and interventions for spiritual care in intensive care unit palliative care. *BMC Palliative Care, 14*(10), 1–8. http://dx.doi.org/10.1186/s12904-015-0008-0

McIntosh, D. N., & Newton, T. (2013). An explicit request for minitheories in the psychology of religion and spirituality. *International Journal for the Psychology of Religion, 23,* 261–270. http://dx.doi.org/10.1080/10508619.2013.795805

McSherry, W., & Jamieson, S. (2013). The qualitative findings from an online survey investigating nurses' perceptions of spirituality and spiritual care. *Journal of Clinical Nursing, 22,* 3170–3182. http://dx.doi.org/10.1111/jocn.12411

McSherry, W., & Smith, J. (2007). How do children express their spiritual needs? *Paediatric Nursing, 19*(3), 17–20.

Meehan, T. C. (2012). Spirituality and spiritual care from a Careful Nursing perspective. *Journal of Nursing Management, 20,* 990–1001. http://dx.doi.org/10.1111/j.1365-2834.2012.01462.x

Meldrum, H. (2012). Humanitarian physicians' views on spirituality. *Implicit Religion, 15,* 167–180. http://dx.doi.org/10.1558/imre.v15.i2.15472

Meredith, P. J. (2010). Has undergraduate education prepared occupational therapy students for possible practice in palliative care? *Australian Occupational Therapy Journal, 57,* 224–232. http://dx.doi.org/10.1111/j.1440-1630.2009.00836.x

Mihalache, G. (2012). The transformational dynamics of becoming forgiving of the seemingly unforgivable: A qualitative heuristic study. *Journal of Spirituality in Mental Health, 14,* 111–128. http://dx.doi.org/10.1080/19349637.2012.671049

Miller, M. M., & Chavier, M. (2013). Clinicians' experiences of integrating prayer in the therapeutic process. *Journal of Spirituality in Mental Health, 15,* 70–93. http://dx.doi.org/10.1080/19349637.2013.776441

Minaye, A. (2012). Trafficked to the Gulf States: The experiences of Ethiopian returnee women. *Journal of Community Practice, 20*(1), 112–133. http://dx.doi.org/10.1080/10705422.2012.649203

Mitchell, M. B., Silver, C. F., & Ross, F. J. (2012). My hero, my friend: Exploring Honduran youths' lived experience of the God–individual relationship. *International Journal of Children's Spirituality, 17*(2), 137–151. http://dx.doi.org/10.1080/1364436X.2012.721752

Morden, P. (2012). The spirituality of C. H. Spurgeon: In establishing communion: A conservative piety. *Baptistic Theologies, 4*(1), 1–26.

Morgan, G. (2010). Independent advocacy and the "rise of spirituality": Views from advocates, service users and chaplains. *Mental Health, Religion and Culture, 13,* 625–636. http://dx.doi.org/10.1080/13674676.2010.488435

Morris, D. N. (2013). Perceptions of spirituality and spiritual care in occupational therapy practice. *Occupational Therapy in Mental Health, 29,* 60–77. http://dx.doi.org/10.1080/0164212x.2013.761109

Mulder, C. (2015). From the inside out: Social workers' expectations for integrating religion and spirituality in practice.

Journal of Religion and Spirituality in Social Work: Social Thought, 34, 177–204. http://dx.doi.org/10.1080/15426432.2014.993106

Muñoz, J. P., Dix, S., & Reichenbach, D. (2006). Building productive roles: Occupational therapy in a homeless shelter. *Occupational Therapy in Health Care, 20*(3/4), 167–187. http://dx.doi.org/10.1080/J003v20n03_11

Murphy, M. M., Begley, T., Timmins, F., Neill, F., & Sheaf, G. (2015) Spirituality and spiritual care-missing concepts from core undergraduate children's nursing textbooks. *International Journal of Children's Spirituality, 20*(2), 114–128. http://dx.doi.org/10.1080/1364436X.2015.1055458

Nabolsi, M. M., & Carson, A. M. (2011). Spirituality, illness and personal responsibility: The experience of Jordanian Muslim men with coronary artery disease. *Scandinavian Journal of Caring Sciences, 25,* 716–724. http://dx.doi.org/10.1111/j.1471-6712.2011.00882.x

Nash, P., Darby, K., & Nash, S. (2012). The spiritual care of sick children: Reflections from a pilot participation project. *International Journal of Children's Spirituality, 18,* 148–161. http://dx.doi.org/10.1080/1364436X.2012.752345

Nesbit, S. G. (2006). Using creativity to experience flow on my journey with breast cancer. *Occupational Therapy in Mental Health, 22,* 61–79. http://dx.doi.org/10.1300/J004v22n02_03

Nicastri, G. R. (2014). Spirituality in medicine: A surgeon's perspective. *Rhode Island Medical Journal, 97*(3), 23–25.

Oakley, E., Katz, G., Sauer, K., Dent, B., & Millar, A. L. (2010). Physical therapists' perception on spirituality and patient care: Beliefs, practices, and perceived barriers. *Journal of Physical Therapy Education, 24,* 45–54.

O'Connor, T., Chow, M., Meakes, E., Young, J., Payne, G., Rivera, M., . . . Howitt, J. (2012). Three doors to spiritual reflection: Ethnographic research on the role of emotion, images, and sacred texts in spiritual reflection done by non-chaplaincy health care professionals. *Journal of Health Care Chaplaincy, 18,* 43–56. http://dx.doi.org/10.1080/08854726.2011.616171

Omu, O., Al-Obaidi, S., & Reynolds, F. (2014). Religious faith and psychosocial adaptation among stroke patients in Kuwait: A mixed method study. *Journal of Religion and Health, 53,* 538–551. http://dx.doi.org/10.1007/s10943-012-9662-1

Orentlicher, M. L., & Gibson, R. (2015). Foundations in transition. In M. L. Orentlicher, S. Schefkind, & R. Gibson (Eds.), *Transitions across the lifespan: An occupational therapy approach* (pp. 21–30). Bethesda, MD: AOTA Press.

Oxhandler, H. K., & Pargament, K. I. (2014). Social work practitioners' integration of clients' religion and spirituality in practice: A literature review. *Social Work, 59,* 271–279. http://dx.doi.org/10.1093/sw/swu018

Parameshwaran, R. (2015). Theory and practice of chaplain's spiritual care process: A psychiatrist's experiences of chaplaincy and conceptualizing trans-personal model of mindfulness. *Indian Journal of Psychiatry, 57,* 21–29. Available from: http://www.indianjpsychiatry.org/text.asp?2015/57/1/21/148511

Park, M., Chesla, C. A., Rehm, R. S., & Chun, K. M. (2011). Working with culture: Culturally appropriate mental health care for Asian Americans. *Journal of Advanced Nursing, 67,* 2373–2382. http://dx.doi.org/10.1111/j.1365-2648.2011.05671.x

Parson, L., & Stanley, M. (2008). The lived experience of occupational adaptation following acquired brain injury for people living in a rural area. *Australian Occupational Therapy Journal, 55,* 231–238. http://dx.doi.org/10.1111/j.1440-1630.2008.00753.x

Pesut, B. (2008). A conversation on diverse perspectives of spirituality in nursing literature. *Nursing Philosophy, 9,* 98–109. http://dx.doi.org/10.1111/j.1466-769X.2008.00341.x

Pesut, B. (2013). Nursings' need for the idea of spirituality. *Nursing Inquiry, 20,* 5–10. http://dx.doi.org/10.1111/j.1440-1800.2012.00608.x

Pitts, J. (2008) Spirituality in the physical therapy curriculum: Effects on the older adult. *Top Geriatric Rehabilitations, 24,* 281–94. http://dx.doi.org/10.1097/TGR.0b013e31818ccfaf

Powell, R. A., Emanuel, L., Handzo, G., Lantos, J., Dunn, L. B., Idler, E. L., . . . Sommer, D. (2015). Transcending differences to study the transcendent: An exploratory study of researchers' and chaplains' reflections on interdisciplinary spiritual care research collaboration. *BMC Palliative Care, 14*(12), 1–6. http://dx.doi.org/10.1186/s12904-015-0004-4

Prentis, S., Rogers, M., Wattis, J., Jones, J., & Stephenson, J. (2014). Healthcare lecturers' perceptions of spirituality in education. *Nursing Standard, 29*(3), 44–52. http://dx.doi.org/10.7748/ns.29.3.44.e8584.

Price, P., Kinghorn, J., Patrick, R., & Cardell, B. (2012). "Still there is beauty": One man's resilient adaptation to stroke. *Scandinavian Journal of Occupational Therapy, 19,* 111–117. http://dx.doi.org/10.3109/11038128.2010.519402

Ramugondo, E. L. (2005). Unlocking spirituality: Play as a health-promoting occupation in the context of HIV/AIDS. In F. Kronenberg, S. A. Algado, & N. Pollard (Eds.), *Occupational therapy without borders: Learning from the spirit of survivors* (pp. 313–325). New York: Elsevier Churchill Livingstone.

Rehnsfeldt, A., & Arman, M. (2012). Significance of close relationships after the tsunami disaster in connection with existential health—a qualitative interpretative study. *Scandinavian*

Journal of Caring Sciences, 26, 537–544. http://dx.doi.org/10. 1111/j.1471-6712.2011.00962.x

Reimer-Kirkham, S., Pesut, B. Sawatzky, R., Cochrane, M., & Redmond, A. (2012). Discourses of spirituality and leadership in nursing: A mixed methods analysis. *Journal of Nursing Management, 20,* 1029–1038. http://dx.doi.org/ 10.1111/j.1365-2834.2012.01480.x.

Reinert, K. G., & Koenig, H. G. (2013). Re-examining definitions of spirituality in nursing research. *Journal of Advanced Nursing, 69,* 2622–2634. http://dx.doi.org/10.1111/jan. 12152

Renz, M., Mao, M. S., Bueche, D., Cerny, T., & Strasser, F. (2012). Dying is a transition. *American Journal of Hospice and Palliative Medicine, 30,* 283–290. http://dx.doi. org/10.1177/1049909112451868

Revheim, N., Greenberg, W. M., & Citrome, L. (2010). Spirituality, schizophrenia and state hospitals: Program description and characteristics of self-selected attendees of a spirituality therapeutic group. *Psychiatric Quarterly 81*(4), 285–292. http://dx.doi.org/10.1007/s11126-010-9137-z

Rogers, M., & Wattis, J. (2015) Spirituality in nursing practice. *Nursing Standard, 29*(39), 51– 57. http://dx.doi. org/10.7748/ns.29.39.51.e9726

Rousseau, D. (2014). A systems model of spirituality. *Zygon, 14,* 476–508. http://dx.doi.org/10.1111/zygo.12087

Rumbold, B. (2013). Spiritual assessment and health care chaplaincy. *Christian Bioethics, 19,* 251–269. http://dx.doi. org/10.1093/cb/cbt027

Saeteren, B., Lindström, U. A., & Naden, D. (2011). Latching onto life: Living in the area of tension between the possibility of life and the necessity of death. *Journal of Clinical Nursing, 20,* 811–818. http://dx.doi.org/10.1111/j.1365-2702. 2010.03212.x

Savin-Baden, M., & Howell Major, C. (2013). *Qualitative research: The essential guide to theory and practice.* Abingdon, UK: Routledge.

Schafer, R. M., Handa, P. J., Brawer, P. A., & Ubinger, M. (2011). Training and education in religion/spirituality within APA-accredited clinical psychology programs: 8 years later. *Journal of Religion and Health, 50,* 232–239. http://dx. doi.org/10.1007/s10943-009-9272-8

Schapmire, T. J., Head, B. A., & Faul, A. C (2012). Just give me hope: Lived experiences of Medicaid patients with advanced cancer. *Journal of Social Work in End-of-Life and Palliative Care, 8,* 29–52. http://dx.doi.org/10.1080/15524256.2012. 650672

Schick Makaroff, K. L., Sheilds, L., & Molzahn, A. (2013). Stories of chronic kidney disease: Listening for the unsayable. *Journal of Advanced Nursing, 69,* 2644–2653. http://dx.doi. org/ 10.1111/jan.12149

Schultz, M., Lulav-Grinwald, D., & Bar-Sela, G. (2014). Cultural differences in spiritual care: Findings of an Israeli oncologic questionnaire examining patient interest in spiritual care. *BMC Palliative Care, 13,* 19. http://dx.doi.org/10. 1186/1472-684X-13-19

Seitz, C. R. (2014). Utilizing a spiritual disciplines framework for faith integration in social work: A competency-based model. *Social Work and Christianity, 41,* 334–354.

Senreich, E. (2013). An inclusive definition of spirituality for social work education and practice. *Journal of Social Work Education, 49,* 548–563. http://dx.doi.org/10.1080/10437 797.2013.812460

Sharpe, T. L., Joe, S., & Taylor, K. C. (2013). Suicide and homicide bereavement among African Americans: Implications for survivor research and practice. *Omega, 66,* 153– 172. http://dx.doi.org/10.2190/OM.66.2.d

Singh, D. K. M., & Ajinkya, S. (2012). Spirituality and religion in modern medicine. *Indian Journal of Psychological Medicine, 34,* 399–402. http://dx.doi.org/10.4103/0253-7176.108234.

Smith, S., & Suto, M. J. (2012). Religious and/or spiritual practices: Extending spiritual freedom to people with schizophrenia. *Canadian Journal of Occupational Therapy, 79,* 77–85. http://dx.doi.org/10.2182/cjot.2012.79.2.3

Smith, T. M., Ludwig, F., Anderson, L. T., & Copolillo, A. (2009). Engagement in occupation and adaptation to low vision. *Occupational Therapy in Health Care, 23,* 119–133. http://dx.doi.org/10.1080/07380570902788782

Svalina, S. S., & Webb, J. R. (2012). Forgiveness and health among people in outpatient physical therapy. *Disability and Rehabilitation, 34*(5), 383–392. http://dx.doi.org/10.3109/ 09638288.2011.607216

Tan, H. M., Wilson, A., Olver, I., & Barton, C. (2011). The experience of palliative patients and their families of a family meeting utilised as an instrument for spiritual and psychosocial care: A qualitative study. *BMC Palliative Care, 10*(7), 1–12. http://dx.doi.org/10.1186/1472-684X-10-7

Tapley, H., Fell, D., & Pitts, D. (2012). Exploration of spirituality in doctor of physical therapy students and graduate students in non-health disciplines. *International Journal of Therapy and Rehabilitation, 19,* 566–574. http://dx.doi. org/10.12968/ijtr.2012.19.10.566

Tate, R. B., Swift, A. U., & Bayomi, D. J. (2013). Older men's lay definitions of successful aging over time: The Manitoba Follow-Up Study. *International Journal of Aging and Human Development, 76,* 297–322. http://dx.doi.org/10.2190/AG. 76.4.b

Taylor, J. J., Hodgson, J. L., Kolobova, I., Lamson, A. L., Sira, N., & Musick, D. (2015), Exploring the phenomenon of spiritual care between hospital chaplains and hospital based healthcare providers. *Journal of Health Care Chaplaincy, 21,* 91–107. http://dx.doi.org/10.1080/08854726.2015.1015302

Teti, M., Martin, A. E., Ranade, R., Massie, J., Malebranche, D. J., Tschann, J. M., & Bowleg, L. (2012). "I'm a keep rising. I'm a keep going forward, regardless": Exploring Black men's resilience amid sociostructural challenges and stressors. *Qualitative Health Research, 22,* 524–533. http://dx.doi.org/10.1177/1049732311422051

Thornton, N., & Pratt Hopp, F. (2011). "So I just took over": African American daughters caregiving for parents with heart failure. *Families in Society: The Journal of Contemporary Social Services, 92,* 211–217. http://dx.doi.org/10.1606/1044-3894.4103

Tiew, L. H., Kwee, J. H., Creedy, D. K., & Chan, M. F. (2013). Hospice nurses' perspectives of spirituality. *Journal of Clinical Nursing, 22,* 2923–2933, http://dx.doi.org/10.1111/jocn.12358

Timmins, F., & McSherry, W. (2012). Spirituality: The Holy Grail of contemporary nursing practice. *Journal of Nursing Management, 20,* 951–957. http://dx.doi.org/10.1111/jonm.12038

Trancik, E. K. (2013). Lost in translation: Spiritual assessment and the religious tradition. *Christian Bioethics, 19,* 282–298. http://dx.doi.org/10.1093/cb/cbt029

Unruh, A., & Hutchinson, S. (2011). Embedded spirituality: Gardening in daily life and stressful life experiences. *Scandinavian Journal of Caring Sciences, 25,* 567–574. http://dx.doi.org/10.1111/j.1471-6712.2010.00865.x

Van Lith, T. (2014). "Painting to find my spirit." Art making as the vehicle to find meaning and connection in the mental health recovery process. *Journal of Spirituality in Mental Health, 16,* 19–36. http://dx.doi.org/10.1080/19349637.2013.864542

Wade, W. (2013). Catholic mass and its healing implications for the addicted person. *Substance Use and Misuse, 48,* 1138–1149. http://dx.doi.org/10.3109/10826084.2013.800744

Welton-Mitchell, C., McIntosh, D. N., & DePrince, A. P. (2013). Associations between thematic content and memory detail in trauma narratives. *Applied Cognitive Psychology, 27,* 462–473. http://dx.doi.org/10.1002/acp.2923

Werdel, M. B., Dy-Liacco, G. S., Ciarrocchi, J. W., Wicks, R. J., & Breslford, G. M. (2014). The unique role of spirituality in the process of growth following stress and trauma. *Pastoral Psychology, 63,* 7–71. http://dx.doi.org/10.1007/s11089-013-0538-4

Wessels, F., & Müller, J. C. (2013). Spirituality in narratives of meaning. *Theological Studies, 69*(2), 1–7. http://dx.doi.org/10.4102/hts.v69i2.1187

Williamson, W. P., & Hood, R. W. (2013). Spiritual transformation: A phenomenological study among recovering substance abusers. *Pastoral Psychology, 62,* 889–906. http://dx.doi.org/10.1007/s11089-012-0502-8

Winter, M. T. (2014). That all may be one. *Journal of Ecumenical Studies, 49*(1), 59–64.

Wu, P., Guo, W., Xia, H., Lu, H., & Xi, S. (2011). Patients' experience of living with glaucoma: A phenomenological study. *Journal of Advanced Nursing, 67,* 800–810. http://dx.doi.org/10.1111/j.1365-2648.2010.05541.x

Yarhouse, M. A., & Carrs, T. L. (2012). MTF transgender Christians' experiences: A qualitative study. *Journal of LGBT Issues in Counseling, 6,* 18–33. http://dx.doi.org/10.1080/15538605.2012.649405

Ybañez-Llorente, K., & Smelser, Q. K. (2014). Client as expert: Incorporating spirituality using the Tree Ring Technique. *Counseling and Values, 59,* 35–48. http://dx.doi.org/10.1002/j.2161-007X.2014.00040.x

Yilmaz, M., & Gurler, H. (2014). The efficacy of integrating spirituality into undergraduate nursing curricula. *Nursing Ethics, 21,* 929–945. http://dx.doi.org/10.1177/0969733014521096

SUBJECT INDEX

Note. Page numbers in *italic* indicate exhibits, figures, and tables.

CITATION INDEX